Experimental and Clinical Interventions in Aging

Experimental and Clinical Interventions in Aging

edited by

Richard F. Walker

Department of Anatomy
and
Sanders-Brown Research Center on Aging
University of Kentucky Medical Center
Lexington, Kentucky

and

Ralph L. Cooper

Center for the Study of Aging and Human Development
and
Division of Medical Psychology
Department of Psychiatry
Duke University Medical Center
Durham, North Carolina

MARCEL DEKKER, INC.   New York and Basel

Library of Congress Cataloging in Publication Data
Main entry under title:

Experimental and clinical interventions in aging.

Includes bibliographical references and index.
1. Geriatrics. 2. Age factors in disease.
3. Endocrine glands—Diseases—Age factors. I. Walker,
Richard F., [date] . II. Cooper, Ralph, L., [date] .
[DNLM: 1. Aging. 2. Geriatrics. WT 104 E966]
RC952.5.E95 1983 618.97 83-17659
ISBN O-8247-7012-9

MARCEL DEKKER, INC.
270 Madison Avenue, New York, New York 10016

Current printing (last digit):
10 9 8 7 6 5 4 3 2 1

PRINTED IN THE UNITED STATES OF AMERICA

Preface

In gerontological research, the term "intervention" is applied to two quite different approaches to the study of aging. To some, intervention implies an attempt to prolong life span, whether at the level of the cell or of the whole organism. To others, intervention means attempting to maintain the function of specific physiological systems into late life, with little concern for the effect of such treatment on the organism's life span. Given the current status of gerontological research, it seems clear that studies emphasizing the latter approach hold the greatest promise for the development of clinical applications and for the advancement of our understanding of the aging process. It is this sense of the term "intervention" that will be the focus of this volume.

Animal model papers address basic issues in aging research and describe several attempts to intervene in the aging process. This research demonstrates that within specific physiological systems the rate of change with age can be manipulated through a variety of treatments instituted at various times of the animal's life. Such studies are crucial to our understanding of how physiological homeostasis and behavioral function can be maintained in late life; they provide the necessary background for clinical research and the development of rational therapy for the elderly patient.

Clinical papers discuss several relevant issues. Geriatric medicine is in its infancy. It is increasingly recognized that the physiological and psychological changes occurring in the elderly make them a unique patient population; thus, treatment of the aged should not necessarily follow procedures established for the young. Clinical intervention in specific aging disorders may include the identification of underlying age-related physiological conditions that predispose the elderly patient to a wide range of physiological or psychological disorders and the selection of drug regimens tailored to these physiological conditions.

Throughout these reports, it is worth noting that the techniques for intervention in the aging process are remarkably simple and straightforward. They have

been developed from the rich background of information available to us from research on the young-adult organism, as a logical extention of this knowledge to
the area of gerontology. Although they do not offer miracle cures for the numerous
maladies afflicting the aged, they do offer assurance that we are headed in the right
direction toward improving physiological and behavioral performance in the elderly.

Richard F. Walker
Ralph L. Cooper

Contributors

Raymond T. Bartus, Ph.D.   Department of CNS Research, Medical Research Division of American Cyanamid Co., Lederle Laboratories, Pearl River, New York

Dan Blazer, M.D., Ph.D.   Head, Division of Social and Community Psychiatry, Department of Psychiatry, Duke University Medical Center, Durham, North Carolina

James R. Brawer, Ph.D.   Departments of Anatomy, Obstetrics, and Gynecology, and the McGill Center for the Study of Reproduction, McGill University School of Medicine, Montreal, Quebec, Canada

William H. Brooks, M.D.   Division of Neurosurgery, University of Kentucky, Lexington, Kentucky

Maurice W. M. Bruwier, M.D.   Department of Neuroendocrinology, Hôpital Geriatrique du Val D'Or, Liege, Belgium

C. Edward Buckley, III, M.D.   Department of Medicine, Duke University Medical Center, Durham, North Carolina

Joy Cavagnaro, Ph.D.*   Department of Pharmacology, Duke University Medical Center, Durham, North Carolina

Vernon J. Choy, Ph.D.†   Department of Physiology-Anatomy, University of California, Berkeley, California

---

Present affiliations
*Hybridoma Technology Section, Hazleton Laboratories America, Inc., Vienna, Virginia
†Postgraduate School of Obstetrics and Gynecology, The University of Auckland, Auckland, New Zealand

John R. Cohn, M.D.* Departments of Medicine, Veteran's Administration and Duke University Medical Centers, Durham, North Carolina

P. Michael Conn, Ph.D. Department of Pharmacology and Center for the Study of Aging and Human Development, Duke University Medical Center, Durham, North Carolina

Ralph L. Cooper, Ph.D. Center for the Study of Aging and Human Development, and Division of Medical Psychology, Department of Psychiatry, Duke University Medical Center, Durham, North Carolina

Richard J. Cross, Ph.D. Department of Medical Microbiology and Immunology, University of Kentucky Medical Center, Lexington, Kentucky

Kenneth L. Davis, M.D. Chief, Psychiatry Service, Department of Psychiatry, Veterans Administration Medical Center, Bronx, New York, and Department of Psychiatry, Mount Sinai School of Medicine, New York, New York

Reginald L. Dean, III Department of CNS Research, Medical Research Division of American Cyanamid Co., Lederle Laboratories, Pearl River, New York

Bernard T. Engel, Ph.D. Laboratory of Behavioral Sciences, National Institute on Aging, National Institutes of Health, Baltimore, Maryland

Bernard A. Eskin, M.D. Department of Gynecology and Obstetrics, The Medical College of Pennsylvania and Hospital, Philadelphia, Pennsylvania

Caleb E. Finch, Ph.D. Department of Biological Science and the Andrus Gerontology Center, University of Southern California, Los Angeles, California

Patricia Gilot Psychoendocrinology Unit, Medical School, University of Liege-Sart-Tilman, Liege, Belgium

Keith V. Kuhlemeier, Ph.D. Departments of Rehabilitation Medicine and Physiology, University of Alabama in Birmingham, Birmingham, Alabama

Jean-Jacques Legros, M.D., Ph.D. Chief, Psychoneuroendocrinology Unit, Medical School, University of Liege-Sart-Tilman, Liege, Belgium

Costas C. Loullis, Ph.D. Department of CNS Research, Medical Research Division of American Cyanamid Co., Lederle Laboratories, Pearl River, New York

William R. Markesbery, M.D. Departments of Pathology and Neurology, and Director, The Sanders-Brown Research Center on Aging, University of Kentucky Medical Center, Lexington, Kentucky

---

Present affiliation
*Departments of Medicine and Pediatrics, Thomas Jefferson University Hospital,., Philadelphia, Pennsylvania

Richard C. Mohs, Ph.D.   Department of Psychiatry, Veterans Administration Medical Center, Bronx, New York, and Department of Psychiatry, Mount Sinai School of Medicine, New York, New York

Thomas L. Roszman, M.D.   Departments of Medical Microbiology, Immunology, and Pathology, University of Kentucky Medical Center, Lexington, Kentucky

Harvey V. Samis, Ph.D.   Veterans Administration Medical Center, Bay Pines, Florida

Stephen W. Scheff, Ph.D.   Department of Anatomy, University of Kentucky Medical Center, Lexington, Kentucky

Wendy A. Smith, Ph.D.*   Department of Pharmacology, Duke University Medical Center, Durham, North Carolina

Gary Thompson, Ph.D.[†]   Center for the Study of Aging and Human Development, Duke University Medical Center, Durham, North Carolina

Martine Timsit-Berthier, M.D.   Departments of Clinical Neurophysiology and Psychopathology, Medical School, University of Liege-Sart-Tilman, Liege, Belgium

Richard F. Walker, Ph.D.   Department of Anatomy and Sanders-Brown Research Center on Aging, University of Kentucky Medical Center, Lexington, Kentucky

Sadao Yamaoka, M.D.   Department of Physiology, Saitama Medical School, Moroyama-cho, Iruma-gun, Saitama, Japan

Leslie A. Zajac-Batell   Veterans Administration Medical Center, Bay Pines, Florida

---

Present affiliations
*Department of Biology, University of North Carolina, Chapel Hill, North Carolina
[†] Psychological Services, Sister Kenny Institute, Minneapolis, Minnesota

Contents

Part I
Aging in the Reproductive System

1

Causes and Consequences of Altered Gonadotropin Secretion in the Aging Rat

Wendy A. Smith* and P. Michael Conn / *Duke University Medical Center, Durham, North Carolina*

INTRODUCTION

Changes in cellular functions that accompany mammalian aging need not arise from irreversible degenerative impairments. Rather, age-related changes in key regulatory systems may lead to suboptimal environments for differentiated cell functions. For example, age-related changes in endocrine function can have profound effects on target tissues, even when those tissues remain capable of normal activity. Reproductive senescence in the rat clearly illustrates the concept of endocrine malfunction as a source of altered cellular activity during aging. Specifically, it appears that changes in the synthesis and release of hormones by the hypothalamopituitary system are primarily responsible for a decline in gonadal activity and reproductive capacity in these animals. In the first section of this review, we will consider the types of endocrine changes that accompany reproductive senescence in the rat and review hypotheses which have been proposed to explain these changes.

Changes in the activity of target tissues can lead to a loss of feedback control in the endocrine system, further disrupting endocrine function. Thus, during reproductive senescence in the rat, alterations in steroid secretion by the gonads appear to perpetuate initial changes in hypothalmic and/or pituitary function. In the second portion of this review, we will consider structural and molecular changes

*Present affiliation: University of North Carolina, Chapel Hill, North Carolina

in the pituitary of senescent rats which may result from a loss of normal feed-back control by the gonads.

BACKGROUND

Normal reproductive functioning in mammals is primarily dependent upon hormones released by the hypothalamus, the pituitary, and the gonads (Fig. 1). In females, activity of the hypothalamopituitary-gonadal axis is cyclic; the result in female rats is a repeated 4 to 5-day estrous cycle. This cycle involves predictable changes in the ovarian functions of germ cell maturation and steroidogenesis, with accompanying changes both in behavior and in the morphology of accessory sexual organs such as the uterus and vagina. Ovarian activity in rats is regulated by three hormones secreted by the pituitary gland: luteinizing hormone (LH), follicle-stimulating hormone (FSH), and prolactin (PRL). During proestrus, circulating levels of all three pituitary hormones undergo a sharp increase. Surges of LH and FSH lead to follicle maturation and also stimulate the secretion of estrogens and progestins. Elevated levels of LH trigger ovulation at estrus, followed by the formation of corpora lutea. In rats, progesterone secretion by the corpora lutea is further stimulated by PRL. If pregnancy does not occur, diestrus ensues during which time the corpora lutea undergo a functional regression, and steroid secretion is curtailed. Unlike females, male rats do not undergo long-term cyclic changes in gonadal activity although diurnal fluctuations in steroid secretion are well-documented. The pituitary hormones LH and FSH regulate reproductive functions in the male as in the female, with FSH initiating gamete maturation (spermatogenesis) and LH stimulating the secretion of androgens by testicular Leydig cells.

In both males and females, the pituitary is in turn regulated by factors released by the hypothalamus. Synthesis and release of LH and FSH are stimulated by gonadotropin-releasing hormone (GnRH),* whereas PRL release appears to be

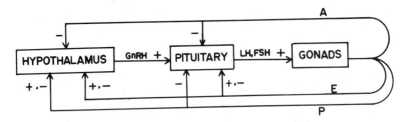

Figure 1 Endocrine regulation of mammalian reproductive function by the hypothalamopituitary-gonadal axis. (+) Stimulation; (−) inhibition; A, androgen; E, estrogen; P, progesterone.

---

*GnRH is variously referred to as luteinizing hormone-releasing hormone (LHRH) and luteinizing hormone-releasing factor (LRF). Since its status as a hormone is unquestionable and it functionally stimulates release of both LH and FSH, we have used the abbreviation GnRH in the present review.

modulated by an inhibiting factor and by thyrotropin-releasing hormone. In addition, hypothalamic neurotransmitters such as norepinephrine, dopamine, and serotonin have been found to influence the secretion of pituitary gonadotropins and PRL.

Recently, functional binding sites for GnRH have been found in extrapituitary locations, including the gonads (Hsueh and Erickson, 1979a, Sharpe, 1980). Occupancy of gonadal GnRH receptors in vitro leads to decreased steroidogenesis (Hsueh and Erickson, 1979a, b). Because hypothalamic GnRH does not reach high levels in the peripheral circulation, the physiological significance of extrapituitary binding sites remains unclear. It is possible that GnRH-like substances released from sites other than the pituitary do exert a direct effect on gonadal function.

Feedback by gonadal steroids plays a critical role in the maintenance of normal patterns of gonadotropin release. It appears that both the hypothalamus and the pituitary are sensitive to feedback regulation by steroids, although the nature of such feedback (positive or negative) is dependent upon a variety of factors including dose and prior exposure to steroids themselves (for a detailed review, see Labrie et al., 1979). For example, in female rats, low levels of estrogen are thought to stimulate the release of GnRH from the hypothalamus as well as cause an increase in the sensitivity of the pituitary to GnRH. High levels of estrogen and progesterone following ovulation exert a negative feedback on the hypothalamopituitary system, inhibiting further surges in gonadotropins and GnRH. In males, high levels of testosterone also exert an inhibitory effect on gonadotropin release.

In both male and female rats, the endocrine control of reproduction is altered with age. We will discuss reproductive changes characteristic of each sex in separate sections that follow.

FEMALES

Changes in Gonadal Function

The mean life spans of common strains of laboratory rats range from 21-24 months; maximal life spans range from 32-40 months (National Academy of Sciences, 1981). However, in all strains of laboratory rats, reproductive senescence begins much earlier. During middle age (8-15 months), the 4 to 5-day estrous cycles characteristic of young rats are often replaced by lengthened cycles of 6 or more days. During this time reproductive capacity declines markedly, as manifested by an increase in embryonic anomalies (Sopelak and Butcher, 1982b) and by a decrease in successfully completed pregnancies (Miller et al., 1979; Miller and Riegle, 1980a). Ovulation occurs less frequently, and fewer eggs are released per ovulation; however, unlike human ovaries, substantial numbers of oocytes remain in the rat ovaries at the time of reproductive failure (Mandl and Shelton, 1959). Alterations in the timing and magnitude of estrogen and progestin secretions appear to accompany the onset of irregular cycles during middle age (Wise, 1982a; Page and Butcher, 1982).

By 17 months of age, most females cease any type of cyclic estrous activity, irregular cycles being replaced by prolonged periods of constant estrus (CE; persistent vaginal cornification) (Ingram, 1959; Huang and Meites, 1975; Lu et al., 1979; Cooper and Walker, 1979) (Fig. 2). In still older animals, a transition is often seen to a series of pseudopregnancies (PP; leukocytic vaginal smears interrupted by periods of estrus) and, finally, to an anestrous (AN; leukocytic smears with no signs of estrus) state (Aschheim, 1961; Mandl, 1961; Huang and Meites, 1975; Lu et al., 1979). Each of the reproductive states of aging female rats is accompanied by characteristic changes in ovarian morphology (Wolfe, 1943; Mandl, 1959; Bloch, 1961; Clemens and Meites, 1971; Huang and Meites, 1975; Aschheim, 1976; Meites and Huang, 1976; Lu et al., 1979). Ovaries of CE rats are polyfollicular and anovulatory; those of PP rats contain well-developed corpora lutea. In AN rats, the ovaries contain only a few small follicles with no corpora lutea. As might be suspected from changes in ovarian and vaginal cytology, aged females show marked changes in the production of ovarian steroids (Huang et al., 1978; Wilkes et al., 1978; Lu et al., 1979; Steger et al., 1979a; Miller and Riegle, 1980b; Lu et al., 1980; Wise and Ratner, 1980a). In particular, cyclic changes in steroid secretion are absent. CE females secrete moderate amounts of estradiol, comparable to those in young females during late diestrus. PP females, by contrast, secrete significantly less of this steroid. However, progesterone levels in CE females are low, whereas those in PP animals are elevated to levels comparable to midproestrous cycling females. In most reports to date, AN females show reduced levels of both estrogen and progesterone.

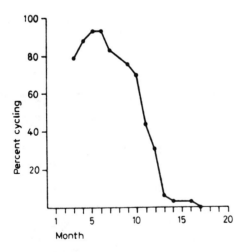

Figure 2   Decline in regular vaginal-ovarian function with age in the Long-Evans rat. Data obtained from animals in the colony of the Duke University Center for the Study of Aging and Human Development. (From Cooper and Walker, 1979).

Changes in Hypothalamopituitary Function

Changes in Gonadotropin Secretion

Changes in the cyclic release of gonadotropins begin during middle age, when the proestrous LH surge becomes both delayed and attenuated (van der Schoot, 1976; Gray et al., 1980; Cooper et al., 1980; Miller and Riegle, 1980b; Wise, 1982b). Cyclic changes in gonadotropin release are entirely absent in CE, PP, and AN females. Basal levels of LH are not altered in senescent females as compared to young cycling animals (Howland and Preiss, 1975; Watkins et al., 1975; Gosden and Bancroft, 1976; Huang et al., 1976a; Huang et al., 1978; Wilkes et al., 1978; Lu et al., 1979; Wise and Ratner, 1980a). However, PRL levels are often extremely high, particularly in PP and AN females (Shaar et al., 1975; Watkins et al., 1976; Huang et al., 1976a; Lu et al., 1979; Damassa et al., 1980). Increases in circulating PRL can be explained in part by the frequent formation of lactotrophic tumors in these groups; however, elevated PRL levels are also observed following elimination of females with tumors from observation (Lu et al., 1979). In addition to changes in total amounts of circulating PRL, alterations in circadian patterns of PRL release have also been found in CE and PP females (Damassa et al., 1980; Gilman et al., 1981).

Altered Response to Ovariectomy, Steroid Treatment, and GnRH

In young, cycling female rats, ovariectomy leads to a dramatic increase in plasma LH and FSH as a result of removal of negative feedback by gonadal steroids on the hypothalamopituitary system. In contrast to young females, increases in plasma LH following ovariectomy are much smaller in all groups of aged female rats, including middle-aged irregularly cycling animals, whereas increases in plasma FSH are comparable to those found in young rats (Shaar et al., 1976a; Peluso et al., 1977; McPherson et al., 1977; Steger et al., 1980; Wise and Ratner, 1980a). Low levels of estradiol benzoate lead to a decrease in LH and FSH following ovariectomy in all groups of aged females, but the decrease in LH is of less magnitude and often of less percent than in ovariectomized young females (Shaar et al., 1975; Howland and Preiss, 1976b; Gosden and Bancroft, 1976; Huang et al., 1976a; Steger et al., 1980). These results indicate that responsiveness of the hypothalamopituitary system to negative feedback by gonadal steroids is retained in aged female rats, but to a lesser degree than in young females.

Responses of ovariectomized females to positive feedback by steroid hormones, particularly treatments known to promote an LH surge in young females, are, in general, lower in aging females. An attenuated LH surge in response to steroid treatments is first seen in middle-aged cycling females, and may be one reason for a subsequent loss of estrous cycles (Gray et al., 1980; Steger et al., 1980). Whereas LH levels in ovariectomized CE or PP females usually increase slightly in response to surge-inducing steroid treatments (Gosden and Bancroft, 1976; Howland, 1976; Lu et al., 1977, 1981; Steger et al., 1980), results vary according to strain of rat tested (Steger et al., 1980) and with length of time following ovariectomy (Lu et al., 1977, 1981). Release of FSH in response to positive feedback by steroids is not altered in senescent rats (Howland, 1976; Steger et al., 1980).

A number of reports indicate that noncycling female rats show a smaller rise in circulating LH following single injections of GnRH than do young controls, suggesting a change in pituitary responsiveness to GnRH with age (Watkins et al., 1975; Howland, 1976; Miller and Riegle, 1978a; Wise and Ratner, 1980b). Responsiveness to GnRH has been enhanced by exposure to estradiol benzoate (Peluso et al., 1977; Lu et al., 1980) or by multiple injections of GnRH (Miller and Riegle, 1978a).

Source of Alterations in Female Reproductive Function

The primary source of reproductive decline in female rats remains to be pinpointed. Ovarian malfunction has long been ruled out on the basis of cross-transplantation experiments between age groups. Ovaries removed from senescent females have been shown to resume normal function in ovariectomized young animals, whereas ovaries from young females take on the functional status of old ovariectomized recipients (Aschheim, 1964/1965; Peng and Huang, 1973). Recently, however, similar experiments have indicated a reduced ability of the senescent ovary to maintain normal cycles in young recipients (Sopelak and Butcher, 1982a). The ovaries of senescent females remain responsive to LH and human chorionic gonadotropin, (hCG; a placental hormone which acts in a manner similar to LH) as measured by the induction of steroid aromatase activity (Erickson et al., 1979) and ovulation (Aschheim, 1965).

Most attention to date has focused on changes in hypothalamic activity as the primary source of reproductive senescence in female rats (for recent reviews, see Riegle and Miller, 1978; Meites et al., 1980; and Walker, this volume). While the content of GnRH in the hypothalamus of senescent females is reduced (Steger et al., 1979a; Wise and Ratner, 1980a), sufficient amounts of this hormone are present to induce LH release in young rats (Miller and Riegle, 1978b; Riegle and Miller, 1978). Agents believed to promote GnRH release by the hypothalamus, such as electrical stimulation, progesterone, adrenocorticotropic hormone, and stress, have been effective in reinitiating estrous cycles in old, CE females (Clemens et al., 1969; Quadri et al., 1973; Huang et al., 1976b; Clemens and Bennett, 1977; Meites et al., 1978; Finch, 1978). Changes in hypothalamic monoamines (catecholamines and serotonin) may contribute to altered gonadotropin levels in senescent females. Catecholamines such as norepinephrine and dopamine are thought to inhibit prolactin secretion and to stimulate the release of gonadotropins. Conversely, serotonin appears to stimulate prolactin and to inhibit gonadotropin secretion. Agents that increase brain catecholamines can reinitiate cycling in aged females (for a review, see Finch, 1978), indicating that an imbalance in hypothalamic monoamines may be one cause of reproductive aging in rats. However, the precise consequences of such an imbalance on gonadotropin secretion remain unclear. In addition, surprisingly little work has been done on changes in hypothalamic mono-amines during middle age, when alterations in gonadotropin secretion first become apparent.

Altered activity of the pituitary glands in senescent female rats may not be caused solely by changes in the hypothalamus. The anterior pituitary glands of senescent female rats, when transplanted to the median eminence region of hypo-physectomized young females, cannot maintain normal estrous cycles to the same degree as similarly grafted glands from young donors (Pecile et al., 1966; Peng and Huang, 1973). Conversely, normal estrous cycling is maintained well into middle age (16 months) when hypophysectomized female rats receive grafts of pituitary glands from young (15-day) male donors (Smith, 1963). Together, these results suggest intrinsic changes in pituitary function with age, a hypothesis supported by recent findings of reduced pituitary responsiveness to GnRH in vitro by the pi-tuitary of middle-aged, cycling females (Smith et al., 1982).

Whereas changes in the hypothalamus and/or pituitary appear to be respon-sible for an initial loss of estrous cycling in senescent females, resultant long-term changes in steroid secretion may perpetuate alterations in hypothalamopituitary function. For example, Lu et al. (1981) have suggested that elevated levels of es-trogens found in CE females may lead to a decreased sensitivity of the hypothal-amopituitary system to the positive feedback effects of ovarian steroids. Five weeks following ovariectomy, treatment with surge-producing steroids produced a significant LH surge in both CE and young females; however, if persistently high levels of estrogen were maintained during the same period with the use of estrogen implants, neither old nor young females showed a significant change in LH levels in response to the steroids. We will consider the relative influence of age vs. endo-crine status in conjunction with alterations in senescent pituitary function.

MALES

Changes in Gonadal Function

Male rats undergo a 50-70% decline in circulating testosterone levels during the second year of life (Ghanadian et al., 1975; Bruni et al., 1977; Chan et al., 1977; Gray, 1978; Miller and Riegle, 1978c; Pirke et al., 1978; Harman et al., 1978; Saksena and Lau, 1979; Bethea and Walker, 1979; Kaler and Neaves, 1981). Where-as a decrease in testicular weight has been observed in aged male rats (Bethea and Walker, 1979; Kaler and Neaves, 1981), the size and number of Leydig (steroid-producing) cells remain comparable to young males (Kaler and Neaves, 1981). Numbers of mature sperm also remain near young-adult levels, although a decrease in the size of litters sired by old males may indicate some change in sperm viability (Saksena et al., 1979). Changes in the activity of certain testicular enzymes in-volved in steroid synthesis have been found to accompany senescence in male rats

(Leathem and Albrecht, 1974; Chan et al., 1977). In addition, aged males show a smaller rise in plasma testosterone following single injections of hCG than do young males (Chan et al., 1977; Miller and Riegle, 1978c). Despite such indications of altered testicular activity in vivo, testes or Leydig cells isolated from aged males show no change in basal levels of testosterone release, or in release of testosterone following stimulation with LH or hCG in vitro (Pirke et al., 1978; Bethea and Walker, 1979; Steger et al., 1979b; Kaler and Neaves, 1981).

Changes in Hypothalamopituitary Function

Declining levels of plasma testosterone in senescent males are accompanied by a reduction in LH and FSH secretion and an increase in PRL (Shaar et al., 1975; Riegle and Meites, 1976; Bruni et al., 1977; Pirke et al., 1978; Saksena and Lau, 1979; Bethea and Walker, 1979; Kaler and Neaves, 1981). Following castration (removal of negative feedback), aged males show a smaller rise in plasma LH than do young-adult males (Shaar et al., 1975). However, injections of testosterone proprionate significantly reduce plasma LH levels in castrated senescent males, indicating that the hypothalamopituitary system remains sensitive to negative feedback by gonadal steroids.

Following single injections of GnRH, plasma LH and FSH levels rise significantly less in aged male rats than in young males (Riegle and Meites, 1976; Bruni et al., 1977; Miller and Riegle, 1978a). According to one report, multiple injections of GnRH have little effect on LH levels in senescent male rats (Bruni et al., 1977), whereas in a second report, multiple injections of GnRH restore LH levels to those of young males (Miller and Riegle, 1978a). Although there are differences in experimental protocols, the reason for such a discrepancy remains unclear.

Sources of Alterations in Male Reproductive Function

Chronic understimulation of the testes in aged males has been suggested as an explanation for decreased plasma testosterone levels. This suggestion has been corroborated by experiments in which plasma testosterone levels were restored to young adult levels by prolonged treatment with hCG (Leatham and Albrecht, 1974; Miller and Riegle, 1978c; Harman et al., 1978). However, the production of testosterone in aged males may not be as severely impaired as has previously been supposed. Kaler and Neaves (1981) have shown that, when the increased blood volume of aged Sprague-Dawley male rats is taken into account, the testes actually release total amounts of steroids comparable to young animals. In this strain, decreased levels of circulating testosterone with age can be explained on the basis of a dilution effect arising from expanding blood volume. The authors have suggested that the fundamental problem in aging males may lie in a failure to compensate for continued adult growth via an increase in gonadotropin secretion and/or testicular production of steroids with age.

As in senescent females, changes in gonadotropin secretion have been attributed to alterations in hypothalamic function. Hypothalamic content of GnRH is reduced in aged males, although sufficient activity is present to stimulate the release of LH from young male pituitaries (Riegle et al., 1977; Riegle and Miller, 1978). A reduced content and turnover of catecholamines and an increased turnover of serotonin have been found in the hypothalamus of senescent males (Simkins et al., 1977; Meites et al., 1978), and such changes in hypothalamic monoamines have been suggested to be responsible for decreases in LH and FSH secretion and increased secretion of PRL. The pituitary of the aged male rat may also be directly altered with age (Riegle and Meites, 1976). Isolated pituitaries of aged males show not only a reduction in LH content, but also a reduced responsiveness to GnRH derived from hypothalamic extracts of young males (Riegle et al., 1977).

CHANGES IN PITUITARY FUNCTION WITH AGE: STRUCTURAL AND MOLECULAR CONSIDERATIONS

Qualitative Changes in the LH Molecule

Most experiments conducted to obtain information about possible sources of reproductive senescence in rats have been performed on intact animals. Whereas such experiments have shown clear changes in plasma gonadotropin levels with age, it is difficult from in vivo studies to distinguish the precise locus where such changes occur. For example, gonadotropins may be cleared at different rates in senescent and young animals, and this could be incorrectly interpreted as a change in rate of secretion. Such a possibility has indeed been proposed by Miller and Riegle (1978a) to explain elevated levels of serum LH in aged females between multiple injections of GnRH. In young females, serum LH drops to basal levels between injection times.

Qualitative molecular changes in LH from senescent rats may be responsible for altered clearance rates in vivo. We have reported an increase in the molecular size of LH (assessed by gel filtration) in the circulation and in pituitaries of old (20-24 month) males (Conn et al., 1980) (Fig. 3). Castration of young males mimics the effect of aging on LH size. LH from senescent males is also cleared more slowly from the circulation of young females than is LH from intact young males (Fig. 4). By injecting testosterone proprionate for 12 days, the LH in senescent males can be restored to the approximate molecular size of LH in young animals. It thus appears that the decreased levels of gonadal steroids in senescent male rats have a qualitative effect on the LH molecule itself. Qualitative changes in LH and FSH have been observed by others following gonadectomy of young-adult rats. These changes include alterations in molecular size (Bogdanove et al., 1974a), clearance rate (Bogdanove et al., 1974b; Weick, 1977), and ratio of biological to immunological activity (Diebel et al., 1973; Mukhopadhyay et al., 1979).

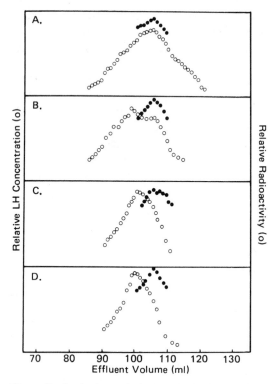

Figure 3 Sephadex gel elution profiles of immunoreactive LH, extracted from pituitaries of male rats aged 5 (a), 10 (b), 13 (c), and 24 (d) months. (●) LH standard; (○) extracted LH. A shift to the left indicates an increase in the Stokes radius (and presumably molecular weight) of the LH molecule. (From Conn et al., 1980.)

In the rhesus monkey, both LH and FSH in gonadectomized males and females show an increase in molecular size that can be reduced or abolished by neuraminidase treatment (Peckham and Knobil, 1976a, b). This indicates that gonadectomy may alter gonadotropin sialic acid content. We have found a similar effect of neuraminidase on the LH of senescent male rats. Whereas sialic acid residues have not been detected in LH from young adult rats (Ward et al., 1971), it is possible that in old rats the sialic acid content of LH is altered. Qualitative changes in LH during the aging process may not be restricted to rats. In human females, postmenopausal changes in serum LH have also been reported. For example, a large form of LH has been found by Prentice and Ryan (1975), and altered biological to immunological activity has been noted by Dufau et al. (1976, 1977).

Morphological Alterations in the Gonadotrope

Secretory proteins are synthesized from mRNAs in a similar fashion within different cell types. Synthesis of the protein molecule occurs in association with the

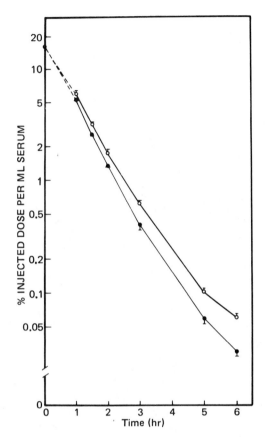

Figure 4 Clearance of immunoreactive LH, extracted from pituitaries of 5-month-old (●) or 24-month-old (○) male rats. Clearance examined in 28-day-old female rats. (From Conn et al., 1981.)

rough endoplasmic reticulum (RER), and further processing (such as glycosylation and assembly) takes place in the Golgi complex. We examined pituitary tissue of aging animals to determine whether or not alterations in hormone synthesis and secretion were correlated with changes in cellular morphology. Electron micrographs were prepared from pituitaries of young (5-month), middle-aged (11-month), and old (24-month) male rats. Figure 5 shows an overview of the pituitary from a young animal with different cell types indicated in the figure caption. The gonadotropes contain a heterogeneous population of granules, a roughly spheroid nucleus, and a large amount of RER. Figure 6 shows a more detailed view of a gonadotrope. The granules are heterogeneous in staining character, and a large number of polysomes can be seen both in association with the RER and free in the cytoplasm.

Figure 7 shows a gonadotrope cell found in an 11-month-old animal. While

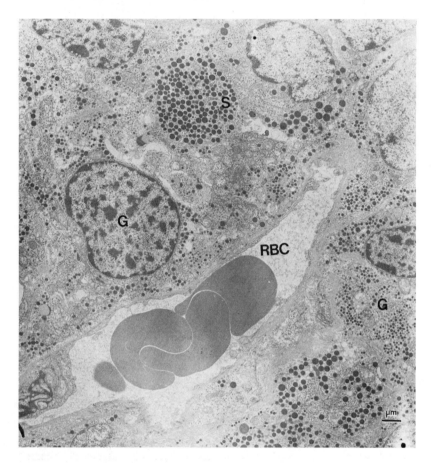

Figure 5 Overview of vascular region of the pituitary from a 6-month-old male rat. The pituitary was removed, fixed, and embedded for electron microscopy. Somatotrope (S), gonadotrope (G), and red blood cells (RBC) are marked.

the secretory granules are still present, large vesicular bodies which appear to be derived from the endoplasmic reticulum (ER), are now visible. These are light-staining and membrane-bound. The vesicles, which appear to be distended ER, are seen to be physically continuous in the 24-month-old animal (Fig. 8). In addition, gonadotropes of the 24-month-old male contain distended Golgi complexes and a paucity of secretory granules. Because such major morphological changes are apparent in the Golgi and RER and because these structures are associated with the protein synthetic and modification machinery, it is tempting to speculate that the molecular changes in the nature of LH during aging might be due to these structural alterations.

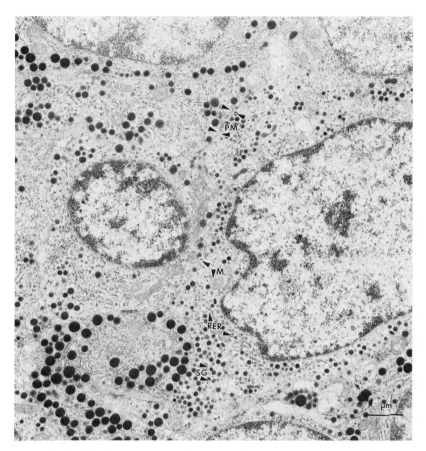

Figure 6   Detailed enlargement of gonadotrope cell from a 6-month-old male rat is shown on the right. The plasma membrane (PM), mitochondria (M), rough endoplasmic reticulum, and characteristic secretory granules (SG) containing gonadotropin are shown.

Whereas, to our knowledge, this is the first report of such morphological changes during aging, a number of other laboratories have described similar changes following ovariectomy in the rat. Farquhar and Rinehart (1954) first showed such vesiculated cells following ovariectomy. After 35 days, an additional cell type appeared which contained bizarre cytoplasmic elements. Several other laboratories have reported similar findings in the pituitaries of ovariectomized animals (DeVirguilus, 1968; Garner and Blake, 1981). These observations suggest that the morphological changes which occur during aging may reflect the endocrine status of the animal more than the age as such. Additional studies which show restora-

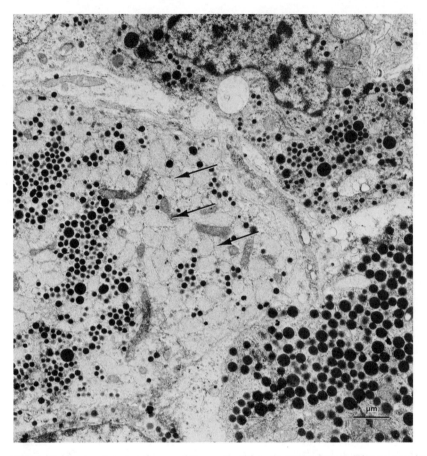

Figure 7 A gonadotrope from a 12-month-old male rat is shown. The arrows indicate the distended membranous sacs containing light-staining material.

tion of the "normal" cell type in old animals by some manipulation such as administration of steroids will be necessary to substantiate this contention.

Changes in GnRH Binding

Considerable progress has been made in recent years on the precise mechanism by which GnRH stimulates release of LH and FSH from the pituitary (for a detailed review, see Conn et al., 1981). Evidence from many laboratories now suggests that the mechanism of action of GnRH may be divided into three parts: (1) GnRH binds to a specific, plasma membrane receptor. Occupancy of this receptor results in mobilization of calcium and (2) a subsequent increase in intracellular calcium

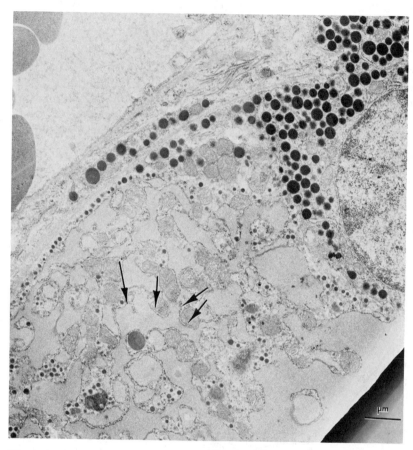

Figure 8 A gonadotrope from a 24-month-old male rat is shown. Note the arrows indicating continuity between the distended areas of membrane. These distended sacs now occupy a major portion of the intracellular space.

which leads to (3) release of the gonadotropins from previously synthesized secretory granules. Accordingly, a molecular "dissection" in which each of these steps is analyzed separately will lead to determination of the precise locus of alterations in pituitary function which occur during aging.

We have recently examined age-related changes in the first step in the action of GnRH on the pituitary, binding to a specific receptor (Marian et al., 1981). Because functional receptor levels can effectively alter target cell sensitivity and because relatively elevated receptor levels appear necessary for maximum LH release, the possibility exists that altered gonadotrope sensivity which occurs during aging is mediated, at least in part, by altered receptor levels. Roth (1978, 1979) has shown that alterations in hormone receptor numbers per cell are a common feature of the aging process in many systems.

We have used a binding assay employing the analogue (^{125}I)-D-Ser(t-butyl)[6]-desGly[10]-ethylamide-GnRH (Buserelin, Hoescht) to determine the number and binding affinity of the GnRH receptor of the pituitary gonadotrope during aging (Marian et al., 1981). Receptor number in pituitaries from PP and CE rats (20-24 months) was compared to that in 30-day-old pups. Since these old animals differ from weanlings both in age and in endocrine status, 6 and 12-month spontaneously CE rats were also examined. For all ages of CE rats, receptor binding was dramatically decreased compared to weanling females. A similar decrease was observed for old PP rats. Receptor affinity was not different between the CE or PP groups, whereas receptor concentration in the CE and old animals was 18-24% of that in the young (Fig. 9). These data suggest that alterations in GnRH receptor number but not binding affinity occur during aging. It does not appear that these alterations are caused by general deterioration of the pituitary, because decreases in

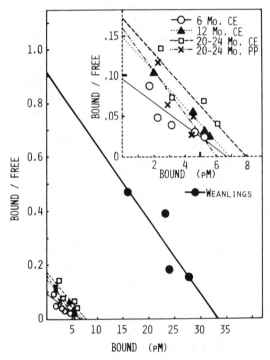

Figure 9 Scatchard analysis of GnRH receptor binding in young precycling and older constant-estrous (CE) and pseudopregnant (PP) rats. Inset is detail of lower left. (From Marian et al., 1981.)

receptor number are apparent in young animals in altered endocrine states. Rather, it appears that changes in endocrine status may indeed be the source of altered pituitary binding of GnRH in senescent females. Whether postreceptor sites are also influenced by the endocrine changes accompanying senescence is a question that will require additional examination of the gonadotrope.

HUMAN REPRODUCTIVE SENESCENCE

A few words may be in order at this point concerning differences between the fundamental causes of reproductive senescence in rats and in humans. In human females, as in rats, irregular cycling, reduced frequency of ovulation, and the formation of cystic follicles are commonly observed prior to a complete loss of cyclic ovarian activity (Talbert, 1978). However, following the onset of menopause, steroid secretion is markedly decreased, and the ovaries become atrophied and fibrotic. In the virtual absence of gonadal steroids, circulating gonadotropin levels rise sharply, yet the ovaries remain unresponsive to such elevated levels of stimulation. This suggests intrinsic ovarian failure to be of primary importance in the loss of reproductive cycles in women.

Age-related changes in reproductive function are more similar in male rats and humans than in females of both species. As in rats, reproductive decline in human males is gradual, with spermatogenesis continuing well past middle age (Harman, 1978). A decline in circulating testosterone levels similar to that seen in rats is also observed in some, but not all, human males during senescence (Vermeulen et al., 1972; Baker et al., 1976). However, unlike rats, aging men show a slight increase in circulating gonadotropin levels (Harman, 1978). Whether reproductive decline in human males arises solely from testicular alterations, or from changes both in the testes and in higher centers, remains unresolved (Harman, 1978).

SUMMARY AND CONCLUSIONS

In both male and female rats, reproductive decline begins during middle age as an apparent result of alterations in the hypothalamopituitary control of gonadotropin secretion. Such changes are manifested as gonadal malfunction, yet the gonads themselves appear potentially capable of normal activity throughout most of adult life. Recent research concerning the primary cause of reproductive senescence in rats has emphasized hypothalamic malfunction, with particular attention being paid to changes in the synthesis of hypothalamic monoamines. However, the initial sources of altered gonadotropin secretion in aging rats have not yet been elucidated.

In this review, we have presented several lines of evidence to indicate that long-term alterations in gonadal activity may in turn have important consequences for pituitary function, leading to changes in the nature of the LH molecule, changes in pituitary structure, and changes in binding of GnRH to the pituitary gonadotropes. These results indicate that care must be taken to separate intrinsic, age-related changes in hypothalamopituitary function from changes induced by the altered steroid environment of the aged animal.

It is clear that a complete understanding of the factors underlying reproductive failure in the rat must come from a careful analysis of both the causes and the consequences of changes in the reproductive endocrine system. Results of investigations using this model may provide insights into the basis for reproductive decline in humans, particularly males. In addition, at the cellular level, reproductive senescence in the rat is likely to be of considerable value as a model for investigating general changes in mammalian endocrine function with age.

ACKNOWLEDGMENTS

During preparation of this manuscript, W. A. Smith was supported by NIA grant 5 T32 AG00029. Research described from our laboratory was supported in part by NIH AG 1204 to P. M. Conn. P. M. Conn is the recipient of NIH RCDA HD 00337. Our thanks to Dr. Don Smith and Dr. Janet Marian for their thoughtful advice and criticism of the manuscript.

REFERENCES

Aschheim, P. (1961). La pseudogestation à repétition chez les rattes séniles. *C. R. Acad. Sci. (Paris) 253*: 1988-1990.

Aschheim, P. (1964/1965). Resultats fournis par la greffe heterochrone des ovaries dans l'etude de la regulation hypothalamo-hyophyso-ovarienne de la ratte sénile. *Gerontologia 10*: 65-75.

Aschheim, P. (1965). La reactivation de l'ovaire des rattes séniles en oestrus permanent au moyen d'hormones gonadotropes de la mise à l'obscurité. *C. R. Acad. Sci. (Paris) 260*: 5627-5630.

Aschheim, P. (1976). Aging in the hypothalamic-hypophyseal-ovarian axis in the rat. In *Hypothalamus, Pituitary and Aging*, A. V. Everitt and J. A. Burgess (Eds.). Charles C Thomas, Springfield, Ill., pp. 376-418.

Baker, H. W., Burger, H. G., De Krester, D. M., and Hudson, B. (1976). Endocrinology of aging: Pituitary testicular axis. *Clin. Endocrinol. 5*: 349-372.

Bethea, C. L., and Walker, R. F. (1979). Age-related changes in reproductive hormones and in Leydig cell responsivity in the male Fischer 344 rat. *J. Gerontol. 34*: 21-27.

Bloch, S. (1961). Untersuchungen uber das genitale altern des Rattenweibschens. *Gerontologia 5*: 55-62.

Bogdanove, E. M., Campbell, G. T., and Peckham, W. D. (1974a). FSH pleomorphism in the rat: regulation by gonadal steroids. *Endoc. Res. Communic. 1*: 87-99.

Bogdanove, E. M., Campbell, G. T., Blair, E. D., Mula, M. E., Miller, A. E., and Grossman, G. H. (1974b). Gonad pituitary feedback involves qualitative change: androgens alter the type of FSH secreted by the rat pituitary. *Endocrinology 95*: 219-228.

Bruni, J. F., Huang, H. H., Marshall, S., and Meites, J. (1977). Effects of single and multiple injections of synthetic GnRH on serum LH, FSH, and testosterone in young and old male rats. *Biol. Reprod. 17*: 309-321.

Chan, S. W. C., Leatham, J. H., and Esashi, T. (1977). Testicular metabolism and serum testosterone in aging male rats. *Endocrinology 101*: 128-133.

Clemens, J. A., and Bennett, D. R. (1977). Do aging changes in the preoptic area contribute to loss of cyclic endocrine function? *J. Gerontol. 32*: 19-24.

Clemens, J. A., and Meites, J. Neuroendocrine status of old constant-estrous rats. *Neuroendocrinology 7*: 249-256.

Clemens, J. A., Amenomori, Y., Jenkins, T., and Meites, J. (1969). Effects of hypothalamic stimulation, hormones, and drugs on ovarian function in old female rats. *Proc. Soc. Exp. Biol. Med. 132*: 561-563.

Conn, P. M., Cooper, R., McNamara, C., Rogers, D. C., and Schoenhardt, L. (1980). Qualitative changes in gonadotropin during normal aging in the male rat. *Endocrinology 106*: 1549-1553.

Conn, P. M., Marian, J., McMillian, M., Stern, J., Rogers, D., Hamby, M., Penna, A., and Grant, E. (1981). Gonadotropin releasing hormone action in the pituitary: a three step mechanism. *Endocrine Rev. 2*: 174-185.

Cooper, R. L., and Walker, R. F. (1979). Potential therapeutic consequences of age-dependent changes in brain physiology. *Interdiscpl. Topics Geront. 15*: 54-76.

Cooper, R. L., Conn, P. M., and Walker, R. F. (1980). Characterization of the LH surge in middle-aged female rats. *Biol. Reprod. 23*: 611-615.

Damassa, D. A., Gilman, D. P., Lu, K. H., Judd, H. L., and Sawyer, C. H. (1980). The twenty-four hour pattern of prolactin secretion in aging female rats. *Biol. Reprod. 22*: 571-575.

DeVirguilus, G. (1968). Ultrastructure des cellules gonadotropes de l'adenohypophyse apres ovarectomie. *Ann. Endocrinol.* (*Paris*) *29*: 553-561.

Diebel, N. D., Yamamoto, M., and Bogdanove, E. M. (1973). Discrepancies between radioimmunoassays and bioassays for rat FSH: evidence that androgen treatment and withdrawal can alter bioassay-immunoassay ratios. *Endocrinology 92*: 1065-1078.

Dufau, M. L., Beitins, I. Z., McArthur, J. W., and Catt, K. J. (1976). Effects of luteinizing hormone releasing hormone (LHRH) upon bioactive and immunoreactive serum LH levels in normal subjects. *J. Clin. Endocrinol. Metab. 43*: 658-667.

Dufau, M. L., Beitins, I., McArthur, J., and Catt, K. J. (1977). Bioassay of serum LH concentrations in normal and LHRH-stimulated human subjects. In *The Testes in Normal and Infertile Men*, P. Troen and H. R. Nankin (Eds.). Raven Press, New York, pp. 309-325.

Erickson, G. F., Hsueh, A. J. W., and Lu, K. H. (1979). Gonadotropin binding and aromatase activity in granulosa cells of young proestrous and old constant estrous rats. *Biol. Reprod. 20*: 182-190.

Farquhar, M. G., and Rinehart, J. F. (1954). Electron microscopic studies of the anterior pituitary gland of castrate rats. *Endocrinology 54*: 516-541.

Finch, C. E. (1978). Reproductive senescence in rodents: Factors in the decline of fertility and loss of regular estrous cycles. In *The Aging Reproductive System*, E. L. Schneider (Ed.). Raven Press, New York, pp. 193-212.

Garner, L. L., and Blake, C. A. (1981). Ultrastructural, immunochemical study of the LH secreting cell of the rat anterior pituitary gland: changes occurring after ovariectomy. *Biol. Reprod. 24*: 461-474.

Ghanadian, R., Lewis, J. G., and Chisolm, G. D. (1975). Serum testosterone and dihydrotestosterone changes with age in rat. *Steroids 25*: 753-762.

Gilman, D. P., Lu, J. K. H., Whitmoyer, D. I., Judd, H. L., and Sawyer, C. H. (1981). Relationship between progesterone and prolactin surges in aged and young pseudopregnant rats. *Biol. Reprod. 24*: 839-845.

Gosden, R. G., and Bancroft, L. (1976). Pituitary function in reproductively senescent female rats. *Exp. Gerontol. 11*: 157-160.

Gray, G. D. (1978). Changes in the levels of luteinizing hormone and testosterone in the circulation of aging male rats. *J. Endocrinol. 76*: 551-552.

Gray, G. D., Tennent, B., Smith, E. R., and Davidson, J. M. (1980). Luteinizing hormone regulation and sexual behavior in middle-aged female rats. *Endocrinology 107*: 187-194.

Harman, S. M. (1978). Clinical aspects of aging of the male reproductive system. In *The Aging Reproductive System*, E. L. Schneider (Ed.). Raven Press, New York, pp. 29-58.

Harman, S. M., Danner, R. L., and Roth, G. S. (1978). Testosterone secretion in the rat in response to chorionic gonadotrophin: Alterations with age. *Endocrinology 102*: 540-543.

Howland, B. (1976). Reduced gonadotropin release in response to progesterone or gonadotropin releasing hormone (GnRH) in old female rats. *Life Sci. 19*: 219-224.

Howland, B. E., and Preiss, C. (1975). Effects of aging on basal serum gonadotropins, ovarian compensatory hypertrophy, and hypersecretion of gonadotropins after ovariectomy in female rats. *Fertil. Steril. 26*: 271-276.

Hsueh, A., and Erickson, G. (1979a). Extrapituitary action of GnRH: direct inhibition of ovarian steroidogenesis. *Science 204*: 854-55.

Hsueh, A., and Erickson, G. (1979b). Extrapituitary inhibition of testicular function by LHRH. *Nature 281*: 66-67.

Huang, H. H., and Meites, J. (1975). Reproductive capacity in aging female rats. *Neuroendocrinology 17*: 289-295.

Huang, H. H., Marshall, S., and Meites, J. (1976a). Capacity of old versus young female rats to secrete LH, FSH, and prolactin. *Biol. Reprod. 14*: 538-543.

Huang, H. H., Marshall, S., and Meites, J. (1976b). Induction of estrous cycles in old non-cyclic rats by progesterone, ACTH, ether stress or L-dopa. *Neuroendocrinology 20*: 21-34.

Huang, H. H., Steger, R. W., and Meites, J. (1978). Patterns of sex steroid and gonadotropin secretion in aging female rats. *Endocrinology 103*: 1855-1859.

Ingram, D. K. (1959). The vaginal smear of senile laboratory rats. *J. Endocrinol. 19*: 182-188.

Kaler, L. W., and Neaves, W. B. (1981). The androgen status of aging male rats. *Endocrinology 108*: 712-719.

Labrie, F., Lagace, L., Beaulieu, M., Ferland, L., De Lean, A., Drouin, J., Borgeat, P., Kelly, P. A., Cusan, L., Dupont, A., Lemay, A., Antakly, T., Pelletier, G. H., and Barden, N. (1979). Mechanisms of action of hypothalamic and peripheral hormones in the anterior pituitary gland. In *Hormonal Proteins and Peptides*, Vol. 7, C. H. Li (Ed.). Academic Press, New York, pp. 206-277.

Leatham, J. H., and Albrecht, E. D. (1974). Effect of age on testes-3-hydroxy-steroid dehydrogenase in the rat. *Proc. Soc. Exp. Biol. Med. 145*: 1212-1214.

Lu, J. K. H., Damassa, D. A., Gilman, D. P., Judd, H. L., and Sawyer, C. H. (1980). Differential patterns of gonadotropin responses to ovarian steroids and to LH-RH between constant-estrous and pseudopregnant states in aging rats. *Biol. Reprod. 23*: 345-351.

Lu, K. H., Gilman, D. P., Meldrum, D. R., Judd, H. L., and Sawyer, C. H. (1981). Relationship between circulating estrogens and the central mechanisms by which ovarian steroids stimulate luteinizing hormone secretion in aged and young female rats. *Endocrinology 108*: 836-841.

Lu, K. H., Hopper, B. R., Vargo, T. M., and Yen, S. S. C. (1979). Chronological changes in sex steroid, gonadotropin and prolactin secretion in aging female rats displaying different reproductive states. *Biol. Reprod. 21*: 193-203.

Lu, K. H., Huang, H. H., Chen, H. T., Kurcz, M., Miodouszewski, R., and Meites, J. (1977). Positive feedback by estrogen and progesterone on LH release in old and young rats. *Proc. Soc. Exp. Biol. Med. 154*: 82-85.

Mandl, A. M. (1959). Corpora lutea in senile virgin laboratory rats. *J. Endocrinol. 22*: 257-268.

Mandl, A. M. (1961). Cyclical changes in the vaginal smears of senile nulliparous and multiparous rats. *J. Endocrinol. 18*: 444-450.

Mandl, A. M., and Shelton, M. (1959). A quantitative study of oocytes in young and old nulliparous laboratory rats. *J. Endocrinol. 18*: 444-450.

Marian, J., Cooper, R. L., and Conn, P. M. (1981). Regulation of the rat pituitary GnRH-receptor. *Mol. Pharmacol. 19*: 399-405.

McPherson, J. C., Costoff, A., and Mahesh, V. (1977). Effects of aging on the hypothalamic-hypophyseal-gonadal axis in female rats. *Fertil. Steril. 28*: 1365-1370.

Meites, J., and Huang, H. H. (1976). Relation of neuroendocrine system to loss of reproductive functions in aging rats. In *Neuroendocrine Regulation of Fertility*, A. Kumar (Ed.). Karger, Basel, pp. 246-258.

Meites, J., Huang, H. H., and Simpkins, J. W. (1978). Recent studies on neuroendocrine control of reproductive senescence in rats. In *The Aging Reproductive System*, E. L. Schneider (Ed.). Raven Press, New York, pp. 213-326.

Meites, J., Steger, R. W., and Huang, H. H. (1980). Relation of the neuroendocrine system to reproductive decline in aging rats and human subjects. *Fed. Proc. 39*: 3168-3172.

Miller, A. E., and Riegle, G. D. (1978a). Serum LH levels following multiple LHRH injections in aging rats. *Proc. Soc. Exp. Biol. Med. 157*: 494-498.

Miller, A. E., and Riegle, G. D. (1978b). Hypothalamic LH-releasing activity in young and aged intact and gonadectomized rats. *Exp. Aging Res. 4*: 145-155.

Miller, A. E., and Riegle, G. D. (1978c). Serum testosterone and testicular response to hCG in young and aged male rats. *J. Gerontol. 33*: 197-203.

Miller, A. E., and Riegle, G. D. (1980a). Temporal changes in serum progesterone in aging female rats. *Endocrinology 106*: 1579-1583.

Miller A. E., and Riegle, G. D. (1980b). Serum progesterone during pregnancy and pseudopregnancy and gestation length in the aging rat. *Biol. Reprod. 22*: 751-758.

Miller, A. E., Wood, S. M., and Riegle, G. D. (1979). The effect of age on reproduction in repeatedly mated female rats. *J. Gerontol. 34*: 15-20.

Mukhopadhyay, A., Leidenberger, F., and Lichtenberg, V. (1979). A comparison of bioactivity and immunoactivity of luteinizing hormone stored in and released *in vitro* from pituitary glands of rats under various gonadal states. *Endocrinology 104*: 925-931.

National Academy of Sciences. (1981). *Mammalian Models for Research on Aging*. National Academy Press, Washington, D.C., pp. 75-132.

Page, R. D., and Butcher, R. L. (1982). Follicular and plasma patterns of steroids in young and old rats during normal and prolonged estrous cycles. *Biol. Reprod. 27*, 383-392.

Pecile, A., Muller, E., and Falconi, G. (1966). Endocrine function of pituitary transplants taken from rats of different ages. *Arch. Int. Pharmacodyn. Ther. 159*: 434-441.

Peckham, W. D., and Knobil, E. (1976a). The effects of ovariectomy, estrogen replacement, and neuraminidase treatment on the properties of the adenohypophyseal glycoprotein hormones of the rhesus monkey. *Endocrinology 98*: 1054-1060.

Peckham, W. D., and Knobil, E. (1976b). Qualitative changes in the pituitary gonadotropins of the male rhesus monkey following castration. *Endocrinology 98*: 1061-1064.

Peluso, J. J., Steger, R. W., and Hafez, E. S. E. (1977). Regulation of LH secretion in aged female rats. *Biol. Reprod. 16*: 212-215.

Peng, M. T., and Huang, H. H. (1973). Aging of hypothalamic-pituitary-ovarian function in the rat. *Fertil. Steril. 23*: 535-542.

Pirke, K. M., Vogt, H. J., and Geiss, M. (1978). *In vitro* and *in vivo* studies on Leydig cell function in old rats. *Acta Endocrinol. (Kph) 89*: 393-403.

Prentice, L. G., and Ryan, R. J. (1975). LH and its subunits in human pituitary, serum, and urine. *J. Clin. Endocrinol. Metab. 40*: 303-312.

Quadri, S. K., Kledzik, G. S., and Meites, J. (1973). Reinitiation of estrous cycles in old constant estrous rats by central-acting drugs. *Neuroendocrinology 11*: 248-255.

Riegle, G. D., and Meites, J. (1976). Effects of aging on LH and prolactin after LRH, L-Dopa, methyl-Dopa, and stress in the male rat. *Proc. Soc. Exp. Biol. Med. 151*: 507-511.

Riegle, G. D., and Miller, A. E. (1978). Aging effects on the hypothalamo-hypophyseal-gonadal control system in the rat. In *The Aging Reproductive System*, E. L. Schneider (Ed.). Raven Press, New York, pp. 159-192.

Riegle, G. D., Meites, J. M., Miller, A. E., and Wood, S. M. (1977). Effect of aging on hypothalamic LH-releasing and prolactin-inhibiting activities and pituitary responsiveness to LHRH in the male laboratory rat. *J. Gerontol. 32*: 13-18.

Roth, G. S. (1978). Hormonal receptor and responsiveness changes during aging: genetic modulation. In *Genetic Effects on Aging*, D. Bergsma and D. H. Harrison (Eds.). Liss, New York, pp. 365-384.

Roth, G. S. (1979). Hormone receptor changes during adulthood and senescence: significance for aging research. *Fed. Proc. 38*: 1910-1914.

Saksena, S. K., and Lau, I. F. (1979). Variations in serum androgens, estrogens, progestins, gonadotropins and Prl levels in male rats from puberty to advanced age. *Exp. Aging Res. 5*: 179-194.

Saksena, S. K., Lau, I. F., and Chang, M. C. (1979). Age dependent changes in the sperm population and fertility in the male rat. *Exp. Aging Res. 5*: 373-381.

Shaar, C. J., Euker, J. S., Riegle, G. D., and Meites, J. (1975). Effects of castration and gonadal steroids on serum luteinizing hormone and prolactin in old and young rats. *J. Endocrinol. 66*: 45-51.

Sharpe, R. M. (1980). Extrapituitary actions of LHRH and its agonists. *Nature 286*: 12-14.

Simpkins, J. W., Mueller, G. P., Huang, H. H., and Meites, J. (1977). Evidence for depressed catecholamine and enhanced serotonin metabolism in aging male rats: Possible relation to gonadotropin secretion. *Endocrinology 100*: 1672-1678.

Smith, P. E. (1963). Postponed pituitary homotransplants into the region of the hypophyseal portal circulation in hypophysectomized female rats. *Endocrinology 73*: 793-806.

Smith, W. A., Cooper, R. L., and Conn, P. M. (1982). Altered pituitary responsiveness to gonadotropin-releasing hormone in middle-aged rats with 4-day estrous cycles. *Endocrinology 111*: 1843-1848.

Sopelak, V. M., and Butcher, R. L. (1982a). Contribution of the ovary versus hypothalamus-pituitary to termination of estrous cycles in aging rats using ovarian transplants. *Biol. Reprod. 27*: 29-37.

Sopelak, V. M., and Butcher, R. L. (1982b). Decreased amount of ovarian tissue and maternal age affect embryonic development in old rats. *Biol. Reprod. 27*: 449-455.

Steger, R. W., Huang, H. H., Chamberlain, D. S., and Meites, J. (1980). Changes in control of gonadotropin secretion in the transition period between regular cycles and constant estrus in aging female rats. *Biol. Reprod. 22*: 595-603.

Steger, R. W., Huang, H. H., and Meites, J. (1979a). Relation of aging to hypothalamic LHRH content and serum gonadal steroids in female rats. *Proc. Soc. Exp. Biol. Med. 161*: 251-254.

Steger, R. E., Peluso, J. F., Bruni, J. F., Hafez, E. S. E., and Meites, J. (1979b). Gonadotropin binding and testicular function in old rats. *Endokrinologie 83*: 1-5.

Talbert, G. B. (1978). Effect of aging of the ovaries and female gametes on reproductive capacity. In *The Aging Reproductive System*, E. L. Schneider (Ed.). Raven Press, New York, pp. 59-83.

van der Schoot, P. (1976). Changing pro-oestrous surges of luteinizing hormone in aging 5-day cyclic rats. *J. Endocrinol. 69*: 287-288.

Vermeulen, A., Rubens, R., and Verdonck, L. (1972). Testosterone secretion and metabolism in male senescence. *J. Clin. Endocrinol. Metab. 34*: 730-735.

Ward, D. N., Reichert, L. E., Fitak, B. A., Nahm, H. S., Sweeney, C. M., and Neill, J. D. (1971). Isolation and properties of subunits of rat pituitary luteinizing hormone. *Biochemistry 10*: 1796-1802.

Watkins, B. E., McKay, D. W., Meites, J., and G. D. Riegle. (1976). L-DOPA effects on serum LH and prolactin in old and young female rats. *Neuroendocrinology 19*: 331-338.

Watkins, B. E., Meites, J., and Riegle, G. D. (1975). Age-related changes in pituitary responsiveness to LHRH in the female rat. *Endocrinology 97*: 543-548.

Weick, R. F. (1977). A comparison of the disappearance rates of luteinizing hormone from intact and ovariectomized rats. *Endocrinology 101*: 157-161.

Wilkes, M. M., Lu, K. H., Fulton, S. L., and Yen, S. S. C. (1978). Hypothalamic-pituitary-ovarian interactions during reproductive senescence in the rat. *Adv. Exp. Med. Biol. 113*: 127-147.

Wise, P. M. (1982a). Alterations in the proestrous pattern of median eminence LHRH, serum LH, FSH, estradiol and progesterone concentrations in middle-aged rats. *Life Sci. 31*: 165-173.

Wise, P. M. (1982b). Alterations in proestrous LH, FSH, and prolactin surges in middle-aged rats. *Proc. Soc. Exp. Biol. Med. 169*: 348-354.

Wise, P. M., and Ratner, A. (1980a). Effect of ovariectomy on plasma LH, FSH, estradiol, and progesterone and medial basal hypothalamic LHRH concentrations in old and young rats. *Neuroendocrinology 30*: 15-19.

Wise, P. M., and Ratner, A. (1980b). LHRH-induced LH and FSH responses in the aged female rat. *J. Gerontol. 4*: 506-511.

Wolfe, J. M. (1943). The effects of advancing age on the structure of the anterior hypophyses and ovaries of female rats. *Am. J. Anat. 72*: 361-383.

2

Pharmacological and Dietary Manipulations of Reproductive Aging in the Rat: Significance to Central Nervous System Aging

Ralph L. Cooper / *Duke University Medical Center, Durham, North Carolina*

INTRODUCTION

Studies of the reproductive system in the female rat offer compelling evidence for the concept of intervention in the aging process. These studies demonstrate that once knowledge is obtained concerning the basic physiological changes that occur during aging, prevention of such changes can be achieved. At times this can be accomplished with rather simple and straightforward procedures. More recent studies demonstrate that it is not only possible to significantly prolong reproductive function, but that it is also possible to delay the development of various pathological conditions that occur as a consequence of reproductive aging.

Reproductive aging in the female rat is usually described in terms of changes in the vaginal cytology that accompany age-related changes in ovarian function. These changes are first noted at approximately 1 year of age when the regular 4 to 5-day cyclical changes in the vaginal smear are replaced by a condition of constant cornification. This transition from regular estrous cycles to constant estrus (CE) may be preceded by a period of irregular cycling in some animals. However, such irregular cycling is not observed in all animals and may be more prevalent in some strains. The CE condition usually lasts from 8-10 months, after which an increased number of females assume a pattern of repetitive pseudopregnancies (RP). The vaginal smear of the RP female is predominantly leukocytic, interrupted occasionally by brief periods of cornification. In the very old female (i.e., ages greater than 24 months), there is an increased incidence of anestrus during which the vaginal smear is permanently leukocytic. The changes in ovarian function and the resultant changes in hormonal status accompanying the various acyclic conditions in the older females have been detailed elsewhere (Huang and Meites, 1975; Huang et al., 1978; Lu et al., 1979; see Smith and Conn chapter for review, this volume).

BRAIN-PITUITARY-OVARIAN FUNCTION IN THE OLD FEMALE RAT

A fundamental question concerning aging within the reproductive system is whether alterations in the brain-pituitary-ovarian axis and associated reproductive organs occur simultaneously as a general aging phenomenon, or whether they are initiated in one particular organ and then spread to other components of this neuroendocrine system. This question has been addressed by a number of recent studies, the results of which indicate that the loss of regular ovarian function in the rat is not primarily the result of ovarian failure, but rather age-dependent changes in the hypothalamohypophyseal complex. Substantial support for this hypothesis is provided by the observation that transplantation of ovaries from old, noncycling female rats into young, ovariectomized rats will result in a resumption of ovarian cycles in the recipient female. The reciprocal transplant of a young female's ovaries into the old female will result in a resumption of CE or RP, depending upon the condition of the aged female prior to ovariectomy (Aschheim, 1965).

Further support for the hypothesis that age-dependent changes in ovarian function occur as a consequence of age-dependent changes in the hypothalamo-hypophyseal complex has been provided by a number of pharmacological studies. Ovulation and/or vaginal cyclicity have been reinitated in the old CE female by systemic injections of luteinizing hormone (LH) (Aschheim, 1976), gonadotropin hormone-releasing hormone (GnRH) (Meites et al., 1978), low doses of progesterone (Everett, 1940), precursors to the central nervous system (CNS) catecholamines (CAs) such as L-tyrosine and L-dopa (Quadri et al., 1973a; Linnoila and Cooper, 1976; Cooper, 1980), and monoamine oxidase inhibitors such as iproniazid (Quadri et al., 1973a). These findings have been interpreted as indicating that the disruption of regular cycles in the aging female is a consequence of age-dependent changes in neurotransmitter regulation of anterior pituitary gland function. Evidence that the effect of such pharmacological manipulations is mediated through the CNS was obtained in studies showing that the ability of systemic L-dopa treatment to reinstate ovarian cycles is enhanced when this CA precursor is administered along with a peripheral dopa decarboxylase inhibitor such as MK 486 or RO 4-4602 (Linnoila and Cooper, 1976). Furthermore, direct placement of L-dopa into the medial preoptic area (MPOA) results in a return to regular vaginal cycling and ovulation (Cooper et al., 1979). Similar treatment with L-dopa into the dorsomedial septum or cortex was ineffective, indicating some degree of specificity for the critical regions involved within the CNS. Clemens et al. (1969) have also shown that ovulation could be induced in the aged CE female by electrical stimulation of the MPOA. These studies demonstrate clearly that some degree of ovarian function can be restored in the old noncycling female rat and that this can be accomplished by treatments designed to affect CNS neurotransmitter function.

The mechanism of action of the CA precursor treatment on ovarian function in the old rat remains to be determined. There is a decrease in CA concentration and turnover in the aged, intact CE female rat (Walker et al., 1980), and the post-ovariectomy rise in CA content, typical of the young female, is not observed in the old, previously CE female after ovariectomy (Wilkes and Yen, 1981). In young rats, systemic treatment with L-tyrosine or L-dopa (Wurtman and Fernstrom, 1972; Gibson and Wurtman, 1977) or direct placement of L-dopa into the brain (Ng et al., 1970) will cause a significant increase in dopamine (DA) and norepinephrine (NE) metabolism. NE receptor stimulation in the MPOA-anterior hypothalamic region (MPOA-AH) facilitates GnRH and LH secretion (see Sawyer, 1975, for review). An increment of dopaminergic activity has been implicated in the reinstatement of vaginal cycling in the old rat, since the response to L-dopa was blocked by pimozide (a dopaminergic receptor blocker), but not by phenoxybenzamine or L-propranolol (a- and β-noradrinergic receptor blockers) (Linnoila and Cooper, 1976). Likewise, treatments with a dopamine receptor agonist such as lergotrile mesylate have also been shown to reinitiate ovarian cyclicity in aging animals (Clemens and Bennett, 1977; Everett, 1980). Thus, the most straightforward explanation of these findings would be that systemic or central treatments of CA precursors restore ovarian function primarily through the effect of these agents on CNS-CA function and subsequent changes in GnRH and LH secretion. However, direct measurements of CA metabolism in the old female subjected to treatment with the various CA precursors have not been made.

Serotonin (5-HT) is also involved in the regulation of gonadotropin hormone secretion. In the young female, enhanced CNS 5-HT metabolism on the afternoon of vaginal proestrus will inhibit LH release and block ovulation (Labhsetwar, 1972; Carrer and Taleisnik, 1970), whereas at other times during the estrous cycle depletion of 5-HT will disrupt regular ovarian function (Kordon et al., 1978) and LH release (Franks et al., 1980). Thus, due to the dynamic interaction of CAs and 5-HT on gonadotropin hormone secretion and the relative changes in the metabolism of these neurotransmitters with age, the suppression of 5-HT may be an important component of the mechanism by which treatment with catecholaminergic agents influences ovarian function in the old rat. The details of this argument have been presented previously (Cooper and Walker, 1979; Cooper and Linnoila, 1980; Cooper, 1980). Briefly, dietary or systemic treatments with the CA precursors L-tyrosine or L-dopa or the CA agonist lergotrile mesylate have been shown to lower CNS 5-HT concentration and metabolism (Fahn et al., 1975; Hutt et al., 1977; Gibson and Wurtman 1977). When administered in the diet, the CA precursors such as L-tyrosine compete with L-tryptophan for entry into the brain at the level of the amino acid transport system (Fernstrom et al., 1975). Its effect on CNS,

CA, and 5-HT may also explain why L-dopa placed into the MPOA reinstated ovulation and vaginal cycling in old rats, whereas centrally administered L-tyrosine did not. Within the CNS, the nonspecificity of the mechanism for uptake of dihydroxylated aromatic amino acids into monoaminergic neurons results in reduced 5-HT neurotransmission after L-dopa is administered (Ng et al., 1970); Tyrosine is not a dihydroxylated aromatic amino acid; unlike L-dopa it is not taken up nonspecifically into both CA and 5-HT neurons (Ng et al., 1970). Thus, L-dopa reduces 5-HT neurotransmission and increases CNS CA synthesis when administered centrally or systemically, whereas L-tyrosine has these effects only when administered systemically.

The possibility that CA precursor treatment affects ovarian function in old rats by suppressing 5-HT neurotransmission is further supported by the results of recently completed studies using zimelidine, a 5-HT reuptake blocker (Cooper, 1980). Treatment with zimelidine results in chronic stimulation of the postsynaptic 5-HT receptors and also prevents the uptake of L-dopa into 5-HT neurons. Subcutaneous injections of zimelidine, 20 mg/kg, dissolved in distilled water [a dose reported to have minimal effects on CA neurotransmission (Rockman et al., 1979)], were administered to young and middle-aged regularly cycling and old CE females for a period of 2 weeks. Treatment to young regularly cycling females resulted in prolonged diestrus or estrous periods (5-7 and 3-5 days, respectively; Table 1) and a delay in the time at which the LH surge occurred on the afternoon of proestrus. This change in the vaginal cycle in young rats following zimelidine treatment resembles the change in the vaginal cycle seen in middle-aged females prior to the appearance of the CE condition. Likewise, the shift in the LH peak to

Table 1   Effect of Zimelidine on Vaginal Cytology of Long-Evans Rats: Vaginal Smear Pattern During 2-Week Treatment Period[a]

Age	Group	Regular cycles	Irregular cycles	Persistent or constant estrus	Predominantly leukocytic or RP
4 months	Zimelidine	2	6	1	1
	Control[b]	10	0	0	0
10 months	Zimelidine	0	2	9	1
	Control[b]	9	0	1	0
19 months	CE control[b]	0	0	10	0
	CE + Sinemet[c]	4	2	4	0
	CE + zimelidine	0	0	0	10
	CE + Sinemet[c] + zimelidine	0	0	0	10

[a]The vaginal smears of all animals were observed for 2 weeks prior to treatment. Numbers indicate animals showing each smear pattern after treatment.
[b]Control rats received 0.5 ml distilled water.
[c]Sinemet (Merck, Sharpe, and Dohme: a combination of carbidopa and levodopa, 1:10) was administered in the diet (Sinemet 500 mg/100 g powdered food).

a later time on the day of proestrus has also been observed in the middle-aged female (Cooper et al., 1980; see subsequent discussion). Finally, we found that treatment of middle-aged regularly cycling females with zimelidine alone produced CE in 9 of 11 rats; 1 female became pseudopregnant, and 2 showed irregular cycles (Table 1). Zimelidine treatment to old CE females receiving L-dopa treatment blocked the reinstatement of vaginal cycles usually observed after treatment with this CA precursor alone. Again, these observations indicate that enhanced 5-HT neuronal activity may be involved in the disruption of regular ovarian function and that reinstatement of ovarian function in the aged female by treatment with CNS CA precursors is mediated in part by their depression of CNS 5-HT metabolism.

The effect of decreasing 5-HT neuronal activity on ovarian function in old CE females was further evaluated using the neurotoxin 5,7-dihydroxytryptamine (5,7-DHT), a compound that causes selective degeneration of central serotonin-containing neurons (Bjorklund et al., 1973). Twenty-four-month-old CE females were treated according to the standard protocol (Bjorklund et al., 1973), in which all animals were given desmethylimipramine (DMI) (25 mg/kg, i.p.) 40-60 min before lesioning with 5,7-DHT. By blocking the uptake of 5,7-DHT into noradrenergic neurons, DMI prevents destruction of that system and enhances the specificity of 5,7-DHT in lesioning serotonergic cells. Rats were anesthetized with pentobarbital (Nembutal), and 5,7-DHT dissolved in 0.05% ascorbic acid was injected into the dorsal and ventral raphe (4 μg/μl vehicle in each area). Old CE control animals received DMI and injections of only ascorbic acid into the raphe nuclei. Young regularly cycling females also received 5,7-DHT lesions. The vaginal smear of each rat was followed for 35 days after surgery. The results of this study are shown in Table 2. Prior to surgery, all old females were CE. During the first 2 postoperative weeks, regular cycles were observed in 23% of the old 5,7-DHT-treated females; between the third and fifth postoperative week, 62% of the old 5,7-DHT-treated females showed regular cycles. None of the sham-operated controls showed regular cycles after surgery; however, the surgery induced long diestrous periods in two rats. Treatment with 5,7-DHT did not disrupt regular cycling in young females. This

Table 2 Effect of 5,7-DHT on Ovarian-Vaginal Condition of Female Rats

Animals/ treatment	No.	Proportion of females revealing regular 4- or 5-day vaginal cycles	
		0-14 days postop	15-30 days postop
Old CE, 5,7-DHT	13	3/13	8/13
Old CE, sham op	4	0/4	0/4
Young, 5,7-DHT	4	4/4	4/4

result agrees with the finding by Meyer (1978) that young-adult females continued to cycle regularly after 5,7-DHT treatment. On the 35th day after surgery, all rats were sacrificed. Corpora lutea were noted in the females that had shown regular vaginal cycles. The ovaries of the control females and the 5,7-DHT-treated females that did not cycle contained follicles but no corpora lutea.

In summary, studies of the aged noncycling female demonstrate that cyclic ovarian function can be restored using pharmacological or dietary manipulations known to alter CNS neurotransmitter function. These studies also indicate that a functional imbalance between CNS CA and 5-HT may be a fundamental aspect of the CNS changes that are responsible for altered ovarian function in the aging female.

BRAIN-PITUITARY-OVARIAN FUNCTION IN THE MIDDLE-AGED FEMALE RAT

The studies discussed in the previous section show that reinstatement of vaginal and ovarian cycles in the old noncycling female is possible and that the effect of these treatments are likely mediated through their influence on CNS neurotransmitter function. However, these studies could be misleading in that old CE and RP females have obviously different endocrine backgrounds than those present in the young-adult cycling female. Thus, it is possible that prolonged exposure to such diverse endocrine conditions per se is responsible for what has been interpreted as an age difference in neurotransmitter function. Accordingly, the relevance of such studies of the old female to our understanding of the mechanisms responsible for the disruption of regular ovarian function could be questioned. More direct evidence concerning the role of the brain and pituitary in age-dependent changes is available from investigations of the middle-aged regularly cycling female.

There is a well-documented decrease in the quantity of LH released by the pituitary of the middle-aged female on the afternoon of vaginal proestrus (van der Schoot, 1976; Miller and Riegle, 1980; Gray et al., 1980; Cooper et al., 1980). The identification of this age difference in hormone secretion prior to the time regular cycling is disrupted has provided further insight into how brain-pituitary-ovarian function changes with age and into the mechanisms responsible for these changes. At least three factors could contribute to changes in LH secretion in the middle-aged female: (1) Altered levels of serum progesterone, (2) decreased responsiveness (i.e., positive feedback) to circulating steroids by the CNS and pituitary, and (3) changes in the CNS mechanisms involved in the LH surge.

Serum progesterone has been reported to be lower in the middle-aged female, and progesterone injections on the morning of proestrus will increase serum LH concentrations in this age group (Miller and Riegle, 1980). We also found the mean serum progesterone values for middle-aged regularly cycling females as a group to be lower than the mean serum progesterone values of the young females (4 months) as a group when measured at 1600, 1800, 2000, and 2200 hr on the day of vaginal proestrus (Fig. 1). The serum for this study was obtained using a serial sampling

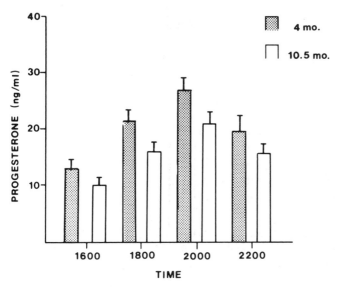

Figure 1 Serum progesterone values obtained from 4-month-old and 10.5-month-old females showing 4-day vaginal cycles. Samples were obtained on the afternoon of vaginal proestrus and are expressed as mean ± one standard of the mean. The concentration of progesterone in the serum of the middle-aged females was significantly lower than that of young females at 1800 and 2000 hr (p < 0.05, Student's t-test).

technique described previously (Cooper et al., 1980). This technique allowed us to also evaluate potential age differences in the pattern of progesterone secretion on proestrus in the two age groups. When individual patterns of progesterone were compared, we found that the time at which peak progesterone levels occurred varied in both age groups, with the majority of animals having peak progesterone values at 2000 hr (Fig. 2). Serum progesterone values peaked in a significant number of young females at 1800 hr. In none of the middle-aged females was the progesterone peak observed at 1800 hr. When the serum progesterone levels in the two age groups were compared according to the time at which the peak occurred, the progesterone values in these two groups were essentially identical, indicating that the difference observed previously (see Fig. 1) was likely the result of the different patterns of progesterone secretion present in the two age groups and not necessarily a difference in the absolute values of progesterone achieved.

The fact that serum progesterone values were not always different between young and middle-aged individuals provides some insight into the role that age-dependent changes in serum progesterone may have on age-dependent changes in LH secretion. Figure 3 depicts the LH concentration observed in the same samples used in this study for only the animals in which the peak progesterone levels occurred at 2000 hr. The LH values are plotted as young or middle-aged group means.

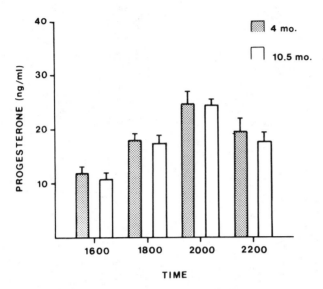

Figure 2 Serum progesterone values from young and middle-aged females in which the progesterone peak was observed at 2000 hr.

Although serum progesterone levels in the animals representing these two age groups were not different, the concentration of LH present in the serum of middle-aged females at 1800, 2000, and 2200 hr on the afternoon of proestrus was significantly below that observed at these times in the young-adult females. Thus, it does not appear that age-dependent changes in progesterone secretion contribute to, or precede, the altered pattern of LH release in the middle-aged female.

The finding that age-related changes in LH secretion precede changes in serum progesterone concentrations indicates that the CNS-pituitary mechanisms controlling LH release may be altered in the middle-aged female. The LH response to GnRH stimulation in middle-aged females is not significantly different than that of the young animals (Steger et al., 1979). However, the increase in serum LH following ovariectomy is less marked in the middle-aged females (Gray et al., 1980), and the LH surge in response to ovarian steroids in the middle-aged female is lower than that observed in similarly treated young females (Gray et al., 1980; Meites et al., 1978). Combined, these observations indicate a decrease in responsiveness of the feedback mechanisms within the CNS. Whether this apparent change in the CNS feedback mechanism is manifest at the level of the steroid receptor, neurotransmitter metabolism, or yet some undefined intracellular change remains to be determined.

The serum LH values depicted in Fig. 3 reveal a significant reduction in the levels of this hormone in the middle-aged animal. However, the way these animals

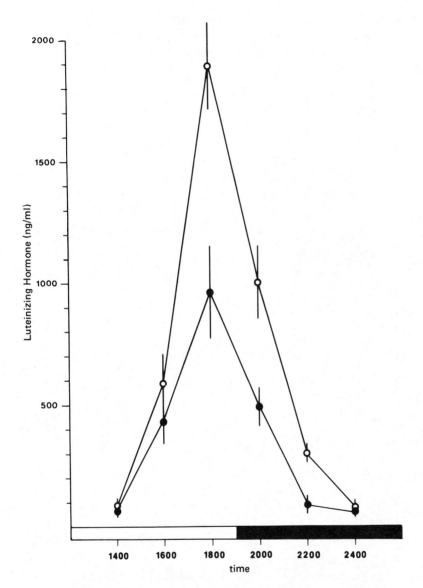

Figure 3 Serum LH values observed in young and middle-aged females in which the peak progesterone values were observed at 2000 hr. LH values are expressed as mean ± one standard error of the mean (SEM).

were grouped for comparison masks another significant difference between the young-adult and middle-aged female. We have shown previously that, in addition to lower peak LH concentrations in the middle-aged female, there is a shift in the time at which the LH surge occurs (Cooper et al., 1980). This difference is shown in Fig. 4. The pattern of LH secretion in the middle-aged female suggests that the

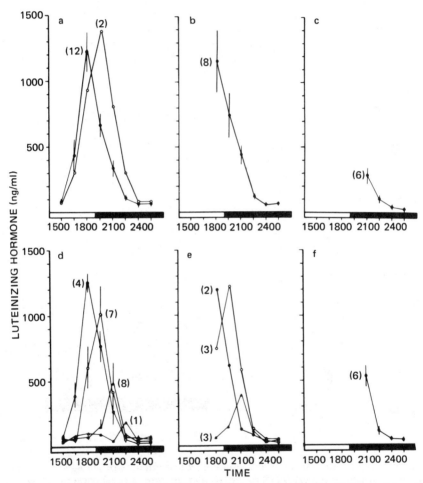

Figure 4 Serum LH (mean ± SEM) in young (top panels) and middle-aged females (lower panels) on the afternoon of vaginal proestrus. Sampling was initiated at 1500 hr (panels A and D), 1800 hr (panels B and E), and 2100 hr (panels C and F). Animals were grouped according to the time their LH peak was observed. The number of animals in each group is indicated in parentheses. (Adapted from Cooper et al., 1980.)

CNS timing mechanisms controlling GnRH secretion and the subsequent onset of the LH surge may be changing with age. This possibility is supported by the finding that the critical period for the pentobarbital blockade of ovulation on the afternoon of vaginal proestrus in the aging female is extended past the normal hours of 1400-1600 hr (van der Schoot, 1976). Age-dependent changes in the periodicity of a variety of behavioral and physiological rhythms have been noted in the female rat (Mosko et al., 1980; Yamaoka, this volume). The suprachiasmatic nucleus of the hypothalamus is a critical component of the central mechanism controlling circadian rhythm generation and entrainment (Pittendrigh, 1974; Moore, 1974), and lesions of this region in young female rats disrupt gonadotropin secretion and ovarian cyclicity (Brown-Grant and Raisman, 1977). Thus, the delay in LH secretion observed in the 10.5-month-old, regularly cycling female may represent one of the first observable consequences of age-dependent changes in the neural timing mechanisms controlling circadian rhythms in general. This possibility is discussed in further detail by Walker (this volume) and Yamaoka (this volume).

TYROSINE DIET AND OVARIAN FUNCTION IN THE AGING FEMALE

As described previously, supplementation of the aged CE female rat's diet with the amino acid L-tyrosine will result in renewed vaginal cycling and ovulation (Cooper and Linnoila, 1980). In subsequent studies (Cooper and Walker, 1979), we found that the age at which regular ovarian cycling was disrupted could be extended significantly by placing females on the L-tyrosine-supplemented diet at a relatively early age (i.e., 7.5 months). In our laboratory, 50% of the females stop cycling by 11.5 months of age and 95% by 13 months. We found that 50% of the females fed the L-tyrosine-supplemented diet continued to cycle regularly until 16.5 months of age; at 19 months of age, 30% of these were still cycling. In two females, regular cycles continued until age 24 months. Thus, it is not only possible to restore ovarian function in the old noncycling female through an L-tyrosine-supplemented diet—this diet significantly prolongs regular ovarian function. The mechanisms by which this diet affects cycling remain to be determined; however, the diet does appear to counter the age-dependent change in LH secretion observed in middle-aged control-fed animals as the amplitude and timing of the proestrous LH surge in the middle-aged females fed this diet was not significantly different from young control animals. These findings suggest that the L-tyrosine-supplemented diet maintains ovarian function in the aging female through some effect on the hypothalamic and pituitary mechanisms governing LH release, perhaps by maintaining the appropriate CA and 5-HT metabolism.

MAMMARY OR PITUITARY TUMOR DEVELOPMENT

Recent studies of the effect of altered amino acid content of the animals' diet have provided some insight into the relationship between diet, the maintenance of

transmitter function, and physiological performance. Concordant with our findings—that a decrease in serotonin function may be a critical component of the
mechanism by which the L-tyrosine-supplemented diet influences reproductive
functions—are the results of studies in which rats were maintained on a diet low
in tryptophan. The tryptophan-deficient diet has been reported to prolong life
span, prolong reproductive function, and decrease the incidence of tumors until
late life (Segall and Timiras, 1976). Likewise, the addition of the CA precursor
L-dopa to the diet has been shown to prolong the life span of mice (Cotzias et al.,
1977) and rats (McNamara et al., 1978), reduce the incidence of mammary tumors
in the rat (McNamara et al., 1978), and cause regression of some tumors already
present in rats (Quadri et al., 1973b) and humans (Frantz et al., 1972). In our
studies, we found that the incidence of mammary gland tumors in females maintained on the L-tyrosine-supplemented diet to be significantly below that observed
in animals maintained on control diets (Cooper and Walker, 1979) (Fig. 5). L-dopa
diets, although producing marked decrements in body weight (i.e., up to 70% of

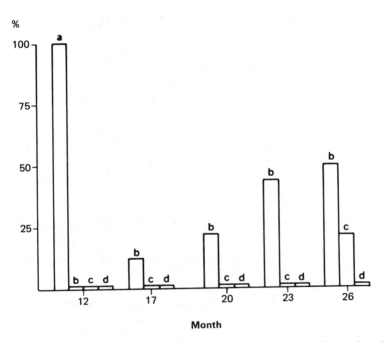

Figure 5 Incidence of mammary tumors observed in Long-Evans females at different ages. Group a: Females received subcutaneous implants of estradiol at 4
months of age. Group b: Control females. Group c: Females maintained on a
tyrosine-supplemented diet beginning 7.5 months of age. Group d: Females ovariectomized at 4 months of age.

control-fed animals) (Cotzias et al., 1977), do not appear to be as deleterious to the animals as tryptophan-deficient diets, which result in more severe weight loss and/or even death in some animals. The body weight of animals maintained on the L-tyrosine-supplemented diet was not different from the body weight of control animals when compared on a short-term (1 to 2-month) or long-term (18 to 19-month) basis.

The delay in the appearance of mammary gland tumors in the L-tyrosine-supplemented animals is likely the direct result of prolonging ovarian function (i.e., the delayed onset of constant estrus). An early appearance of mammary tumors in young female rats will result from subcutaneous implants of Silastic tubing containing estrogen which produces a chronic elevation of serum estrogen (see Fig. 5). This prolonged exposure to elevated serum estrogen (and concomitant elevated prolactin levels) closely approximates the hormonal changes observed in the aging, spontaneously CE female (Huang et al., 1978). In contrast, maintaining very low serum estrogen levels throughout life by ovariectomizing the female at an early age will lead to significantly reduced occurrences of mammary gland tumors (Fig. 5).

The extension of the animal's life span was not a primary concern of our studies investigating the effect of the L-tyrosine-supplemented diet on reproductive function. However, we have found that this diet may indeed influence life span. The mean life span of the Long-Evans females in our colony is 27.5 months. The primary cause of death in these females is pituitary tumors. Pituitary tumors have been observed in a few females as early as 18 months of age, but are present in a significant number of animals (i.e., more than 68%) sacrificed or dying after 24 months of age (Fig. 6). We found that pituitary tumors were present in only 9% of the females maintained on the L-tyrosine-supplemented diet and sacrificed at 32 months of age. Thus, it appears that the development of pituitary tumors is significantly delayed in females maintained on the tyrosine diet. Importantly, 72% of the animals maintained on the L-tyrosine-supplemented diet survived to 32 months of age.

The majority of pituitary tumors are hemorrhagic and prolactin secreting. They range in size from 5-8 mm in diameter and cause significant compression atrophy of the base of the brain, the extent of which varies as a function of the size of the tumor. Physical symptoms are present prior to death and include decreased appetite, lethargy, extreme loss of weight, and motor disturbances. The argument that these tumors are the result of prolonged exposure to elevated serum estrogen levels is supported by the observation that Silastic estrogen implants to the 4-month-old female will result in large tumors (i.e., 10-12 mm) at 10-12 months of age. The development of pituitary tumors is also delayed in females that have been ovariectomized at 4 months of age (Fig. 6). A number of studies have shown that estrogen treatment will induce pituitary tumors in the rat (Nakagawa et al., 1980). Results similar to these have also been reported for the mouse (Felicio et al., 1980; also see Brawer and Finch, this volume).

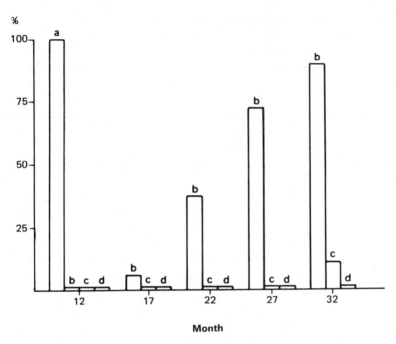

Figure 6 Incidence of pituitary tumors observed in Long-Evans females sacrificed or dying at different ages. Animals were grouped as described in Fig. 5.

These observations address only two pathological conditions associated with the disruption of regular ovarian cycling. However, these studies indicate that mammary and pituitary tumors develop in the aging female as a consequence of the altered estrogen and prolactin levels present in the aging female and that treatments that delay or prevent the development of the CE condition will in turn delay and possibly prevent the development of these age-associated pathologies. Further studies investigating the consequences of prolonged exposure to estrogen on CNS morphology are presented by Brawer and Finch (this volume).

CONCLUSION

The studies discussed in this chapter address several questions concerning aging in the female rat's reproductive system. Aging in this neuroendocrine axis does not appear to occur in all organs simultaneously. Rather, the disruption of regular ovarian function is likely the result of selective changes in the hypothalamic (CNS) mechanisms controlling LH release. An important component of these neuronal changes appears to be alterations in the CNS CA and 5-HT control of LH release such that the ability of the middle-aged female's pituitary to secrete this hormone is compromised. More studies are needed to reveal the exact nature of these changes and to reveal how they bring about alterations in the timing and amount of LH release in the middle-aged female.

Related to the theme of this book, the studies discussed in this chapter indicate clearly that age-dependent changes in ovarian function can be reversed or delayed by pharmacological treatments or dietary modifications designed to increase CNS CA and decrease CNS 5-HT metabolism. The fact that the efficacy of such treatments is markedly improved when treatment is initiated at a relatively early age indicates that early intervention should be a primary focus of future gerontological and geriatric research (i.e., identifying and preventing those conditions which precede the anomalous conditions present in the older organism). Findings supporting the usefulness of this approach have been presented by Bartus (1980) in studies investigating the effect of feeding animals diets supplemented with acetylcholine precursors. Such diets are reported to prevent the age-related decline in behavioral performance observed in rodents. Similar observations in humans suggest that the functional decline observed in Alzheimer patients can be slowed if such patients are identified and treated with acetylcholine precursors or stimulants in the early stages of this disease (Christie, cited in Wurtman et al., 1981).

The studies discussed in this chapter also indicate that the occurrence of the tumors typically associated with age-dependent changes in reproductive function are also affected by pharmacological or dietary manipulations that delay the disruption of regular ovarian function. These tumors appear as a consequence of the altered endocrine milieu present in the noncycling older female. The fact that the incidence of such tumors can be reduced, or their occurrence delayed, by maintaining regular ovarian function, again stresses the importance of understanding the conditions that precede the development of such pathologies. Such an understanding can only be achieved by investigating changes that develop in the organism throughout its life span. When such an understanding is achieved, improved techniques for intervention can be developed.

ACKNOWLEDGMENTS

The unpublished studies presented in this chapter were conducted in collaboration with Dr. Markku Linnoila and Dr. Colleen McNamara. The excellent technical assistance of Karen Wacome, Suzie Dakin, Grace Wojno, Jennifer LeFever, Scott Gabel, and Mary Eye is also gratefully acknowledged.

Portions of this research were supported by a Public Health Service Grant from the National Institute on Aging (00566) and a research award from the Josiah Trent Foundation.

REFERENCES

Aschheim, P. (1965). Resultats fournis par la greffe heterochrome des ovaires dans l'etude de la regulation hypothalamo-hypophyso-ovarienne de la ratte senile. *Gerontologia 10*: 65-75.

Aschheim, P. (1976). Aging in the hypothalamic-hypophyseal ovarian axis in the rat. In *Hypothalamus, Pituitary and Aging*, A. V. Everitt and J. A. Burgess (Eds.). Charles C Thomas, Springfield, Ill., pp. 376-418.

Bartus, R. (1980). Cholinergic drug effects on memory and cognition in animals. In *Aging in the 1980s: Psychological Issues*, L. Poon (Ed.). American Psychological Press, Washington, D.C., pp. 163-180.

Bjorklund, A., Nobin, A., and Stenevi, T. (1973). The use of neurotoxic dihydroxytryptamines as tools for morphological studies and localized lesions of central indolamine neurons. *Z. Zellforsch. Mikrosk. Anat. 145*: 479-484.

Brown-Grant, K., and Raisman, G. (1977). Abnormalities in reproductive function associated with the destruction of the suprachiasmatic nuclei in female rats. *Proc. R. Soc. Lond. [Biol] 198*: 279-296.

Carrer, H. F., and Taleisnik, S. (1970). Effect of mesencephalic stimulation of the release of gonadotropins. *J. Endocrinol. 48*: 527-539.

Clemens, J. A., and Bennett, D. R. (1977). Do aging changes in the preoptic area contribute to loss of cyclic endocrine functions? *J. Gerontol. 32*: 19-24.

Clemens, J. A., Amenomori, Y., Jenkins, T., and Meites, J. (1969). Effect of hypothalamic stimulation, hormones and drugs on ovarian function in old female rats. *Proc. Soc. Exp. Biol. Med. 132*: 561-563.

Cooper, R. L. (1980). Brain serotonin and ovarian function in the aged rat. In *Progress in Psychoneuroendocrinology*, F. Brambilla, G. Racagni, and D. De-Wied (Eds.). Elsevier-North Holland, Amsterdam, pp. 523-529.

Cooper, R. L., and Linnoila, M. (1980). Effect of centrally and systemically administered L-tyrosine and L-leucine on ovarian function in the old rat. *Gerontology 26*: 270-275.

Cooper, R. L., and Walker, R. F. (1979). Potential therapeutic consequences of age-dependent changes in brain physiology. In *CNS Aging and Its Neuropharmacology*, W. Meier-Ruge (Ed.). Karger, Basel, pp. 54-76.

Cooper, R. L., Brandt, S., Linnoila, M., and Walker, R. F. (1979). Induced ovulation in aged female rats by L-dopa into the medial preoptic area. *Neuroendocrinology 30*: 15-19.

Cooper, R. L., Conn, P. M., and Walker, R. F. (1980). Characterization of the LH surge in middle-aged female rats. *Biol. Reprod. 23*: 611-615.

Cotzias, C. G., Miller, S. T., Tang, L. C., and Papavasiliou, P. S. (1977). Levodopa, fertility, and longevity. *Science 196*: 549-550.

Everett, J. (1940). The restoration of ovulatory cycles and corpus luteum formation in the persistent-estrous rat. *Endocrinology 27*: 681-686.

Everett, J. (1980). Reinstatement of estrous cycles in middle-aged spontaneously persistent-estrous rats: Importance of circulating prolactin and the resulting facilitative action of progesterone. *Endocrinology 106*: 1691-1696.

Fahn, S., Snider, S., Prasad, A. L. N., Lane, E., and Makadon, H. (1975). Normalization of brain serotonin by L-tryptophan in levodopa-treated rats. *Neurology 25*: 861-865.

Felicio, L. S., Nelson, J. F., and Finch, C. E. (1980). Spontaneous pituitary tumorigenesis and plasma oestradiol in aging female C57BL/6J mice. *Exp. Gerontol. 52*: 139-143.

Fernstrom, J. D., Faller, D. V., and Shabshelowitz, H. (1975). Acute reduction of brain serotonin and 5-HIAA following food consumption: Correlation with the ratio of serum tryptophan to the sum of competing amino acids. *J. Neural Trans. 36*: 113-121.

Franks, S., McElhone, J., Young, S. N., Kroulis, I., and Ruf, K. B. (1980). Factors determining the diurnal variation in progesterone-induced gonadotropin release in the ovariectomized rat. *Endocrinology 108*: 353-358.

Frantz, A. G., Habif, D. V., Hyman, G. A., and Suh, H. K. (1972). Remission of metastatic breast cancer after reduction of circulating prolactin in patients treated with L-dopa. *Clin. Res. 20*: 864.

Gibson, C. J., and Wurtman, R. J. (1977). Physiological control of brain catechol synthesis by brain tyrosine concentration. *Biochem. Pharmacol. 26*: 1137-1142.

Gray, G. D., Tennent, B., Smith, E. R., and Davidson, J. (1980). Luteinizing hormone regulation and sexual behavior in middle-aged female rats. *Endocrinology 107*: 187-194.

Huang, H. H., and Meites, J. (1975). Reproductive capacity in aging female rats. *Neuroendocrinology 17*: 289-295.

Huang, H. H., Steger, R. W., Bruni, J. F., and Meites, J. (1978). Patterns of sex steroid and gonadotropin secretion in aging female rats. *Endocrinology 103*: 1855-1859.

Hutt, C. S., Snider, S. R., and Fahn, S. (1977). Interaction between bromocryptine and levodopa: Biochemical basis for improved treatment for Parkinsonism. *Neurology 27*: 505-510.

Kordon, C., Hery, M., Gogan, F., and Rotsztein, W. H. (1978). Circadian pattern of secretion of hormones by the anterior pituitary gland with particular reference to the involvement of serotonin in their rhythmic regulation. In *Environmental Endocrinology*, I. Assenmacher and D. S. Farner (Eds.). Springer, New York, pp. 163-171.

Labhsetwar, A. P. (1972). Role of monoamines in ovulation: Evidence for a serotonergic pathway for inhibition of spontaneous ovulation. *J. Endocrinol. 54*: 169-175.

Linnoila, M., and Cooper, R. L. (1976). Reinstatement of vaginal cycles in aged female rats. *J. Pharmacol. Exp. Ther. 199*: 477-482.

Lu, K. H., Hopper, B. R., Vargo, T. M., and Yen, S. C. N. (1979). Chronological changes in sex steroid, gonadotropin and prolactin secretion in aging female rats displaying different reproductive states. *Biol. Reprod. 21*: 193-203.

McNamara, C. M., Miller, A. T., and Libby, C. B. (1978). Levodopa prevents mammary lipomas in rats. *J. Am. Aging Assoc. 1*: 83-84.

Meites, J., Huang, H. H., and Simpkins, J. W. (1978). Recent studies on neuroendocrine control of reproductive senescence in rats. In *The Aging Reproductive System*, E. L. Schneider (Ed.). Raven, New York, pp. 213-235.

Meyer, D. C. (1978). Hypothalamic and raphe serotonergic systems in ovulation control. *Endocrinology 103*: 1067-1074.

Miller, A., and Riegle, G. D. (1980). Temporal changes in serum progesterone in aging female rats. *Endocrinology 106*: 1579-1583.

Moore, R. Y. (1974). Visual pathways and the central neural control of diurnal rhythms. In *The Neurosciences Third Study Edition*, F. O. Schmitt and F. G. Worden (Eds.). MIT Press, Cambridge, Mass., pp. 537-542.

Mosko, S. S., Erickson, G. F., and Moore, R. Y. (1980). Dampened circadian rhythms in reproductively senescent female rats. *Behav. Neural Biol. 28*: 1-14.

Nakagawa, K., Obera, T., and Tashiro, K. (1980). Pituitary hormones and prolactin-releasing activity in rats with primary estrogen-induced pituitary tumors. *Endocrinology 106*: 1033-1039.

Ng, K. Y., Chase, T. N., Colburn, R. N., and Kopin, I. J. (1970). L-dopa-induced release of cerebral monoamines. *Science 170*: 76-77.

Pittendrigh, C. S. (1974). Circadian oscillations in cells and the circadian organization of multicellular systems. In *Neurosciences Third Study Edition*, F. O. Schmitt and F. G. Worden (Eds.). MIT Press, Cambridge, Mass., pp. 437-458.

Quadri, S. K., Kledzik, G. S., and Meites, J. (1973a). Reinitiation of estrous cycles in old constant estrous rats by central acting drugs. *Neuroendocrinology 11*: 248-255.

Quadri, S. K., Kledzik, G. S., and Meites, J. (1973b). Effect of L-dopa and methyldopa on growth of mammary cancers in rats. *Proc. Soc. Exp. Biol. Med. 142*: 759-761.

Rockman, G. W., Amit, Z., Carr, G., Brown, Z. W., and Ogren, S.-O. (1979). Attenuation of ethanol intake by 5-hydroxytryptamine uptake blockade in the mediation of the positive reinforcing properties of ethanol. *Arch. Int. Pharmacodyn. Ther. 241*: 245-259.

Sawyer, C. H. (1975). Some recent developments in brain-pituitary-ovarian physiology. *Neuroendocrinology 17*: 97-124.

Segall, P. E., and Timiras, P. S. (1976). Patho-physiologic findings after chronic tryptophan deficiency in rats. A model for delayed growth and aging. *Mech. Age. Dev. 5*: 109-124.

Steger, R. W., Huang, H. H., Chamberlain, D. S., and Meites, J. (1979). Changes in control of gonadotropin secretion in the transition period between regular cycles and constant estrus in aging female rats. *Biol. Reprod. 22*: 595-603.

van der Schoot, P. (1976). Changing pro-oestrous surges of luteinizing hormone in aging 5-day cyclic rats. *J. Endocrinol. 69*: 287-288.

Walker, R. F., Cooper, R. L., and Timiras, P. S. (1980). Constant estrus: Role of rostral hypothalamic monoamines in development of reproductive dysfunction in aging rats. *Endocrinology 107*: 249-255.

Wilkes, M. M., and Yen, S. S. C. (1981). Attenuation during aging of the post-ovariectomy rise in median eminence catecholamines. *Neuroendocrinology 33*: 144-147.

Wurtman, R. J., and Fernstrom, J. D. (1972). L-tryptophan, L-tyrosine, and the control of brain amine biosynthesis. In *Perspectives in Neuropharmacology. A Tribute to Julius Axelrod*, S. Snyder (Ed.). Oxford, New York, pp. 143-200.

Wurtman, R. J., Growdon, J. H., Corkin, S., Reinstein, D., and Zeisel, S. (1981). Meeting report of the International Study Group on the Pharmacology of Memory Disorders Associated with Aging. *Neurobiol. Aging 2*: 149-151.

3

Normal and Experimentally Altered Aging Processes in the Rodent Hypothalamus and Pituitary

James R. Brawer / *McGill University School of Medicine, Montreal, Quebec*

Caleb E. Finch / *University of Southern California, Los Angeles, California*

INTRODUCTION

Recent data indicate that some major events in the aging of the female rodent reproductive hypothalamus and pituitary are influenced by ovarian hormones. Actions of gonadal steroids, particularly estradiol, are well established in the sexual differentiation of the hypothalamus and induce apparently irreversible changes in brain circuitry of neonatal rodents. Such long-lasting actions of steroids during development have been termed "organizational effects," in contrast to the short-term and reversible "activational effects" of steroids, as exemplified by the positive and negative feedback regulation of gonadotropins. Work from our laboratories now suggests that estradiol exerts long-term effects on the *adult* rodent hypothalamus which may be irreversible. Comparison of the effects of estradiol on young female rodents with the changes seen during normal reproductive aging indicates that it is possible to accelerate or to intervene in some reproductive neuroendocrine aging processes.

GONADOTROPIN-REGULATING CIRCUITRY

Briefly, the circuitry may be considered as a two-neuron chain. The cyclic drive is initiated in the anterior hypothalamus (medial preoptic area and/or suprachiasmatic nucleus) and is transmitted by way of axonal connections to putative luteinizing

hormone-releasing hormone (LHRH) neurosecretory cells in the medial basal hypothalamus (Sawyer, 1975). It should be emphasized, however, that this is only a
simplified working model. It is known, for example, that LHRH immunoreactive
cells actually occur throughout the entire periventricular hypothalamus, medial
preoptic area, and even in nonhypothalamic structures such as the septal nuclei
and paraolfactory area (Zimmerman, 1976). LHRH immunoreactive axons have
been traced from the medial preoptic area itself to the median eminence, although
the biological significance of this projection is unclear, since transection of this
pathway increases rather than diminishes tonic LH secretion (Kalra, 1976). Furthermore, the amygdala, hippocampus, and the lower brain stem all project to the
hypophysiotropic hypothalamus and have the capability of influencing patterns
of gonadotropin release under a variety of conditions. Nevertheless, a hypothalamic
island consisting only of medial preoptic area, medial basal hypothalamus, median
eminence, and pituitary is, by itself, capable of maintaining cyclic surges of LH
with subsequent ovulation in the female rat (Tejasen and Everett, 1967; Halasz,
1969; Taleisnik et al., 1970), whereas disruption of the connections between the
medial preoptic area and the medial basal hypothalamus abolishes cyclicity (Halasz,
1969; Blake et al., 1973).

Thus, other regions of the brain that influence gonadotropin secretion in the
female rat do so in large measure by way of the medial preoptic area and medial
basal hypothalamic circuitry. Impairment of this region will, therefore, result in
concomitant alterations in the gonadotropin secretory patterns independent of
the functional status of other gonadotropin-influencing regions of the central nervous system.

EFFECT OF ESTRADIOL ON THE IMMATURE HYPOTHALAMUS

There is now extensive documentation of steroid-induced changes in hypothalamic
structures which are causally linked to the onset of functional neuroendocrine
changes in immature rats. For example, the sex differences in synaptic organization of the preoptic region and arcuate nucleus depend on differing paranatal exposure to steroids (Raisman and Field, 1973; Gorski et al., 1978; Matsumoto and
Arai, 1980). Exposure of the neonatal hypothalamus to aromatizable androgen
(or free estrogen) will result in male synaptic patterns, regardless of the genetic
sex of the animal. The diminishing sensitivity of the neonate to the sexually differentiating effects of steroids by about the 10th postnatal day led to the concept
of a critical paranatal period for hypothalamic differentiation. The existence of
such a critical period does not, however, preclude further influences of steroids on
synaptic populations.

For example, the onset of puberty is also associated with steroid influences
on synaptogenesis. Treatment of 28-day-old female rats with pregnant mare serum
gonadotropins (PMSG) not only advances puberty, but also sharply increases the

number of mature synapses in the hypothalamic arcuate nucleus, as compared to normal untreated or ovariectomized-treated controls (Matsumoto and Arai, 1977). Because PMSG does not facilitate synaptogenesis in the absence of ovaries, this effect is probably mediated by ovarian estrogens.

Additionally, 45 days of postnatal life are required for the development of the final adult complement of synapses in the female hypothalamic arcuate nucleus (Matsumoto and Arai, 1976). During this time, the hypothalamus retains some plasticity, and steroids may act by modifying normal growth and developmental processes that ultimately fashion the adult hypothalamic circuitry. After puberty, however, the reproductive hypothalamic circuitry has generally been considered as fixed and, therefore, not subject to organizational influences. Matsumoto and Arai (1979) have shown, for example, that estradiol is not capable of stimulating synaptogenesis in the normal adult arcuate nucleus. In the extensive literature on activational effects of gonadal steroids on the hypothalamus, it has been tacitly assumed that organizational (long-lasting) effects of steroids are no longer possible in adults.

LONG-LASTING EFFECTS OF ESTRADIOL ON THE ADULT HYPOTHALAMUS

Estradiol-Induced Hypothalamic Pathogenesis and Anovulation

In contrast to the traditional view, recent studies indicate that gonadal steroids can continue to exert potent, long-lasting effects on the adult hypothalamus. Furthermore, these effects may be important causes of various anovulatory states, including that of normal aging.

If young-adult rodents are injected with estradiol, regular ovulatory cycles disappear within a span of days to weeks, and are replaced by a persistent vaginal cornification (PVC) syndrome (Brawer et al., 1978; Mobbs et al., 1981). Typically, the ovary is anovulatory but contains cohorts of large follicles which produce substantial estradiol. A similar polyfollicular PVC syndrome spontaneously occurs during aging in mice (Nelson et al., 1981) and rats (Lu et al., 1979), and is also associated with impaired hypothalamic responses to the steroid-mediated induction of the gonadotropin surge (Finch et al., 1980). The possibility that estrogen injections act at the hypothalamic level was first suggested by observations of the effects of estradiol valerate (EV) on cytology of the arcuate nucleus in the adult female rat (Brawer and Sonnenschein, 1975). Following several monthly injections of 2 mg EV, the arcuate nucleus contains multiple, histopathological foci exhibiting degenerating axons and dendrites. The degenerative foci are most apparent in the lateral regions of the nucleus. The neuronal degeneration is accompanied by reactive microglia containing engorged debris and reactive astrocytes that contain numerous pleomorphie pools of dense material and large bundles of fine filaments. The microglial response is a long-established marker for neuronal degeneration. It has been documented in degenerating nervous tissue in a variety of pathologies such as that induced by mechanical lesions (Dunkerley and Duncan, 1969; Matthews and Kruger, 1973), or in diseases involving neuronal death such as Huntington's chorea and Parkinson's disease (Bernheimer et al., 1973). The astrocytic reaction is somewhat unusual. The development of dense inclusions may be a peculiar property of periventricular astrocytes, and it is not yet clear whether these cells are responding to neuronal degeneration or directly to the hormone treatment.

These results lead to the question of whether the progressive development of the lesion in the arcuate nucleus requires constant exposure to grossly elevated circulating estradiol (as would be expected from the monthly injections). If the injected EV were the cause, some signs of remission should appear upon cessation of the EV treatment. Accordingly, rats were given a 2 mg-dose of EV, (which induced PVC in about 1 month) and were studied 6 months later. The changes in the arcuate nucleus progressed with the same time course, intensity, and distribution as those seen in rats given monthly injections of 2 mg EV (Brawer et al., 1978). Hormone levels were also measured. Circulating estradiol was very high immediately after injection ($\sim$125 pg/ml), but dropped by 6 weeks to a steady state of about 30 pg/ml plasma, which is at the upper limit of the physiological range. Similar results are obtained in mice (Mobbs and Finch, unpublished.) Plasma prolactin levels rose sharply immediately following injection, but then declined to control levels within 1 month. Plasma LH was maintained at a steady level in the high-normal range, whereas plasma FSH declined to a steady low-normal level. The onset of the PVC syndrome, the slightly elevated LH, and the reduced FSH closely paralleled the first appearance of histologically identifiable glial changes in the arcuate nucleus 3-6 weeks after injection.

Functional Significance of the Estradiol Lesion

The constellation of reproductive and endocrine features induced by EV injections in young rodents strikingly resembles the anovulatory syndrome resulting from surgical anterior deafferentation of the medial basal hypothalamus (Blake et al., 1972, 1973; Halasz, 1969). In view of the degeneration within the neuropil of the arcuate nucleus in the EV-treated animals, it was hypothesized (Brawer et al., 1978) that EV treatment may cause a functional-anatomical disconnection of the arcuate nucleus from the more anterior hypothalamic regions associated with the preovulatory surge mechanism, such as the medial preoptic area (MPOA), producing a type of anovulation equivalent to that of the surgical deafferentation syndrome.

The patency of connections between the MPOA and the medial basal hypothalamus was assessed by measuring plasma LH and FSH following electrochemical stimulation of the MPOA in anovulatory PVC rats 3.5 months after the EV treatment (Brawer et al., 1980a). Parallel studies of pituitary responsiveness to an LHRH analogue in EV-lesioned rats were also undertaken to evaluate possible changes in pituitary function, independent of the hypothalamus. EV-treated rats in PVC exhibiting the hypothalamic lesion released significantly less LH 1 hr following electrochemical stimulation of the MPOA than did proestrous controls. Plasma LH levels were similar in controls and treated rats 1 hr after injection of LHRH analogue, suggesting that the reduced LH surge following preoptic stimulation in the EV-treated group resulted from a hypothalamic rather than a pituitary defect.

Further support for the conclusion of hypothalamic change is derived from EV-lesioned C57BL/6J mice, which showed marked impairments of the estradiol-induced gonadotropin surge, but exhibited a normal LH response to exogenous LHRH with peaks 20 min after injection (Mobbs et al., 1981). Since, in this study, both EV-treated and control mice were ovariectomized for 60 days before testing for hormonal responses, differences in gonadotropin regulation due to the immediate effects of the PVC condition are minimized. It is of interest that the elevation of LH 30 days postcastration was significantly lower in the mice previously treated with EV (100 ng/ml) than in untreated controls (150 ng/ml). These results support the hypothesis that the histologically identifiable arcuate lesion caused by a single EV treatment leading to PVC represents a disruption of connections between the medial preoptic area and medial basal hypothalamus, resulting in partially impaired transmission of LH-releasing stimuli emanating from the medial preoptic area.

Pathophysiology of the Estradiol-Induced Arcuate Lesion

How can a single EV treatment produce such an irreversible progressive neuropathological change? The answer may lie in the fact that 2 months after a single dose of EV, plasma estradiol levels remain somewhat elevated, but within psysiological values. (Brawer et al., 1978; Mobbs and Finch, unpublished). It was hypothesized that the arcuate lesion could develop in response to this chronic (albeit mild) elevation of plasma estradiol. More specifically, the initial dose of EV may act by upsetting some, yet unknown, mechanism within the brain-pituitary-gonadal axis, thereby resulting in a cycle of hypothalamic impairment which causes an increased tonic output of gonadotropins. This, in turn, would produce elevated tonic secretion of ovarian estradiol producing increased hypothalamic impairment. A corollary to this hypothesis is that other manipulations leading to PVC with only mildly elevated plasma estradiol should show arcuate lesions. If such were the case, it would indicate that the gonadotropin-regulating circuitry within the arcuate nucleus is exquisitely sensitive to effects of estradiol.

In order to test this possibility, female rats were exposed to constant illumination which induces a PVC syndrome with polycystic ovaries and stable plasma levels of estradiol in the physiological range. These features are very similar to those produced by a single large dose of EV. Rats kept under constant illumination for 3 months exhibited the same enhanced glial reactivity as did the EV-treated animals (Brawer et al., 1980b) (Fig. 1). Thus, arcuate damage may be a

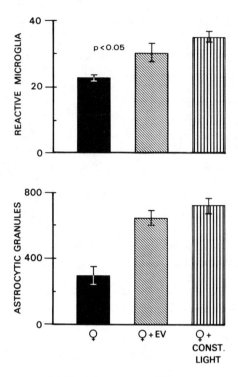

Figure 1 Glial response to EV treatment and to constant light exposure. All of the animals in both of these experimental groups showed an extended period of persistent estrus. Both the astrocytic and microglial reactivity was significantly greater in the two experimental groups than in controls of the same age. Furthermore, there was no statistical difference in glial responses between these two experimental groups, that is, constant light exposure was as effective in generating a glial response as EV treatment. The Y axis represents total counts of four fields of arcuate nucleus per animal. N = 5. (Adapted from Brawer et al., 1980b.)

general consequence of the polyfollicular ovarian-PVC syndrome, regardless of how the condition is induced. Since ovariectomy prior to either EV injection or constant light exposure prevented the glial reaction (Fig. 2), it appears that the hypothalamic damage is ovary-dependent and is probably due to the sustained exposure during PVC to ovarian steroids. That the ovarian product responsible for the lesion may be estradiol is suggested by the fact that the arcuate lesion can be produced in intact male rats by several monthly injections of 0.02 mg EV (Brawer et al., 1980b). The histological characteristics of this estrogen lesion in the male are indistinguishable from those produced in females by a single injection of EV or by exposure to constant illumination. Thus, estradiol is the most likely candidate as the ovarian product directly responsible for the hypothalamic lesion.

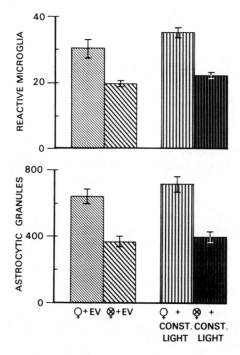

Figure 2   Effect of ovariectomy on the glial response to EV and to constant light. Ovariectomy prior to treatment significantly diminished the astrocytic and microglial responses to both EV treatment and constant light. Furthermore, the degree of reduction was similar for both experimental groups, indicating that the influence of the ovaries is the same in both experimental systems (EV treatment and constant light). N = 5. (Adapted from Brawer et al., 1980b.)

A phenomenon related to these experimentally induced changes may occur in sheep which are exposed to continuous estrogen in their diet by grazing on the estrogenic "Dinnin up" clover. It has been long known by sheep raisers in Australia that permanent infertility results from grazing of sheep on certain types of clover. It is now recognized that such clovers contain phytoestrogens which result in damage to hypothalamic neurons, but not to those in the hippocampus or cortex (Adams, 1977). The major neuroendocrine disturbance resulting from this exposure to phytoestrogens thus suggests that adults of other mammals, as well as rodents, may be susceptible to long-term effects of estrogens.

In summary, pathological changes in the arcuate nucleus of young rodents occur in the presence of constant physiological levels of estradiol. This damage may reflect partial disconnection of the arcuate nucleus from the MPOA, resulting in the PVC syndrome with acyclicity, anovulation, and polyfollicular ovaries.

ROLE OF ESTROGEN IN HYPOTHALAMIC AGING

The sensitivity of the arcuate nucleus to neurotoxic effects of ovarian estradiol in the adult female rat appears to be involved in the process of normal reproductive senescence leading to PVC and anovulation. It has long been suspected that early age-associated reproductive failure in female rats involves hypothalamic changes. Most female rodents have lengthening, irregular cycles by 8-12 months and exhibit PVC (12-15 months), at an age at which the pituitaries and ovaries maintain at least some responses to their characteristic hormonal stimuli (Aschheim, 1976; Meites et al., 1978; Riegle and Miller, 1978). Despite major oocyte depletion to 5-10% of that in the young, normal numbers of ova may still be spontaneously ovulated (Talbert, 1977; Gosden et al., 1983). Further evidence supporting pituitary and ovarian patency during early senescent anovulation is that ovulatory cycles can be transiently reinitiated in sexually senescent PVC rats by injections of various agents, including progesterone, tyrosine, epinephrine, L-dopa, and monoamine oxidase inhibitors, or by direct hypothalamic stimulation (Clemens et al., 1969; Quadri et al., 1973; Meites et al., 1978; Cooper et al., 1979). However, in C57BL/6J mice, ovarian depletion is far advanced at the time cycles cease (Gosden et al., 1983).

Furthermore, the loss of hypothalamic responsiveness during aging in the female rodent is ovary-dependent. The role of an ovarian product in the development of senescent hypothalamic anovulation was first demonstrated by Aschheim (1964/1965). If young cyclic rats are ovariectomized and allowed to age to 24 months, cycles will resume upon receipt of ovarian grafts from young rats. These striking results were recently confirmed with C57BL/6J mice (Nelson et al., 1980) and suggest that the chronic absence of an ovarian product (presumably estrogen) delayed or interrupted hypothalamic aging.

It seems likely that the ovary-dependent, PVC syndromes of aging described previously and the PVC syndromes induced in young rodents by EV or constant light (see preceding section) share a common mechanism at the hypothalamic level. The link between the experimentally induced PVC models and the normally aging female is suggested by observations that microglial and astrocytic activity normally increase in the arcuate nucleus with age in rats and mice (Brawer et al., 1980b; Schipper et al., 1981). The arcuate nucleus of a senescent PVC rodent exhibits a glial profile which resembles that of young females in PVC as the result of EV treatment or constant light exposure, indicating that both EV and constant light treatments may produce their effects by accelerating some hypothalamic aging processes. The possibility of a common etiology is further supported by the fact that the experimentally induced anovulatory rats exhibit the same reproductive features as senescent anovulatory females (anovulation, polycystic ovaries, PVC). Furthermore, as already stated, these experimentally induced anovulatory conditions, as well as normal aging of the hypothalamus, are ovary-dependent.

The role of ovarian estradiol in the aging process was further examined by studies on chronically ovariectomized rodents. The normal increases in glial reactivity in the arcuate nucleus of female rats from 6-14 months is almost completely suppressed by early ovariectomy (Schipper et al., in press). Similarly, ovariectomy attenuates histological aging of the hypothalamus in the C57BL/6J mouse. Aging of the hypothalamus, as reflected by glial activity, is restored in ovariectomized rats given Silastic implants of estradiol that maintain plasma E_2 in a physiological range (< 50 pg/ml), indicating that estradiol itself is the ovarian product responsible for aging (Brawer et al., unpublished results). These observations suggest at least two different types of mechanisms which are discussed next.

Mechanisms Involving Cumulative Effects of Estrous Cycles

Each preovulatory elevation of plasma estradiol might destroy a fraction of the axonal connections between the preoptic region and the medial basal hypothalamus. The numbers of synaptic contacts may be reduced independently (noncontingently) of neuronal cell death. During the 30-60 ovarian cycles usually experienced during the life span of the laboratory rodent, the gradual erosion of connections between the preoptic area and medial basal hypothalamus may lead to a critical deficit, disrupting neuronal circuitry that mediates the steroid-induced gonadotropin surges; the rodent would then enter the PVC state. Impairments of the spontaneous and experimentally induced LH surge in mice showing age-related lengthening cycles, or those in PVC (Finch et al., 1980), are consistent with this model. This hypothesis could also explain the similarity of impairments of the steroid-induced LH surge observed in the PVC status of the EV-treated mice (Mobbs et al., 1981), in PVC rodents during normal aging (Finch, 1979), and in young rats sustaining preoptic lesions (Wiegand et al., 1980).

Steroid Imbalance Mechanisms

Since the studies to date have focused primarily on the end points of reproductive aging, it can not yet be excluded that the morphological correlates (even if irreversible) represent damage inflicted by the major imbalances of sex steroids in the noncycling PVC or irregularly cycling states in which the estradiol:progesterone ratio is elevated (Nelson, 1981). Such effects of steroid imbalance might be independent of the number of cycles, as well as independent of chronological age.

ROLE OF GONADAL STEROIDS IN AGING OF THE MALE HYPOTHALAMUS

In contrast to the hypothalamic changes caused by E_2, the effects of testosterone (T) appear to be relatively mild. Four monthly injections of 2 mg testosterone propionate in male rats were required to produce significant reactive gliosis, whereas four monthly injections of only 0.02 mg EV were quite effective. The relative ineffectiveness of exogenous T in generating an arcuate lesion is also reflected in aging of the male hypothalamus. Although both astrocytic and microglial indices increase with age in the male rats, the rate of increase is significantly less than in the female (Schipper et al., 1981). Furthermore, males gonadectomized at 2 months of age showed no significant retardation in the development of the arcuate lesion from 6-14 months of age (although there may be a trend in this direction). Thus, T may not contribute significantly to hypothalamic aging.

EXPERIMENTAL INTERVENTIONS

Progesterone

The possibility was considered in the previous section that the elevated estrogen: progesterone ratio that occurs with age contributes to the hypothalamic damage. Progesterone is known to act directly on the hypothalamus where it binds to neurons in the arcuate nucleus and elsewhere (Sar and Stumpf, 1973; Warembourg, 1978). Hypothalamic cytosols contain binding proteins with steroid specificities for progestins which are clearly distinct from the estrogen receptors (Lee et al., 1979). Progesterone is long recognized for its ability to modify or antagonize the actions of estradiol in the uterus (Brenner and West, 1975). Moreover, in the uterus, progesterone appears to influence the retention of the nuclear estrogen receptor by mechanisms dependent on RNA and protein synthesis (Evans and Leavitt, 1980). In the brain, progesterone does not compete with estradiol for binding to estradiol receptors (Davies et al., 1975), nor does it influence the recycling of estrogen receptors after a single injection of estradiol (Pavlik and Coulson, 1976). Interactions of estrogen and progesterone in the brain may occur in different cells that communicate by way of synaptic connections, rather than in the same target cell, as in the case of the uterus.

The possibility that progesterone may interact in the EV lesion process was investigated in our laboratory. Normally cycling Wistar rats were injected with 2 mg of EV and left for 4 months. Other females received the single dose of EV, but were treated simultaneously with 25 mg of medroxyprogesterone acetate (Depoprovera) given intraperitoneally and 25 mg medroxyprogesterone acetate given intramuscularly (a total of 50 mg medroxyprogesterone acetate given at the time of EV injection). Subsequently, each rat received 25 mg medroxyprogesterone acetate intramuscularly per week for 4 months. A third group receiving no EV was maintained on a schedule of medroxyprogesterone acetate treatment identical to the second group. As expected, all EV-treated rats went into persistent estrous at about 1 month. However, rats given EV plus medroxyprogesterone acetate showed irregular changes in cyclicity for 4 months, whereas the medroxyprogesterone-acetate-treated animals exhibited persistent diestrus after about 45 days. The rats which entered PVC as a result of the EV injection exhibited high levels of glial reactivity in the arcuate nucleus. Strikingly, the glial reactivity was completely suppressed in EV-treated rats that also received the progestin (Brawer and Schipper, unpublished results).

These results indicate that progestins can inhibit the neuropathogenic effects of estradiol and suggest that progesterone may play a significant role in attenuating estradiol-dependent hypothalamic aging. The exact location and mechanism of the progestin effect remain to be determined.

Androgens

Since the increase in glial activity with aging of the male hypothalamus proceeds at the same rate in gonadectomized and intact male rats, T does not appear to influence the aging process. Preliminary results indicate a paradoxical effect of T on hypothalamic histology. Injections of normally cycling rats with testosterone propionate (TP) (2 mg per month for 4 months) slightly, but significantly, *reduced* microglial reactivity in the arcuate nuclei while leaving pituitary weights and cyclicity unaffected (Brawer and Schipper, unpublished results). This result indicates that not only is T nonpathogenic in rodents, but it may inhibit the ability of endogenous estrogen to induce hypothalamic lesions. In contrast, TP given to gonadectomized female rats restored microglial activity (normally very low in gonadectomized females) to the nongonadectomized control level. Thus, in the normal female rat, T may inhibit arcuate pathogenesis, whereas in the gonadectomized female it contributes to it. Four monthly injections of TP produced only a slight, but significant, increase in arcuate glial activity in the male (Brawer and Schipper, unpublished results). Any hypothesis explaining these paradoxical observations must take into account that the hypothalamus can produce estradiol by aromatizing the A ring of T (see Naftolin et al., 1976). Therefore, whatever neuropathogenic effect T exerts on the arcuate nucleus may require prior conversion to E_2. The weak pathogenicity of T may be explained by a low rate of hypothalamic aromatization.

In order to determine whether ring-A aromatization is necessary for the weak pathogenic effect of T, ovariectomized female rats were implanted with Silastic capsules containing cholesterol (controls), capsules containing crystalline unconjugated T, or capsules containing crystalline $5a$-DHT, a ring-A-reduced metabolite of T which can not be aromatized to estradiol by hypothalamic enzymes. The size of these capsules were selected to maintain the physiological plasma levels of these androgens. Preliminary results indicate that T was ineffective in generating reactive gliosis in the arcuate nucleus above castration control levels. DHT, on the other hand, significantly *suppressed* the astrocytic reaction, and a similar (albeit statistically insignificant) trend was seen with respect to microglial reactivity (Brawer and Schipper, unpublished results).

These results suggest that ring-A-reduced metabolites of T may be powerful inhibitors of arcuate neuropathogenesis, thus adding an additional dimension to the explanation for the effects of T. The hypothalamus is not only capable of aromatizing the A ring of T, but also contains 5a-reductase and, therefore, can produce 5a-DHT (Massa et al., 1972). If ring-A-reduced steroids were inhibitory to the estradiol pathogenesis, one could envision that a fraction of T (endogenous or exogenous) is metabolized to E, whereas another fraction goes to 5a-DHT, and the effects of these two steroids would tend to cancel one another. The relative activities of the hypothalamic aromatase and reductase would then account for the different effects of T under the different experimental conditions previously described. This hypothesis is being tested further by examining the effect of ring-A-reduced androgens (5a-DHT; 5a,17β-androstan,3a-diol) on estradiol-facilitated hypothalamic aging.

In summary, since aging of the reproductive hypothalamus is so dependent upon exposure to estradiol, it is not surprising that steroids which have the capacity to inhibit the effect of estradiol in other target tissues should also be powerful inhibitors of estradiol-dependent hypothalamic aging.

PITUITARY CHANGES DURING AGING

Pituitary Tumors

Pituitary tumors that contain prolactin (PRL) occur spontaneously during aging in many strains of mice (Felicio et al., 1980) and rats (Duchen and Schurr, 1976), and are also a late consequence of EV injections. Since PRL appears to interact with the hypothalamus, the relationship of these tumors to the age-related abnormalities in estrous cycles needs careful consideration. In rodents, for example, exogenous PRL accelerates dopamine turnover in the median eminence (Annunziato and Moore, 1978) and increases dopamine content of pituitary-stalk blood (Gudelsky and Porter, 1980). Elevated PRL also inhibits the postcastration rise of LH (Grandison et al., 1976) and impairs the pulsatile release of LH (Beck et al., 1977). Since PRL release is augmented by elevated plasma estrogens, the effects of EV injections in young rats and the effects of constant "unopposed" E_2 in the aging PVC animals could involve some action of PRL.

Plasma Prolactin in Aging Mice

A detailed analysis of reproductive hormones in aging C57BL/6J mice detected abnormalities in 11 to 12-month-old mice that were still cycling. At this age, the estrous-cycle length has become longer (mode of 5 days) though some 4-day cycles still occur (Nelson et al., 1981). At proestrous, 11 to 12-month-old mice have striking deficits of their plasma PRL surge; the onset of the PRL surge begins and ends at the same time, but the elevations at proestrous are about 50% smaller (Flurkey et al., unpublished data) (Fig. 3). Similarly, the proestrous LH and P surges are smaller by 30-50%. Although plasma E_2 elevation at proestrous (peak) is normal in the older mice, the gradual rise of E_2 (from its nadir at estrus) takes

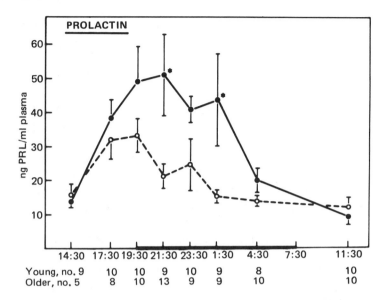

Figure 3 Proestrous plasma prolactin in C57BL/6J mice aged 5-7 months (●——●) and 11-12 months (o----o). (Adapted from Flurkey et al., in preparation).

about 1 day longer to reach an equivalent of the young level (Nelson et al., 1981). Because elevated E_2 is required for the proestrous gonadotropin surge (Schwartz, 1969), it is possible that the smaller elevations of PRL at proestrous are related to the *slower* rise of E_2 before proestrous. Alternatively, age may affect the control of PRL at the hypothalamic level independently of the altered time course of the E_2 rise. The hypothalamic factors which normally control PRL secretion are poorly understood, but may include dopamine, serotonin, enkephalins (Meites, 1980), and vasoactive intestinal peptide (Kato et al., 1978). In any case, in mice which are still cycling at 12 months, when there are clear impairments in gonadotropin regulation, there is no evidence for an increased output of PRL. Further support for the view that elevated PRL is not the cause of dysfunctions in LH regulation in the aging rodent derive from studies in aging female rats in which the elevations of PRL were suppressed by injections of dopamine agonist lergotrile; however, in spite of the normalization of PRL levels, the LH postcastration rise and the E_2-induced LH surge remained impaired (Clemens et al., 1978). It remains possible that the (presumably longstanding) pituitary tumors which caused elevated PRL had also damaged the contiguous gonadotropes, possibly by compression or constriction of blood supply, or that chronic elevations of PRL induced irreversible effects on the brain.

The moderate elevations of PRL which occur at 12 months in noncycling PVC mice are most likely due to the noncycling, polyfollicular PVC state in which plasma E_2 is maintained at a level close to estrous, whereas plasma P is very low

(Nelson et al., 1981). Elevations of prolactin are rare in humans. In a large sample of Tokyo men and women without evidence of endocrine disorders, serum PRL did not increase with age (Yamaji et al., 1976).

The Onset of Tumors

By 12-14 months, most C57BL/6J mice have ceased cycling and have entered PVC. Concurrently, pituitary weight increases by about 20% (Felicio et al., 1980), and microscopic foci of hypertrophied mammotropes (microadenomas) can be detected (Schechter et al., 1981). Microscopically visible tumors are found occasionally by 14 months but increase steadily thereafter (Fig. 4). By 24 months, nearly 50% of living mice had gross tumors at autopsy. The tumors contained predominantly hypertrophied mammotropes and some somatotropes (Schechter et al., 1981). Although it is not known how much of the tumor growth represents cell proliferation as distinct from cell hypertrophy, mitotic figures are seen in the tumors, particularly in the periphery (Schechter et al., 1981). Although the growing tumor mass may press up into the brain and extend beyond the sella, human histopathological studies suggest that metastasis is rare in human pituitary tumors (reviewed in Berry and Kaplan, 1979).

Plasma PRL (obtained from rapidly decapitated, nonstressed mice) was generally low (less than 35 ng/ml) in 25-month-old mice without tumors. In mice with medium-sized or grossly enlarged tumors, PRL tended to be somewhat elevated (50-200 ng/ml). Only in an occasional mouse did PRL reach higher levels (greater than 300 ng/ml) (Nelson et al., 1980), such as often found in aging female rats

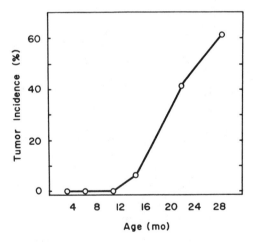

Figure 4 Incidence of gross pituitary tumors in female C57BL/6J mice during aging. (Adapted from Felicio et al., 1980.)

with pituitary tumors (Huang et al., 1976). It is of interest that about 30% of older mice with grossly enlarged, suprasellar tumors still had PRL of less than 50 ng/ml, that is, in the range of those without tumors. In humans, nonsecreting pituitary tumors represent a major pituitary tumor category, and are often detected because they compress the optic chiasm, leading to visual impairments, or because they compress the pituitary itself, leading to hypopituitarism (Berry and Kaplan, 1979). The generally low values of PRL in mice with small mammotropic tumors suggest that the onset of prolactinemia is an independent and later event in tumorigenesis. The reduced PRL surge at proestrous in 12-month-old mice (see previous discussion) also supports the concept that PRL hypersecretion is a later rather than earlier event in tumorigenesis.

During the studies of the effects of long-term ovariectomy and ovarian transplants of reproductive aging, the incidence of pituitary tumors was also evaluated. Long-term ovariectomy strikingly reduced tumor incidence; intact mice given young ovarian grafts at 17 months and killed at 25 months had greater than 80% incidence of gross pituitary tumors (medium or large size). In contrast, in mice ovariectomized at 5 months and deprived of ovaries until 17 months, when they were then given ovarian grafts, at sacrifice (25 months) only 30% had visible tumors (Nelson et al., 1980). These data strongly suggest the ovarian dependency of the mammotropic tumor. It is pertinent that in male C57BL/6J mice pituitary tumors are extremely rare throughout the life span (less than 0.1%) (Finch, 1973).

The ability of estrogen treatment to induce mammotropic pituitary tumors is well established in rodents (Nakagawa et al., 1980; Brawer and Sonnenschein, 1975, McEwen et al., 1936); the EV treatments which rapidly lead to precocious PVC in young rats and mice also appear to lead to mammotropic adenomas, but this effect remains to be fully evaluated. In the human condition of polycystic ovarian disease, which is associated with elevated estrone but not estradiol (Baird et al., 1977), hyperprolactinemia can occur in association with mammotropic adenomas (Futterweit and Krieger, 1979). Our working hypothesis is that the initial EV injections in young rats indirectly cause tumorigenesis by establishing preconditions of acyclicity with constant moderate levels of plasma E_2 and low levels of plasma P. Future studies may define the duration of PVC required to promote and maintain the stages of mammotrope hypertrophy and hyperplasia, and the role of changes in hypothalamic influences which may have different time courses of response to EV or PVC. There is some evidence for altered brain catecholamine metabolism (van Loon, 1978) and defective regulation of prolactin in hyperprolactinemic states in humans (Tucker et al., 1980). Moreover, in 2-year-old male rats direct measurements showed reduced dopamine in hypophyseal-stalk blood of animals with elevated plasma PRL (Gudelsky et al., 1981); since elevated PRL increases hypothalamic dopamine turnover and output into stalk blood in young rats (Annunziato and Moore, 1978; Gudelsky and Porter, 1980), the elevated PRL and reduced portal blood dopamine in old rats imply age changes in regulation of hypothalamic dopamine metabolism, possibly through a decoupling of PRL action on the hypothalamus. It is noteworthy in 28-month-old C57BL/6J mice that hypothalamic dopamine turnover is slowed (Osterburg et al., 1981) with no evidence of elevated PRL in this age group (determined in a previous study, Finch et al., 1977). Thus, reduced hypothalamic dopamine turnover is not inevitably associated with elevated PRL.

IMPLICATIONS FOR HUMANS

These studies on rodents suggest that sex steroids can have unexpected actions on the brain and pituitary which may be irreversible. The widespread, relaxed use of steroids in all age groups (oral contraceptives, postmenopausal steroid replacement, and antiinflammatory steroids) alerts us to the possibility of major side effects and interactions with aging processes which could not have been revealed by the conventional drug-screening procedures. Adverse side effects of unopposed estrogens have been detected in epidemiological studies showing increased incidence of endometrial carcinoma (Mack et al., 1976). There is also evidence for increased pituitary tumors in association with oral contraceptives (Sherman et al., 1978), but not all studies agree (discussed in Martinez et al., 1980). Other anticipated correlates of steroid usage may emerge as well. Adult rodent brains show clear susceptibility to steroids, suggesting new classes of steroid effects which might interact with aging changes in memory loss and cognitive function [through glucocorticoid action on the hippocampus (Landfield, 1978, Landfield et al., 1978)] and on the many other vital functions regulated in the hypothalamus, limbic system, and brain stem where sex-steroid-sensitive neurons are located.

REFERENCES

Adams, N. R. (1977). Morphological changes in the organs of ewes grazing oestrogenic subterranean clover. *Res. Vet. Sci. 22*: 216-221.

Annunziato, L., and Moore, K. E. (1978). Prolactin in CSF selectively increases dopamine turnover in the median eminence. *Life Sci. 22*: 2037-2042.

Aschheim, P. (1964/1965). Résultats fournis par la greffe heterochrone des ovaires dans l'étude de la régulation hypothalamo-hypophyso-ovarienne de la ratte sénile. *Gerontologia 10*: 65-75.

Aschheim, P. (1976). Aging in the hypothalamic-hypothyseal ovarian axis in the rat. In *Hypothalamus, Pituitary and Aging*, A. V. Everitt and J. A. Burgess (Eds.). Charles C Thomas, Springfield, Ill., p. 376.

Baird, D. T., Corker, C. S., Davidson, D. W., Hunter, W. M., Michie, E. A., and van Look, P. S. A. (1977). Pituitary-ovarian relationship in the polycystic ovary syndrome. *J. Clin. Endocrinol. Metab. 45*: 798-809.

Beck, W., Engelbart, S., Gelato, M., and Wuttke, W. (1977). Antigonadotrophic effect of prolactin in adult castrated and in immature female rats. *Acta Endocrinol. 84*: 62-71.

Bernheimer, H., Berkmayer, W., Hornykiewicz, O., Jellinger, K. S., and Eitelberger, F. (1973). Brain dopamine and the syndrome of Parkinson and Huntington: clinical morphological and neurochemical correlation. *J. Neurol. Sci. 20*: 415-255.

Berry, R. G., and Kaplan, H. J. (1979). An overview of pituitary tumors. *Ann. Clin. Lab. Sci. 9*: 94-102.

Blake, C., Scaramuzzi, R., Hilliard, J., and Sawyer, C. (1973). Circulating levels of pituitary gonadotropins and ovarian steroids in rats after hypothalamic de-afferentation. *Neuroendocrinology 12*: 86-97.

Blake, C., Weiner, R., Gorski, R., and Sawyer, C. (1972). Secretion of pituitary luteinizing hormone and follicle stimulating hormone in female rats made persistently estrous or diestrous by hypothalamic deafferentation. *Endocrinology 90*: 855-861.

Brawer, J. R., and Sonnenschein, C. (1975). Cytopathological effects of estradiol on the arcuate nucleus of the female rat: a possible mechanism for pituitary tumorigenesis. *Am. J. Anat. 144*: 57-89.

Brawer, J. R., Naftolin, F., Martin, J., and Sonnenschein, C. (1978). Effects of a single injection of estradiol valerate on the hypothalamic arcuate nucleus and on reproductive function in the female rat. *Endocrinology 103*: 501-512.

Brawer, J. R., Ruf, K. B., and Naftolin, F. (1980a). The effects of estradiol-induced lesions of the arcuate nucleus on gonadotropin release in response to preoptic stimulation in the rat. *Neuroendocrinology 30*: 144-149.

Brawer, J. R., Schipper, H., and Naftolin, F. (1980b). Ovary-dependent degeneration in the hypothalamic arcuate nucleus. *Endocrinology 107*: 274-279.

Brenner, R. M., and West, N. B., (1975). Hormone regulation of the reproductive tract in female mammals. *Ann. Rev. Physiol. 37*: 273-302.

Clemens, J. A., Amenomori, Y., Jenkins, T., and Meites, J. (1969). Effects of hypothalamic stimulation, hormones, and drugs on ovarian function in old female rats. *Proc. Soc. Exp. Biol. Med. 132*: 561-563.

Clemens, J. A., Fuller, R. W., and Owen, N. V. (1978). Some neuroendocrine aspects of aging. In *Parkinson's Disease II. Aging and Neuroendocrine Relationships*, C. E. Finch, D. E. Potter, and A. D. Kenny (Eds.). Plenum, New York, pp. 77-100.

Cooper, R. L., Brandt, S. J., Linnoila, M., and Walker, R. F. (1979). Induced ovulation in aged female rats by L-dopa implants into the medial preoptic area. *Neuroendocrinology 28*: 234-240.

Davies, I. J., Sin, J. Naftolin, F., and Ryan, K. J. (1975). Cytoplasmic binding of steroids in brain tissues and pituitary. In *Advances in the Biosciences*, G. Raspe (Ed.). Pergamon Press, Oxford, pp. 89-108.

Duchen, L. W., and Schurr, P. H. (1976). In *Hypothalamus, Pituitary and Aging*. A. V. Everitt and J. A. Burgess (Eds.). Charles C Thomas, Springfield, Ill., pp. 137-156.

Dunkerley, G. B., and Duncan, D. (1969). A light and electron microscopic study of the normal and degenerating corticospinal tract in the rat. *J. Comp. Neurol. 137*: 155-183.

Evans, R. W., and Leavitt, W. W. (1980). Progesterone inhibition of uterine nuclear receptor: dependence on RNA and protein synthesis. *Proc. Natl. Acad. Sci. USA 77*: 5856-5860.

Felicio, L. S., Nelson, J. F., and Finch, C. E. (1980). Spontaneous pituitary tumorigenesis and plasma oestradiol in aging female C57BL/6J mice. *Exp. Gerontol. 15*: 139-143.

Finch, C. E. (1973). Catecholamine metabolism in the brains of aging male mice.
Brain Res. 52: 261-276.

Finch, C. E. (1977). Neuroendocrine and autonomic aspects of aging. In *Handbook
of the Biology of Aging*, C. E. Finch and L. Hayflick (Eds.). Van Nostrand,
New York, pp. 262-280.

Finch, C. E. (1979). Neuroendocrine metabolisms and aging. *Fed. Proc. 38*: 178-
183.

Finch, C. E., Felicio, L. S., Flurkey, K., Gee, D. M., Mobbs, C., Nelson, J. F., and
Osterburg, H. H. (1980). Studies on ovarian hypothalamic-pituitary interactions during reproductive aging in C57BL/6J mice. *Peptides 1* (Suppl. 1):
163-175.

Flurkey, K., Gee, D. M., Sinha, Y. N., and Finch, C. E. (1900). Age effects on luteinizing hormone, progesterone, and prolactin in proestrus and acyclic
C57BL/6J mice. *Biol. Reprod. 26*: 835-846.

Flurkey, K., Gee, D. M., Sinha, Y. N., Wisner, J. R., Jr., and Finch, C. E. (in press).
Age effects on luteinizing hormone, progesterone, and prolactin in proestrous
and acyclic C57BL/6J mice. *Biol. Reprod.*

Futterweit, W., and Krieger, D. T. (1979). Pituitary tumors associated with hyperprolactinemia and polycystic ovarian disease. *Fertil. Steril. 31*: 608-613.

Gorski, R. A., Gordon, J. H., Shryne, J. E., and Southam, A. M. (1978). Evidence
for a morphologic sex difference within the medial preoptic area of the rat
brain. *Brain Res. 148*: 333-346.

Gosden, R. G., Liang, S. C., Felicio, L. S., Nelson, J. F., and Finch, C. E. (1983).
Imminent oocyte exhaustion and reduced follicular recruitment mark the
climacteric in ageing mice. *Biol. Reprod.*, in press.

Grandison, L. J., Hodson, C. A., Chen, H. T., Advis, J., Simkins, J., and Meites, J.
(1977). Inhibition by prolactin of post-castration rise in LH. *Neuroendocrinology 23*: 312-322.

Gudelsky, G. A., and Porter, J. C. (1980). Release of dopamine from tuberoin-
fundibular neurons into pituitary stalk blood after prolactin or haloperidol
administration. *Endocrinology 106*: 526-529.

Gudelsky, G. A., Nansel, D. N., and Porter, J. C. (1981). Dopaminergic control of
prolactin secretion in the aging male rat. *Brain Res. 204*: 446-450.

Halasz, B. (1969). The endocrine effects of isolation of the hypothalamus from
the rest of the brain. In *Frontiers in Neuroendocrinology*, W. F. Ganong, and
L. Martini (Eds.). Oxford University Press, New York, p. 301.

Huang, H. H., Marshall, S., and Meites, J. (1976). Capacity of old versus young female rats to secrete LH, FSH, and prolactin. *Biol. Reprod. 14*: 538-543.

Kalra, S. (1976). Tissue levels of luteinizing hormone releasing hormone in the
preoptic area and hypothalamus, and serum concentrations of gonadotropins
following anterior hypothalamic deafferentation and estrogen treatment of
the female rat. *Endocrinology 99*: 101-107.

Kato, Y., Iwasaki, Y., Iwasaki, J., Abe, H., Yanaihara, N., and Imura, H. (1978).

Prolactin release by vasoactive intestinal peptide in rats. *Endocrinology 103*: 554-558.

Landfield, P. W. (1978). An endocrine hypothesis of brain aging and studies on brain-endocrine correlations and monosynaptic neurophysiology during aging. In *Parkinson's Disease II*, C. E. Finch, D. E. Potter, and A. D. Kenny (Eds.). Plenum, New York, pp. 179-199.

Landfield, P. W., Waymire, J. E., and Lunch, G. (1978). Hippocampal aging and adrenocorticoids: quantitative considerations. *Science 202*: 1098-1102.

Lee, H., Davies, I., and Ryan, K. (1979). Progesterone receptor in the hypothalamic cytosol of female rats. *Endocrinology 104*: 791-800.

Lu, K. H., Hopper, B. R., Vargo, T. M., and Yen, S. S. C. (1979). Chronologic changes in sex steroid, gonadotropin and prolactin secretion in aging female rats displaying different reproductive states. *Biol. Reprod. 21*: 193-203.

Mack, T. M., Pike, M. C., and Henderson, B. E. (1976). Estrogen and endometrial cancer in a retirement community. *N. Engl. J. Med. 284*: 878-881.

Martinez, A. J., Lee, A., Moossey, J., and Maroon, J. C. (1980). Pituitary adenomas: clinical and immunohistochemical study. *Ann. Neurol. 7*: 24-36.

Massa, R., Stupnika, E., Kniewald, Z., and Martini, L. (1972). The transformation of testosterone into dihydrotestosterone by the brain and the anterior pituitary. *J. Steroid Biochem. 3*: 385-399.

Matthews, M. R., and Kruger, L. (1973). Electron microscopy of non-neuronal cellular changes accompanying neuronal degeneration in thalamic nuclei of the rabbit. II. Reactive elements within the neuropil. *J. Comp. Neurol. 148*: 313-346.

Matsumoto, A., and Arai, Y. (1976). Developmental changes in synaptic formation in the hypothalamic arcuate nucleus of female rats. *Cell Tiss. Res. 169*: 143-156.

Matsumoto, A., and Arai, Y. (1977). Precocious puberty and synaptogenesis in the hypothalamic arcuate nucleus in pregnant mare serum gonadotropin (PMSG) treated immature female rats. *Brain Res. 129*: 375-378.

Matsumoto, A., and Arai, Y. (1979). Synaptogenic effect of estrogen on the hypothalamic arcuate nucleus of the adult female rat. *Cell Tiss. Res. 198*: 427-433.

Matsumoto, A., and Arai, Y. (1980). Sexual dimorphism in "wiring pattern" in the hypothalamic arcuate nucleus and its modification by neonatal hormonal environment. *Brain Res. 190*: 238-242.

McEwen, C. S., Selye, H., and Collip, J. B. (1936). Some effects of prolonged administration of oestrin in rats. *Lancet 230*: 775-776.

Meites, J. (1980). Controls of prolactin secretion. In *Growth Hormone and Other Biologically Active Peptides*. Excerpta Medica, Amsterdam, *Int. Cong. Ser. 495*, pp. 258-266.

Meites, J., Hwang, H., and Simkins, J. (1978). Recent studies on neuroendocrine controls of reproductive senescence in rats. In *The Aging Reproductive System*, E. L. Schneider (Ed.). Raven Press, New York, pp. 213-235.

Mobbs, C., Flurkey, K., Gee, D., and Finch, C. E. (1981). Estradiol-induced acyclicity in mice: a model of reproductive aging? *63rd Annual Meeting of the Endocrine Society*, p. 159.

Naftolin, F., Ryan, K. J., and Davies, I. J. (1976). Androgen aromatization by neuroendocrine tissues. In *Subcellular Mechanisms in Reproductive Neuroendocrinology*, F. Naftolin, K. J. Ryan, and I. J. Davies (Eds.). Elsevier, Amsterdam, pp. 347-355.

Nakagawa, K., Obara, T., and Tashiro, K. (1980). Pituitary hormones and prolactin-releasing activity in rats with primary estrogen-induced pituitary tumors. *Endocrinology 106*: 1033-1039.

Nelson, J. F., Felicio, L. S., and Finch, C. E. (1980). Ovarian hormones and the etiology of reproductive aging in mice. In *Aging, Its Chemistry*, A. Kietz, (Ed.). American Society for Clinical Chemistry, Washington, D.C. pp. 64-81.

Nelson, J. F., Felicio, L. S., Osterburg, H. H., and Finch, C. E. (1981). Altered profiles of estradiol and progesterone associated with prolonged estrous cycles and persistent vaginal cornification in aging C57BL/6J mice. *Biol. Reprod. 24*: 784-794.

Nelson, J. F., Felicio, L. S., Osterburg, H. H., and Finch, C. E. (1981). Altered profiles of estradiol and progesterone associated with prolonged estrous cycles and persistent vaginal cornification in aging C57BL/6J mice. *Biol. Reprod. 24*: 784-794.

Nelson, J. F., Felicio, L., Sinha, Y. N., and Finch, C. E. (1980). An ovarian role in the spontaneous pituitary tumorigenesis and hyperprolactinemia of aging female mice. *The Gerontologist* (part II) abstract, 20: 171.

Osterburg, H. H., Donahue, H. G., Seaverson, J. A., and Finch, C. E. (1981). Catecholamine levels and turnover during aging in brain regions of male C57BL/6J mice. *Brain Res. 213*: 337-252.

Pavlik, E. J., and Coulson, P. B. (1976). Modulation of estrogen receptors in four different target tissues: different effects of estrogen and progesterone. *J. Steroid Biochem. 7*: 369-376.

Quadri, S. K., Kledzik, G. S., and Meites, J. (1973). Reinitiation of estrous cycles in old constant-estrous rats by central-acting drugs. *Neuroendocrinology 11*: 248-255.

Raisman, G., and Field, P. (1973). Sexual dimorphism in the neuropil of the preoptic area of the rat and its dependence on neonatal androgen. *Brain Res. 54*: 1-29.

Reigle, G. D., and Miller, A. E. (1978). Aging effects on the hypothalamic-hypophyseal-gonadal control system in the rat. In *The Aging Reproductive System, Aging*, Vol. 4, E. L. Schneider (Ed.). Raven Press, New York, pp. 159-192.

Sar, M., and Stumpf, W. (1973). Neurons of the hypothalamus that concentrate (^{3}H) progesterone or its metabolites. *Science 182*: 1266-1268.

Sawyer, C. (1975). Some recent developments in brain-pituitary-ovarian physiology. *Neuroendocrinology 17*: 97-124.

Schechter, T. E., Felicio, L., Nelson, J., and Finch, C. E. (1981). Pituitary tumorigenesis in aging female C57BL/6J mice: a light and electron microscopic study. *Anat. Rec. 199*: 423-432.

Schipper, H., Brawer, J. R., Nelson, J. F., Felicio, L. S., and Finch, C. E. The role of the gonads in histologic aging of the hypothalamic arcuate nucleus. *Biol. Reprod. 25*: 413-419.

Schwartz, N. B. (1969). A model for the regulation of ovulation in the rat. *Rec. Prog. Horm. Res. 25*: 1-55.

Sherman, B. M., Schlechte, J., and Halmi, N. S. (1978). Pathogenesis of prolactin-secreting pituitary adenomas. *Lancet 2*: 1019-1021.

Talbert, G. (1977). Aging of the female reproductive system. In *Handbook of the Biology of Aging*, C. E. Finch and L. Mayflick (Eds.). Van Nostrand, New York, pp. 318-356.

Talesnik, S., Velasco, M., and Astrada, J. (1970). Effect of hypothalamic deafferentation on the control of luteinizing hormone secretion. *J. Endocrinol. 46*: 1-7.

Tejasen, T., and Everett, J. (1967). Surgical analysis of the preoptico-tuberal pathway controlling ovulatory release of gonadotropins in the rat. *Endocrinology 81*: 1387-1396.

Tucker, G. H. St., Lankford, H. V., Gardner, D. F., and Blackward, W. G. (1980). Persistent defect in regulation of prolactin secretion after successful pituitary tumor removal in women with the galactorrhea-amenorrhea syndrome. *J. Clin. Endocrinol. Metab. 51*: 968-971.

van Loon, G. R. (1978). A defect in catechol neurons in patients with prolactin-secreting adenomas. *Lancet 2*: 868-871.

Warembourg, M. (1978). Uptake of ^{3}H-labeled synthetic progestin by rat brain and pituitary: a radioautographic study. *Neurosci. Lett. 9*: 329-332.

Wiegand, S. J., Terasawa, E., Bridson, W. E., and Goy, R. E. (1980). Effects of discrete lesions of preoptic and suprachiasmatic structures in the female rat. *Neuroendocrinology 31*: 147-157.

Yamaju, T., Shimamoto, K., Ishibashi, M., Kosaka, K., and Orimo, H. (1976). Effect of age and sex on circulating and pituitary prolactin levels in human. *Acta Endocrinol. 83*: 711-719.

Zimmerman, E. (1976). Localization of hypothalamic hormones by immunochemical techniques. In *Frontiers in Neuroendocrinology*, Vol. 4, L. Martini and W. F. Ganong, (Eds.). Raven Press, New York, pp. 25-62.

4

Animal Models for Aging of the Reproductive System

Richard F. Walker / *University of Kentucky Medical Center, Lexington, Kentucky*

INTRODUCTION

Gerontological research entered a logarithmic growth phase during the past 15 years. During this time, the majority of research was descriptive; that is, old and young animals were observed in the laboratory, with hopes that comparative study of their cells, tissues, and systems would provide a key to understanding the process of age transformation. Although this expectation has not been realized, descriptive gerontological research provided a broad base of comparative literature upon which contemporary studies are being built. Now, more experimental approaches are used to enhance our understanding of the mechanism(s) of aging and, thereby, to promote future interventive therapy for and/or prophylaxis against degenerative diseases of senescence.

It is becoming quite clear that the answer to the riddle of aging will not be found in old animals, which are really the products of process(es) which began well before those individuals were old. In fact, the obvious infirmaties of age are really the sum of more subtle deficits which begin earlier in life and accumulate over time.

To understand the aging process, it is imperative to recognize the preliminary and subtle aspects of postmaturational change which precede frank senescence. To this end, we can exploit carefully selected models for given aging phenomena. With these, selected mechanisms may be isolated from the more complex mosaic of total organismal aging, subjected to rigorous examination, and eventually understood. This type of systematic analysis may lead to greater understanding of the total syndrome.

Certain considerations should precede the use of models in gerontological research. In the first place, the phenomenon being studied should be conducive to modeling; and, second, the model should simulate those events which occur naturally in the aging animal, or at least it should allow accurate extrapolation to the true aging process.

MODEL SYSTEMS FOR STUDYING AGING IN THE FEMALE REPRODUCTIVE SYSTEM

One example of a system well suited for experimental gerontological research is the reproductive system of the female rat. Several factors defend this choice, not the least of which is an extensive literature on normal function in the young adult. This resource provides a substantial background for understanding aberrant function in the old animal. Second, the primary characteristics of female reproductive senescence are unambiguous, occur in the absence of pathology, and are easily quantifiable. For example, chronic anovulation is the hallmark of aging in this neuroendocrine axis and represents an end point in the animal's reproductive life span. It is generally held that in the rat changes intrinsic to the brain, not the gonad, are responsible for ovulatory dysfunction with advancing age (Peng and Huang, 1972; Aschheim, 1976). These changes are characterized by suboptimal integrating signals, especially involving the preovulatory secretion of gonadotropin, and promote a functional decline of the total reproductive axis over time. For example, in rats approaching 1 year of age, phasic secretion of luteinizing hormone (LH) loses its temporal relationship with the light:dark cycle, resulting in delayed onset of LH release and reduced serum content of the hormone at the peak of the surge (Cooper et al., 1980). As timing of the LH surge progressively deteriorates, the estrous cycle becomes irregular, characteristically prolonged within the estrous interval. Finally, the LH surge is lost completely, and aging female rats become acyclic, entering constant estrous (CE) (Steger and Peluso, 1979), an endocrine condition in which the ovarian production of estrogen is practically continuous (Huang et al., 1978). The ovaries of CE rats do not produce progesterone; therefore, these animals experience a relatively unopposed estrogenic steroid milieu. Since estrogen elicits LH surges in young rats, the absence of surges in CE rats implies that the CNS mechanism for positive feedback is defective. Since degeneration of the LH surge precedes and predicates deterioration of the estrous cycle, it is possible that the CNS site controlling steroid-positive feedback is a primary locus for propagation of more general age lesions in the reproductive system of the female rat. For this reason, it is logical to examine model systems which target on mechanisms controlling the temporal characteristics of the LH surge, as well as those which allow detailed study of the positive feedback response to estrogen.

There are at least two experimental treatments suitable for studying these parameters, including (1) the use of altered photoperiod and (2) administration of supraphysiological doses of estrogen. For example, temporal desynchronization of phasic LH secretion, which characterizes the initial and subtle age changes in middle-aged rats, also occurs in young animals kept in constant light for a few days (McCormack and Sridaran, 1978; Daane and Parlow, 1971; Watts and Fink, 1981). Both groups of rats show phase-shifted LH surges which are delayed in onset and attenuated. Age-type changes also occur in ovariectomized rats bearing subcutaneous pellets of estrogen. Legan and Karsch (1975) showed that young rats chronically exposed to estrogen lose their ability to produce LH surges. Daily LH surges begin about 2 days after Silastic capsules containing estradiol are surgically implanted under the skin of ovariectomized rats. However, the surges do not continue indefinitely. Instead, they attenuate gradually and finally cease approximately 2 weeks after the estrogen is first implanted (Chazal et al., 1977). Extinction of daily LH surges represents the spontaneous development of estrogen insensitivity with regard to the ability of these rats to show a positive feedback response. In the same sense, aged CE rats are estrogen-insensitive and lack the ability to release an LH surge, even in response to supraphysiological levels of estrogen (Lu et al., 1980). Since these apparent similarities exist between aging and young experimental rats, these models were investigated in more depth to evaluate their potential to serve in experiments designed to elucidate the mechanisms of reproductive system aging.

METHODS

Alteration by Light of the Temporal Characteristics of LH Secretion

Since the effects of light upon reproductive function must be mediated through the central nervous system, it is conceivable that constant light alters, in some way, the neural signal for the LH surge. Since the LH surge is a circadian rhythm (Chazal et al., 1977; McCormack and Sridaran, 1978), it is also logical that the neural signal which triggers the surge occurs intermittently and coincides with the surge. Hypothalamic monoamines are known to influence phasic secretion of LH, though relative contributions to the total signal, made by catecholamines and serotonin, are still not established. However, several factors suggest that a major timing contribution is made by serotonin. First, serotonin shows a circadian rhythm whose acrophase occurs during the critical period for activation of the LH surge (Quay, 1968). Thereafter, and during active secretion of LH under the influence of its neural signal, hypothalamic serotonin content falls. Basal serotonin levels are reached during early evening when the LH surge terminates. If the reduction of hypothalamic serotonin content represents depletion of the neurotransmitter during a period of enhanced utilization, then increased activity in serotoninergic circuits coincides with the rising phase of the LH surge. This idea is supported by the fact that abolition of the serotonin rhythm with p-chlorophenylalanine (pCPA) blocks the LH surge, whereas drugs which block serotonin neurotransmission given during the LH surge cause it to terminate prematurely (Hery et al., 1976; Walker, 1980). Based upon this logic, temporal characteristics of the hypothalamic serotonin rhythm were measured on proestrus in middle-aged rats and in young rats exposed to constant light for 3 days preceding proestrus. Both of these groups of rats are reported to show similar alteration in LH surge patterns (Cooper et al., 1980; Watts and Fink, 1981), compared with young female rats kept in standard photoperiod (14:10) that show normally phased LH surges.

To determine if the serotonin and gonadotropin rhythms are functionally related, rats were given treatments designed to alter patterns of serotonin metabolism. 5-Hydroxytryptophan (5-HTP), which enhances the synthesis of serotonin, was injected during the evening of diestrus day 2 in young rats showing regular estrous cycles and normal patterns of LH secretion on proestrus. They were then bled on proestrus to characterize the LH surge. Others were killed at several time points on proestrus, and hypothalamic serotonin content and turnover were determined, so as to evaluate the effect of treatment on the serotonin circadian rhythm. As an alternative to this experiment, middle-aged rats showing irregular cycles were placed in photoperiods with reduced light exposure. Such treatment has been shown to reinstate cycles in constant estrous rats (Everett, 1942), presumably by reinstating the LH surge mechanism. It was reasoned that such treatment might also restore normal LH surge profiles in middle-aged rats showing aberrant preovulatory LH secretion. Therefore, these rats were placed in 10:14 hr photoperiods (lights on 0500-1500 hr) beginning on diestrus 1, and were bled for LH determinations on the following proestrus. Rats were killed at several times during the afternoon and evening of proestrus and their brains assayed for content and turnover of serotonin in the hypothalamus.

Loss of Positive Feedback in Female Rats Exposed Chronically to Estrogen

Brawer and Finch (Chap. 3) suggested that exposure of rodents to endogenous estrogen during estrous cycles causes neural changes to accumulate over their reproductive life span and promote ovarian senescence. Presumably, estrogen (E) alters neurotransmitter homeostasis in the hypothalamus, and these perturbations are reflected primarily as the loss of LH surges. Interestingly, Legan and Karsch (1975) found that daily LH surges occur when estrogen capsules are implanted in ovariectomized (OVX) rats. These surges gradually attenuate and finally cease after about 2 weeks. Extinction of the daily LH surges represents the development of estrogen insensitivity in these young rats and is not unlike that occurring spontaneously with advancing age (Lu et al., 1980). Therefore, the estrogen-insensitive rat might provide a good model for studying certain types of reproductive system aging, since it resembles, endocrinologically, the old CE rat in many ways. Therefore, this preparation was examined with regard to selected neuroendocrine parameters, so as to determine if it might adequately serve as a model for CE and its sequelae, particularly those concerning loss of positive feedback in response to estrogen. In the course of this investigation, the following considerations were made: (1) Do monoamine changes in the hypothalamus of OVX + E rats resemble those seen in CE rats? (2) Are endocrine profiles in pituitary and serum of both groups comparable? (3) Is the acquired estrogen insensitivity of OVX + E rats reversible, as in aged rats? (4) Do both groups respond comparably to pharmacological therapy involving monoaminergic neuroleptics?

Initially, content and turnover of hypothalamic monoamines were determined, before and after extinction of daily LH surges in OVX + rats bearing estrogen implants. The purpose was to characterize changes in neurotransmitter profiles which occur coincident with loss of the estrogen-positive feedback effect, and to see if monoamine profiles in these rats are comparable to those in CE rats which are also estrogen-insensitive. Furthermore, the changes provided a rationale for subsequent pharmacological treatments used in attempts to reinstate the LH surge.

Hypothalamic monoamines were measured by radioenzymatic assay in three groups including OVX (empty implants, no estrogen), OVX + E (estrogen-sensitive, implants for 3 days), and OVX + E (estrogen-insensitive, implants $>$ 30 days). Rats were decapitated, and their brains were rapidly frozen on dry ice and stored at -80°C until they were dissected and assayed. As each group was killed, the rats were exsanguinated and the pituitaries were collected. Both tissues were then measured for content of gonadotropins and prolactin, and the data were compared with established values for aged CE rats to determine if the endocrinology of the insensitive rat is comparable to the old animals.

Since it has been shown that estrogen sensitivity returns to aged rats if they are tested 4-5 weeks after ovariectomy, similar evaluation was made in estrogen-insensitive rats. To determine if loss of estrogen-positive feedback is reversible, the pellets were removed from insensitive rats. Four weeks later, each animal was given a single injection of estrogen, followed 2 days later by progesterone (0.5 mg), since this steroid treatment reinstates LH surges in the old CE, OVX rat. The test rats were bled from their tail veins during the afternoon and evening of the day of progesterone injection to determine if estrogen sensitivity was restored after a 30-day hiatus from the steroid. Last, certain neuroleptics were administered to old and young estrogen-insensitive rats in an attempt to normalize neurotransmitter balance in both groups and restore positive feedback. All rats used in this series of experiments initially showed daily LH surges after implantation of estrogen; however, all were acyclic at the time of treatment. Estrogen implants were in situ in excess of 30 days preceding drug administration. Neuroleptics were administered by subcutaneous injection according to the following schedule: (1) p-Chlorophenylalanine (pCPA; 250 mg/kg + L-dihydroxyphenylalanine (L-dopa; 200 mg/kg). The rationale for using both of these drugs was to depress serotonin and enhance catecholamine synthesis in an attempt to favor catecholamine influence on gonadotropin secretion. pCPA, which blocks serotonin synthesis, was given at 1830 hr, day 1. L-dopa, which enhances catecholamine synthesis, was administered concomitant with pCPA, and at 1100 hr on the next 2 days, days 2 and 3. Blood samples for LH determination were taken at 1200 and 1800 hr on each day of L-dopa treatment. (2) 5-Hydroxytryptophan (5-HTP; 70 mg/kg) or L-dopa (200 mg/kg). One or the other amino acid was administered at 1100 hr to test the effect of enhanced catecholamine (L-dopa) or serotonin (5-HTP) metabolism in the estrogen-insensitive rat. Blood was taken at 1200 and 1800 hr of the day preceding and the day of drug treatment. (3) pCPA (250 mg/kg + 5-HTP (70 mg/kg). These drugs were used to experimentally normalize hypothalamic serotonin metabolism which was enhanced in estrogen-insensitive rats (see section on results). Since pCPA abolishes daily changes in serotonin and also blocks the LH surge, 5-HTP was also provided in an attempt to reinstate both the serotonin circadian rhythm, as well as phasic secretion of the gonadotropin. pCPA was given at 1830 hr, day 1. 5-HTP was given the next day (day 2) and/or at 1100 hr 2 days later (day 3). Blood samples for LH determination were taken at 1200 and 1800 hr.

LH was assayed in duplicate, using materials provided in the double-antibody NIAMDD rat LH kit. The gonadotropin concentrations are, therefore, expressed in nanograms per milliliter, with reference to LH-RP 1. Sensitivity of the assay is 1 ng LH, whereas intra- and interassay variances are 7 and 12% respectively.

Hypothalamic tissue was dissected and extracted in 10 volumes of ice-cold 0.1 N perchloric acid. Then, monoamine content in 10 μl of the acid extract was determined by radioenzymatic methods and expressed as nanograms per milliliter wet weight of tissue, as previously described (Walker et al., 1980). Data were statistically evaluated using Student's t-test, and $p < 0.05$ was taken as the level of significance.

RESULTS

As seen in Fig. 1, LH surges in young rats exposed to constant light show changes in secretory patterns which resemble those occurring spontaneously in aging rats. Since aging is not a synchronized process, all middle-aged rats did not show the same degree of change occurring in light-exposed rats. However, patterns were comparable among the groups. Typically, the onset of the surge was delayed, and peak LH values were significantly lower than those seen in young rats kept in a standard photoperiod. Figure 2 shows that similar changes in hypothalamic serotonin metabolism occurred in middle-aged rats and in constant light-exposed young rats as a concomitant of altered LH secretion. These changes are characterized by a reduction in the differences in serotonin turnover during the LH surge, that is, differences in hypothalamic content of serotonin after paygyline are reduced when comparing values at 1400 and 2100 hr. On the other hand, highly significant differences are seen at these two time points in young rats showing high-amplitude

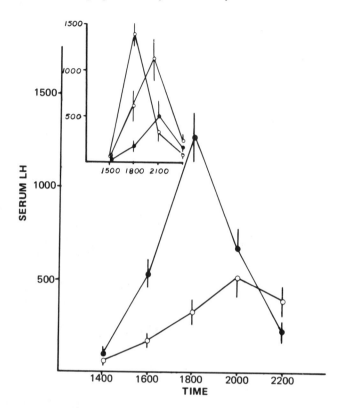

Figure 1 Effect of constant light exposure on LH surge profiles in young rats previously showing regular estrous cycles in a photoperiod with 14 hr of light (14:10). Beginning on diestrus 1, lights were kept on 24 hr per day for 3 days until proestrus, when blood samples were taken for LH determinations. Rats in constant light showed LH surges with delayed onset and attenuated peaks. LH values at 1600 and 1800 hr were significantly different between constant light (——○——) and alternating (14:10) photophase (——●——) groups. N = 6 rats per group. Inset: LH surge profiles in middle-aged rats showing regular (——○——) and irregular (——●——) estrous cycles. Spontaneous changes in phasic secretion of LH occurring with advancing age resemble those resulting from exposure to constant light in young rats. Serum LH is expressed as X = SEM (ng/ml).

LH surges. Aged, constant estrous rats are sensitive to reduced light exposure (Everett, 1942), showing restored LH surges when the photophase is changed from 14 to 10 hr. As seen in Fig. 3, CE rats kept in the shortened photoperiod showed changes in hypothalamic serotonin content which resembled those seen in young, cycling rats, that is, serotonin content fell during the rising phase of the LH surge. On the other hand, CE rats kept in 14 hr of light failed to show LH surges, and hypothalamic content remained high throughout the day.

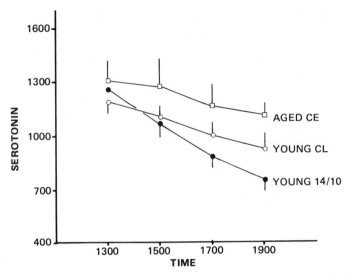

Figure 2 Comparison of serotonin turnover in hypothalami of aged rats showing constant estrus (CE) and young rats exposed to constant light (CL). Hypothalamic serotonin content 30 min after pargyline treatment is expressed as $\overline{X}$ = SEM (ng/g wet weight hypothalamic tissue). Values at 1300 and 1900 hr are significantly different (p < 0.02) in young rats (14:10), but the difference between values at these time points are not significant in aged CE or young CL rats.

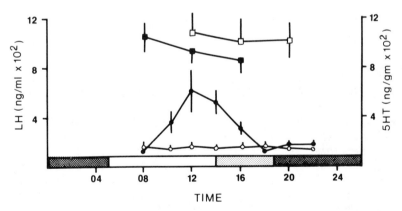

Figure 3 Changes in hypothalamic serotonin content associated with restored LH surges resulting from reduced light exposure in constant estrous rats. When the photoperiod was changed to 10:14 (light:dark), LH surges occurred in aged rats previously showing constant estrus. Hypothalamic serotonin content (□ ■) was reduced as the result of the altered photoperiod. Serotonin metabolic changes resembled those seen in younger rats showing regular estrous cycles with LH surges. Gonadotropin values represent $\overline{X}$ = SEM for six rats per group. Serotonin values represent $\overline{X}$ = SEM for rats from each photoperiod. Six were killed at each time point.

74

The flattening of the hypothalamic serotonin rhythm seems to be directly correlated with damped LH surges. Support for this hypothesis is presented in Fig. 4. The administration of 5-HTP on the evening of diestrus caused the proestrus LH surge to attenuate and shift after constant light exposure. As seen in Fig. 4, 5-HTP caused the day:night change in hypothalamic serotonin content after pargyline to be less pronounced than usual.

Table 1 shows that significant changes in monoamine content and turnover accompanied loss of the LH surge in rats chronically exposed to estrogen from subcutaneous implants. During early exposure to estrogen, when daily LH surges occur spontaneously, levels of all hypothalamic monoamines which were measured were depressed. However, differential turnover of serotonin persisted between 1400 and 2200 hr. As estrogen insensitivity developed, with attenuation and final cessation of spontaneous LH surges, turnover of hypothalamic serotonin increased. As seen in Fig. 5, this effect obliterated the serotonin rhythm, resulting in uniformly high levels of the amine throughout the day. Comparable profiles of

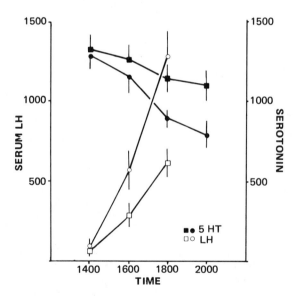

Figure 4 Relationship between changes in hypothalamic serotonin and serum LH in rats treated with 5-HTP. A single injection of 5-HTP (50 mg/kg) on diestrus 2 accelerated the synthesis of serotonin on the afternoon of proestrus. This metabolic change reduced the decline in hypothalamic serotonin between 1400 and 2000 hr, thereby flattening its circadian rhythm. The rising phase of the LH surge was significantly lower (p < 0.05, 1800 hr) in 5-HTP-treated rats. These findings suggest a functional correlation between the characteristics of the serotonin and LH circadian rhythms. LH surge (——□——) and serotonin content (——■——) in rats treated with 5-HTP in diestrus 2 are shown.

Table 1 Effect of Estrogen on LH Secretion and Hypothalamic Monoamines in Ovariectomized Rats[a]

Duration of estrogen exposure (days)	Serum LH	Monoamine content					
		Serotonin		Norepinephrine		Dopamine	
		A	B	A	C	A	C
0	Castration levels	937 ± 75 p < 0.05	1209 ± 93	1921 ± 139 p < 0.05	1217 ± 88	817 ± 52	637 ± 48
3	LH surge	676 ± 41 p < 0.05	855 ± 73	1569 ± 81	1109 ± 67	737 ± 50	591 ± 44
30	Basal levels	849 ± 67	1215 ± 110	1543 ± 75	1128 ± 70	766 ± 53	595 ± 50

[a]Young rats previously showing regular estrous cycles were ovariectomized. Two weeks later they received subcutaneous implants of estrogen, and were killed before daily LH surges began (day 0), during the period of spontaneous LH surges (3 days), and after daily surges ended (30 days). Monoamine content is expressed as $\overline{X} \pm$ SEM, ng/g wet weight hypothalamic tissue for six rats. A = content of tissue without drug pretreatment. B = content 30 min after pargyline (75 mg/kg body weight). C = content 60 min after α-MT (200 mg/kg body weight).

hypothalamic serotonin are also present in aged rats showing constant vaginal estrus (Fig. 2). When the steroid capsules were removed from the young, acyclic rats, or the ovaries removed from aged, constant estrous rats, estrogen sensitivity eventually returned, and the ability to produce a positive feedback response returned in both groups. As seen in Table 2, serum LH was significantly elevated 5 hr after progesterone in estrogen-primed rats. Although the response was attenuated in these animals, its presence demonstrates that the circuits which generated the neural signal for phasic secretion of LH have not degenerated completely, though they are nonfunctional during the early stages of CE. Again, hypothalamic serotonin rhythms return as a concomitant of renewed cyclicity, further suggesting a functional relationship between the neurotransmitter and gonadotropin rhythms (Table 2).

As seen in Table 3, serum and pituitary gonadotropin and prolactin in the chronic estrogen-implanted rat resemble those seen in aged CE rats. Generally, hormone content of the serum was higher in rats exposed to estrogen, whether endogenous (CE) or exogenous. Serum LH and follicle-stimulating hormone (FSH) were slightly elevated in both groups, while prolactin was two to three times higher than in controls. On the other hand, pituitary content of these hormones differed from serum profiles. Although FSH and prolactin content was elevated, LH content of the pituitary was significantly lower than controls. These hormonal profiles

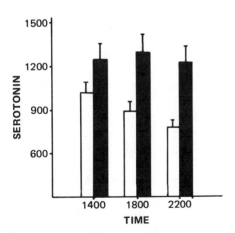

Figure 5 Effect of chronic exposure to estrogen on daily changes in hypothalamic serotonin content in rats treated with estrogen for 3 (□) and 30 (■) days. Serotonin content 30 min after pargyline treatment is significantly higher ($p < 0.05$) at 1400 vs. 2200 hr; however, these temporal differences are not present after 30 days of estrogen exposure. Increased serotonin synthesis throughout the day obliterates circadian serotonin changes in rats treated chronically with estrogen. Values represent the X = SEM for six rats per group. Serotonin content is expressed as ng/g wet weight of hypothalamic tissue.

Table 2 Effect of Estrogen and Progesterone Injections on Serum LH and Hypothalamic Monoamines in Young and Old Rats with Different Histories of Estrogen[a] Exposure

Treatment	Serum LH 1700 hr	Hypothalamic serotonin (30 min after pargyline 75 mg/kg) (pg/mg wet weight)	
		1300 hr	2000 hr
Young OVX	1130 ± 189	1006 ± 131	704 ± 70[b]
Young OVX + E	163 ± 51	1396 ± 297	1180 ± 179
Young + E, - E	955 ± 110	966 ± 104	725 ± 100[b]
Old CE	96 ± 21	1144 ± 199	1300 ± 244
Old CE OVX	633 ± 97	991 ± 76	780 ± 84[b]

[a]Young rats previously showing regular estrous cycles and old rats in constant estrus were ovariectomized. After 30 days they received single subcutaneous injections of estrogen (50 μg), followed 2 days later by progesterone. (0.5 mg, 1200 hr). The purpose was to determine the effect of these hormones on plasma LH and hypothalamic monoamines after a 30-day hiatus from the influence of ovarian steroids. Similar tests were made in young OVX rats bearing subcutaneous estrogen pellets for 30 days and also 30 days after the pellets were removed. +E = estrogen pellets for 30 days; -E = estrogen pellets removed for 30 days; CE = constant estrus; OVX = ovariectomy.
[b]Values represent the a ± SEM for determinations using six rats per group.

resulting from chronic exposure to estrogen resemble those occurring spontaneously in female rats as they age.

Table 4 shows that LH surges can be restored pharmacologically in young and old estrogen-insensitive rats. Despite the presence of a stable steroid environment maintained by the estrogen capsule, LH surges occurred following treatment with drugs altering brain monoamine metabolism.

The combined effects of pCPA (to depress serotonin metabolism) and L-dopa (to enhance catecholamine metabolism) did not restore daily surges. On the other hand, a small number of rats showed LH surges after treatment with precursors of catecholamines or serotonin. Two out of ten rats treated with L-dopa showed plasma LH levels at 1800 hr, which were significantly higher (p < 0.05) than values at 1200 hr. Similarly, the plasma from 4 out of 14 rats given 5-HTP at 1100 hr, contained surge levels of LH at 1800 hr. No significant, spontaneous increases in plasma LH occurred in 15 control rats for the same time interval. The LH changes in drug-treated rats represent restoration of gonadotropin surges in 20 and 29% of the L-dopa- and 5-HTP-treated rats, respectively.

In contrast to the modest stimulatory effect of monoamine precursors alone, the combined effect of pCPA + 5-HTP restored surges in the majority (88%) of

Table 3 Effect of Estrogen on Pituitary and Serum Gonadotropins and Prolactin[a]

Group	LH		FSH		Prolactin	
	S (ng/ml)	P (µg/mg)	S (ng/ml)	P (µg/mg)	S (ng/ml)	P (µg/mg AP)
Young intact (control)	29 ± 9	8.9 ± 0.9	116 ± 21	1.8 ± 0.4	163 ± 40	1.1 ± 0.3
Young OVX + E	47 ± 15	4.4 ± 0.6[c]	166 ± 21[b]	3.9 ± 0.5[b]	296 ± 73[b]	3.9 ± 0.5[b]
Old CE	64 ± 27[b]	2.7 ± 0.3[c]	196 ± 47[b]	6.2 ± 0.9[b]	331 ± 99[b]	4.2 ± 0.7[c]

[a]Young rats previously showing regular estrous cycles were ovariectomized and given subcutaneous pellets. Thirty days later serum and pituitary content of gonadotropins and prolactin from these animals was determined and compared with values derived from old constant-estrus and young intact rats in vaginal estrus. [b]p < 0.05 when compared with intact controls. [c]p < 0.01 when compared with intact controls. OVX = ovariectomized; E = estrogen implants for 30 days; CE = constant estrus; S = serum; P = pituitary.

Table 4 Pharmacological Reinstatement of LH Surges in Young and Old Rats Lacking the Positive-Feedback Response to Estrogen

Treatment	Number treated/ number responding	Serum LH (ng/ml) (responders)	
		1200 hr	1800 hr
Young rats			
Saline	15/0	–	–
pCPA + L-dopa	8/0	–	–
L-dopa	10/2	99 ± 18	315 ± 66^b
5-HTP	14/4	117 ± 25	418 ± 71^b
pCPA + 5-HTP (1800 hr day 2; 1100 hr day 3)	6/0	–	–
pCPA + 5-HTP (1100 hr day 3)	16/14	83 ± 12	1410 ± 223^b
Old rats			
Saline	10/0	–	–
L-dopa	13/4	39 ± 5	295 ± 59^b
pCPA + L-dopa	12/1	45	377
pCPA + 5-HTP	13/10	34 ± 5	699 ± 115^c

[a]Drugs were administered according to the schedule reported in the section on methods. Rats were considered responding to drug treatment with serum LH values at 1800 hr were significantly higher than at 1200 hr. Blood was assayed for LH content at 1200 and 1800 hr after drug treatment. Values represent x ± SEM.
[b] $= p < 0.05$.
[c] $= p < 0.01$, when comparing values at 1200 vs. 1800 hr in the same group.

estrogen-insensitive rats tested. However, this response was dependent upon the time when 5-HTP was administered. The effectiveness of 5-HTP was maximal when it was administered at 1100 hr, 2 days after pCPA. In contrast, 5-HTP was ineffective when given at 1830 hr 1 day after pCPA and at 1100 hr 2 days after pCPA.

DISCUSSION

In this study, experimental procedures altering the positive feedback response to estrogen were evaluated for their potential to be used as tools to investigate mechanisms of reproductive senescence in rats. Exposure to constant light or to supraphysiological doses of estrogen causes changes in the LH surge resembling those accompanying advancing age. The first changes involve timing of LH release. After 2 days of continuous light exposure, the onset of phasic LH secretion is delayed and the surge becomes attenuated (Watts and Fink, 1981; Daane and Parlow, 1971;

this study), changes which closely resemble those occurring in middle-aged rats during presenescence when estrous cycles become irregular. The changes in both the model and the aged animal precede cessation of cycles and the development of constant estrous. These similarities imply a common mechanism at play and suggest that light exposure might be a useful tool for understanding how LH surge mechanisms become nonfunctional in old animals.

The second age change amenable to modeling is loss of positive feedback to estrogen. In the aging female rat, persistent growth of ovarian follicles in the absence of ovulation and corpora lutea formation produces a relatively unopposed estrogenic milieu. Since estrogen is required for expression of the neural signal for LH release in young rats, the absence of LH surges in this environment implies the development of estrogen insensitivity with advancing age. A similar loss of positive feedback in the presence of estrogen occurs when ovariectomized rats carry, for 2 or 3 weeks, subcutaneous implants of estrogen-containing capsules. The initial effect of these implants is to stimulate phasic release of LH; however, the induced LH surges do not persist indefinitely. Instead, they gradually attenuate and finally end after the capsules are in situ for about 15-20 days. Interestingly, the LH surges shift in phase with regard to the light:dark cycle in a manner resembling changes induced by constant light or age. This implies a common underlying mechanism for degeneration and ultimate loss of the LH surge in these seemingly different conditions.

Recent studies have implicated serotonin in the neural control for LH secretion (Walker, 1980; Marco and Fluckiger, 1980). Since the metabolism of this amine shows a circadian rhythm whose integrity seems to be essential for signaling the LH surge (Coen and MacKinnon, 1979), it was prudent to determine how light and age affect temporal patterns of its content and apparent turnover in the hypothalamus. In the young castrate female kept in a standard photoperiod, absolute levels of serotonin before and after pargyline treatment at 1300 hr were significantly higher than at 2200 hr, while values at 1500 and 1800 hr were intermediate between the two extremes. These temporal differences persisted when the rats received estrogen pellets, but the absolute amount of serotonin diminished at each time point. This effect was due apparently to estrogen-enhanced sensitivity of serotonin circuits which triggered negative feedback on the synthesis of the monoamine (Macon et al., 1971; Robson et al., 1954). During the early period of estrogen exposure, daily LH surges occurred. However, with increasing time after implantation of the estrogen pellets, serotonin synthesis increased at each time point, especially during the evening hours. These metabolic changes resulted in a gradual abolition of the serotonin rhythm and correlated with temporal changes in phasic secretion of LH. When estrogen sensitivity was lost and LH surges no longer occurred, serotonin content and turnover were no longer statistically different at 1300 and 2200 hr. These changes in the dynamics of serotonin metabolism are attributed to a compensatory hypersynthesis induced by prolonged estrogen exposure. Paradoxically, estrogen initially causes LH secretion, perhaps by stimulating serotonin receptors to couple the neural signal to the LH secretory apparatus.

A similar phenomenon occurs with light exposure which, unlike estrogen treatment, does not stimulate an initial negative feedback on serotonin synthesis. Instead, light exposure for several days causes hypersynthesis of serotonin aroung the clock, and thereby obliterates the serotonin circadian rhythm. The rapid development of this effect correlates with and may cause changes in the temporal pattern of LH secretion under the same environmental conditions (Watts and Fink, 1981).

These findings are particularly relevant when considering that temporal deficits in serotonin metabolism begin during middle age, when rats start showing irregular estrous cycles with altered LH surges. The day:night changes in serotonin turnover become more ambiguous with advancing age, such that the natural decline begins later and nadir values are reached later, correlating with delayed onset and attenuated levels of LH during the surge. If the steepness of the line representing day:night changes in serotonin can be translated into intensity of a neural signal, then the steeper drop would correlate with an earlier and sharper rise phase for LH secretion. On the other hand, a smaller change between 1300 and 2200 hr would represent a less significant signal for LH release.

I propose that loss of the serotonin rhythm represents actual loss of the intermittent signal for the LH surge and results in constant estrus. This idea is supported by the fact that reducing light exposure in constant estrus rats reinstates cycles (Everett, 1942) and also restores the serotonin rhythm. Furthermore, the serotonin rhythm disappears as young rats become estrogen-insensitive, but reappear 4 weeks after estrogen capsules are removed, when LH surges are again inducible by estrogen and progesterone injections.

These findings support the proposal of Brawer and Finch (Chap. 3) that estrogen, which is essential for phasic LH secretion, actually causes degeneration of the neural trigger for the LH surge. The data suggest that exposure to estrogen during the reproductive life span causes the compensatory hypersynthesis of serotonin as seen accelerated in the Legan-Karsch model, and leads to obliteration of the neural signal. The data suggest that the estrogen exposure model more closely resembles the true aging condition because loss of the serotonin rhythm occurs after homeostatic control mechanisms degenerate (e.g., prolonged negative feedback leading to changes in regulatory control). On the other hand, light exposure simply drives serotonin synthesis. producing the same endocrine effect but, in this case, the effect is reversible since damage on the control mechanism is not imposed by the treatment.

This idea is supported by the finding that constant estrous rats are unresponsive to estrogen + progesterone injections given immediately after ovariectomy, whereas the same treatment, delayed 4-5 weeks after surgery, stimulates LH surges. Correlated with the return of the positive feedback response is reemergence of the serotonin circadian rhythm in the hypothalamus, which was absent in the CE rat before and immediately after ovariectomy. However, the amplitude of the restored serotonin rhythm is reduced when compared with young rats. This difference is also correlated with a smaller LH surge in the old rat which has been ovariectomized for greater than 1 month. Further evidence that an intermittent signal for LH release is generated by the serotonin circadian rhythm derives from the fact that the most effective treatment for restoration of LH surges in the estrogen-insensitive rat was pCPA + 5-HTP. In effect, pCPA may have provided a pharmacological brake on serotonin synthesis by blocking the action of tryptophan hydroxylase. Then, the properly timed, secondary injection of 5-HTP given 2 days later circumvented the block, presumably reestablished the endogenous serotonin rhythm, and thereby provided the neural trigger for phasic LH secretion on that day.

The studies reported herein demonstrate the value of using carefully selected models for investigating mechanisms of senescence in specific animal systems. Interventive gerontology seeks to understand mechanisms of senescence, in order that prophylactic and/or therapeutic treatments may be used to prevent or reverse, respectively, the sequelae of advancing age. In order to gain this capability, we must go beyond simple observations and descriptions of anatomical and physiological changes in old animals and humans. Carefully designed experiments to accelerate or retard the aging process will transcend the limitations of descriptive studies and enhance our ability to understand those factors which actually facilitate senescent change, the onset of specific lesions of aging, and determine life span itself. Since ethical and moral restrictions prevent such experiments in humans, interventive gerontology will be built upon animal systems which can be used as appropriate models for aging in humans. This presentation describing rodent models for manipulation and analysis of the mechanisms of female reproductive system aging demonstrates the validity of that assumption.

REFERENCES

Aschheim, P. (1976). Aging in the hypothalamic-hypophyseal-ovarian axis in the rat. In *Hypothalamus, Pituitary and Aging*, A. V. Everitt and J. A. Burgess (Eds.). Charles C Thomas, Springfield, Ill., pp. 376-418.

Chazal, G., Faudon, M., Gogan, F., Hery, M., Kordon, C., and LaPlante, E. (1977). Circadian rhythm of luteinizing hormone secretion in the ovariectomized rat implanted with oestradiol. *J. Endocrinol. 75*: 251-260.

Coen, C. W., MacKinnon, P. C. B. (1979). Serotonin involvement in the control of phasic luteinizing hormone release in the rat: evidence for a critical period. *J. Endocrinol. 82*: 105-113.

Cooper, R. L., Conn, P. M., and Walker, R. F. (1980). Characterization of the LH surge in middle-aged female rats. *Biol. Reprod. 23*: 611-615.

Daane, T. A., and Parlow, A. F. (1971). Serum FSH and LH in constant light-induced persistent estrus: short-term and long-term studies. *Endocrinology 88*: 964-968.

Everett, J. W. (1942). Certain functional interrelationships between spontaneous persistent estrus, "light estrus" and short day anestrus in the albino rat. *Anat. Rec. 82*: 409.

Hery, M., LaPlante, E., and Kordon, C. (1976). Participation in serotonin in the phasic release of LH. I. Evidence from pharmacological experiments. *Endocrinology 99*: 496.

Huang, H. H., Steger, R. W., Bruni, J. F., and Meites, J. (1978). Patterns of sex steroid and gonadotropin secretion in aging female rats. *Endocrinology 103*: 1855-1859.

Legan, S. J., and Karsch, F. J. (1975). A daily signal for the LH surge in the rat. *Endocrinology 96*: 57.

Lu, J. K. H., Gilman, D. P., Meldrum, D. R., Judd, H. L., and Sawyer, C. H. (1980). Relationship between circulating estrogens and the control mechanisms by which ovarian steroids stimulate luteinizing hormone secretion in aged and young female rats. *Endocrinology 108*: 836.

Macon, J. B., Sokoloff, L., and Glowinski, J. (1971). Feedback control of rat brain 5-hydroxytryptamine synthesis. *J. Neurochem. 18*: 323-331.

Marko, M., and Fluckiger, E. (1980). Role of serotonin in the regulation of ovulation. *Neuroendocrinology 30*: 228-231.

McCormack, C. E., and Sridaran, R. (1978). Timing of ovulation in rats during exposure to continuous light: evidence for a circadian rhythm of luteinizing hormone secretion. *J. Endocrinol. 76*: 135-140.

Peng, M. T., and Huang, H. O. (1972). Aging of hypothalamic-pituitary-ovarian function in the rat. *Fertil. Steril. 23*: 635-542.

Quay, W. B. (1968). Differences in circadian rhythms in 5-hydroxytryptamine according to brain region. *Am. J. Physiol. 215*: 1448.

Robson, J. M., Trounce, J. R., and Didcock, K. A. H. (1954). Factors affecting the response of the uterus to serotonin. *J. Endocrinol. 10*: 129-132.

Steger, R. W., and Peluso, J. J. (1979). Hypothalamic-pituitary function in the old irregularly cycling rat. *Exp. Age. Res. 5*: 303-317.

Walker, R. F. (1980). Serotonin neuroleptics change patterns of preovulatory secretion of luteinizing hormone in rats. *Life Sci. 27*: 1063.

Watts, A. G., and Fink, G. (1981). Effects of short-term constant light on the proestrous luteinizing hormone surge and pituitary responsiveness in the female rat. *Neuroendocrinology 33*: 176-180.

5

Menopause: Hormones and Drug Therapy During Reproductive Senescence

Bernard A. Eskin / *The Medical College of Pennsylvania and Hospital, Philadelphia, Pennsylvania*

INTRODUCTION

Reproductive aging in women has only recently received proper attention. When life expectancy was only a few years beyond menopause, cessation of cyclic vaginal bleeding was considered as physical evidence of an aging woman. It has taken many years for this myth to be dispelled. With the advent of proper obstetrical and gynecological care, the life span of the female has lengthened to a point, in the United States, where she is expected to outlive the male. It has long been considered that the loss of reproduction is responsible for a reduction in the quality of life during these climacteric years. Because of this hypothesis, intervention with sex hormones and other related medications has been advocated. This chapter will discuss the relationship that reproductive senescence has to clinical changes and and advisability of therapeutics.

A functional reproductive system is limited to a specific period in a woman's lifetime. In 1975, E. C. Jones published evidence that longevity is not related to the length of reproductive life or activity in women (Jones, 1975). Studying various animal models, she showed that the length of reproductive years to life span is specific in most mammals, although by genetic experimentation in mice, the relative reproductive period can be changed by inbreeding. The present trend for American women shows that the span of potential fertility has increased as longevity has lengthened (Eisdorfer, 1972). This may be related to diet, health, and exercise. With longevity has come a need to improve the quality of life during the postreproductive period.

The fertile period in women has been limited, possibly because of the severe physiological strain of childbearing. We can project that a prolongation of gestational potential would considerably decrease life expectancy and present many other health hazards to the older women and their fetuses (Schneider, 1980). In contrast, in men procreation continues to an older age than women. However, the ability to perform sexually requires a continuation of male hormonal secretion which is coupled with physiological testicular activity (Fig. 1).

It is important to recognize that while the years of reproductive activity are limited, the physiological and anatomical changes before and after this era may provide many medical complaints which come to the attention of physicians who attend women. As more information becomes apparent, we recognize that reproductive senescence is not limited to the ovaries, but involves the total response of hormones secreted from the ovary, pituitary, hypothalamus, and the central nervous system. Additionally, end-organ receptor systems and target cells throughout the body are affected by reproductive aging, resulting in multidisciplinary clinical modifications.

In this chapter, I will describe briefly the insidious process of reproductive aging which occurs from the onset of puberty to the postmenopausal period. Reproductive aging causes a series of changes which are initially heralded by minor abnormalities in cyclicity and anatomy, but soon show evidence of recognizable medical changes. Some of the most distressing problems derive from the menopausal mythology about women developed over the years. In recent years, marked

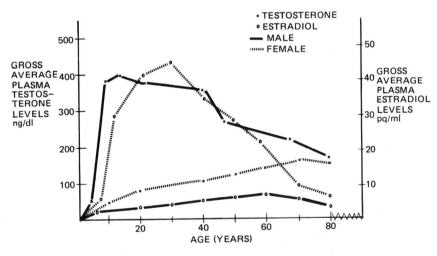

Figure 1   Plasma levels of total estrogens and testosterone in men and women according to age. (From Eskin, 1980a.)

improvement in the acceptance of many of the changes brought on by reproductive senescence has been seen. A new approach to intervention of reproductive senescence with hormones and other therapies has provided qualitative improvement in the symptomatology of the postmenopausal woman.

STAGES OF REPRODUCTION

The aging processes first appear in reproduction about the mid-20s when a mild downturn in the rate of ovulatory cycles has been observed (Collett et al., 1954). The various divisions of the reproductive epoch of women are shown in Fig. 2. These stages are described on the basis of endocrine secretions and feedback activated primarily by estrogen.

From birth to approximately 8 years of age estrogen buildup is functionally dependent on secretions resulting from ovarian maturation. Puberty (ages 8-13) evolves when a maturing hypothalamopituitary axis is adjusted to a feedback from active ovarian follicles. The onset of ovulation at menarche is the cyclic secretion of gonadotropic hormones. The active reproductive periods (ages 13-36) with an ascent (ages 13-27) and partial descent (ages 27-36) of cyclic function follow. However, the decelerating reproductive stage (ages 36-42) is characterized by cyclic adverse bleeding events as well. By 42, symptoms of perimenopause with evident estrogen deficiency predicate a decreased fertility potential and lead to the menstrual demise of menopause at 51. Postmenopausal manifestations mount with specific symptomatology when physiological reproduction is over (Fig. 2).

ESTROGEN RESPONSE DURING PHASES OF THE LIFE CYCLE OF WOMEN

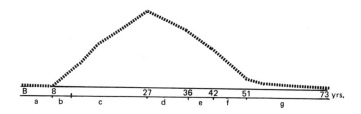

A. PREPUBERTAL

B. PUBERTY

C & D. ACTIVE REPRODUCTIVE

E. DECELERATING REPRODUCTIVE

F. PERIMENOPAUSE (PREMENOPAUSE)

G. POSTMENOPAUSE

Figure 2   Estrogen response during phases of the life cycle of women.

Prepuberty

The ovary matures during this period. Initially filled with thousands of potential ova, the number dwindles through atresia and stroma proliferate surrounding the preovular sac. The capabilities for steroid secretion increase, and estradiol (E_2) and estrone (E_1) titers are similar to those in the follicular phase (Table 1). A two-cell theory has been advanced which shows that both granulosa and theca cells are required in tandem to produce the estrogen. Estrogen intracellular receptors increase, and estrogen-effective tissues become active.

Prepuberty begins after early childhood (4 years) and features endocrine changes at the level of the hypothalamopituitary axis. Gonadotropic (peptide) hormones are secreted due to the feedback mechanism of the estrogens, primarily from the ovary to the pituitary and hypothalamus. Characteristically, an increased negative feedback threshhold in the hypothalamopituitary area occurs, so that even a small amount of estrogen prevents cyclic gonadotropin release of luteinizing hormone (LH) and follicular-stimulating hormone (FSH). Maturation of the higher centers results in both negative and positive feedback mechanisms required for ovulation (Fig. 3), which are appropriate to the response later seen in the menopause. The onset of ovulation is the sum of growth and development of both the ovary and the hypothalamopituitary axis (Boyar et al., 1972; Winter and Faiman, 1979).

Reproduction

With ovarian secretion of estrogens, the remarkably efficient intracellular receptor system of the secondary sexual tissues and central nervous system responds. After the menarche, the hypothalamopituitary-ovarian axis fully matures and monthly ovulatory cycles provide gestational opportunities. Hormonal activity is not limited only to the control of menses but for cyclic changes which may be seen in the central nervous system, breast tissues, skin, and probably in the various parts of the

Table 1 Serum Levels of Ovarian Steroids in Physiological Condition (pg/ml)

	Estrone (E_1)	Estradiol (E_2)	Estriol (E_3)	Progesterone
Normal women				
Follicular phase	50	60	–	50
Midcycle	200	400	150	–
Luteal phase	140	250	120	12,000
Postmenopausal	30	10	7	5
Pregnancy (third month)	1100	2600	970	35,000
Normal men	60	20	10	120

Source: Deghenghi (1980).

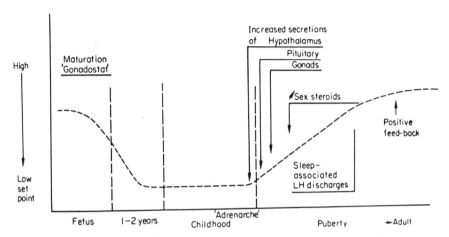

Figure 3 Diagram of current concepts of the regulatory factors in gonadal function divided into the fetal, perinatal, pubertal, and adult stages of sexual development. (From Forest et al., 1976.)

body where there may be estrogen receptors. The cycle becomes more consistent during the late teens and early 20s, reaching an apex about ages 26-28, at which time ovulation is most predictable.

Decelerating Reproduction

Irregularity of menses is the first symptom recognized as a result of early aging of the ovary which causes aberrations in the hypothalamopituitary-ovarian axis because of a relative decline in estrogen secretion.

Irregularities of the menstrual cycle that occur include a range of clinical dysfunctional bleeding from amenorrhea to menorrhagia. These abnormalities become sufficiently disturbing that many diagnostic minor surgical procedures are done. Aging of oocytes is considered the prime cause of many genetic abnormalities in pregnancies in this age group. Serum estrogen levels alone cannot account for this reduced response, but the combination of several dynamic endocrine factors seems to be included. One endocrine effect is that a weaker estrogen may be produced such as estrone. Studies have shown that peripheral conversion of androstenedione to estrone increases in this age group and that the estrone:estradiol ratio increases (Hemsell et al., 1974). Whereas the acceleration of intermediate androgens is not as marked as that seen in the perimenopause or postmenopausal era, the change is significant, and peripheral conversion of these steroids becomes meaningful (Fig. 4).

Data are accruing that show that during decelerating reproduction the aging process is not only related to ovarian secretions but also the higher centers and end-organ receptor systems. Follicular number and size decrease subsequently as

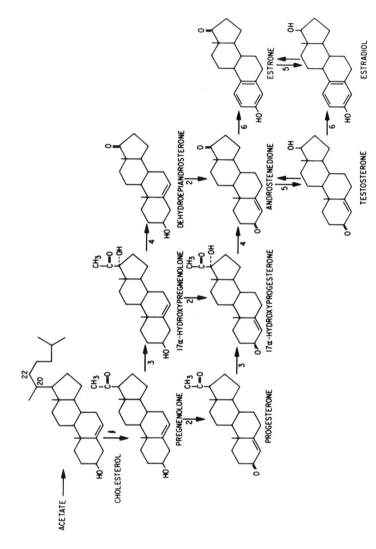

Figure 4 Steroid biosynthetic pathways. The following enzymes are required where indicated: (1) 20-hydroxylase, 22-hydroxylase, and 20,22-desmolase; (2) 3β-ol-dehydrogenase and Δ^4 Δ^5-isomerase; (3) 17-α-hydroxylase; (4) 17,20-desmolase; (5) 17-β-ol-dehydrogenase; (6) aromatizing enzyme system. (From Goebelsmann, 1979.)

PHYSIOLOGY OF THE AGING OVARY

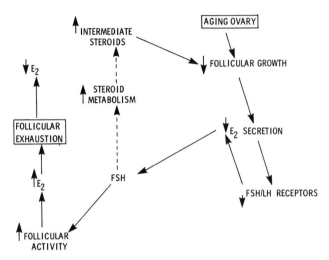

Figure 5 Physiology of the aging ovary. Endocrine responses leading to follicular exhaustion.

less estrogen is secreted (Fig. 5), which could be related to gonadotropin receptor aging defects. Reduced estrogen has been shown to cause both a decrease in available estrogen and gonadotropin receptors, with curtailed negative feedback to the pituitary as the prime result (Chan and O'Malley, 1976; Channing and Tsafriri, 1977). Following the sequence of events outlined in Fig. 5, follicle-stimulating hormone (FSH) increases follicular activity, and estrogen is released until exhaustion of the follicle occurs. The increased FSH can increase secretions of intermediate steroids which diminish follicular growth even further.

There are indications that subtle changes in hormone receptors may cause adverse tissue reactions to therapy (Roth and Adelman, 1975). The controversy of whether surgery or persistent hormonal treatment is best remains. Recent popularity of laparoscopic or minilap bilateral tubal ligation for sterilization has increased the number of women leaving the birth control pill and presumably the protection it provided in regulating vaginal bleeding.

Perimenopause

During the perimenopause (ages 42-51) the deceleration of endocrine cyclicity (Fig. 5) leads towards final ovarian failure at the menopause. The perimenopause is a period of decline in the efficiency of ovum growth and granulosa-thecal cell development. The aging process has reduced the effectiveness of follicular receptor action to the gonadotropins with resulting minimal estrogen release. Since estrogen

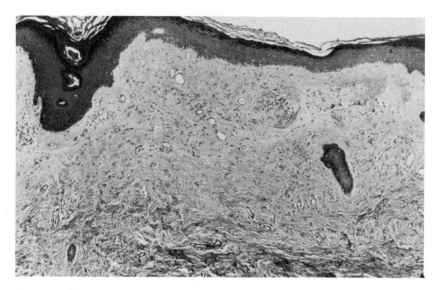

Figure 6 Microphotograph of perivulvar atrophy. There is an increase in the density and thickness of dermal collagen. Skin appendages are absent. Hematoxylin and eosin, reduced from X 60. (From Krouse, 1980.)

is required for FSH and LH receptor response this results in double jeopardy to the sequence (Sherman and Korenman, 1975; Aksel and Jones, 1975). Additionally, aging may reduce the responsiveness of the granulosa-theca estrogen pathway.

Estrogen secretion is the result of a complex series of well-orchestrated events through the androgens moderated by enzymes. When the two-cell pathway is impaired and aromatization to estrogens does not occur, many intermediate products are secreted, and these have biological responses which can be undesirable (Fig. 6). When ovulation decreases, more ovarian stroma forms from atresia, and from this precursors of the estrogens are formed. Most prominent are dihydroepiandrosterone (DHEA) and androstenedione (A_4). These androgenic substances can cause hirsutism or mild virilization.

Androgens can be converted in several extragonadal tissues to form both estrogens, mostly estrone (E_1), or testosterone. The secretions by the perimenopausal woman begin to favor estrone (E_1) over estradiol (E_2) (Table 1), and this reversal of the $E_2:E_1$ ratio has been viewed as a cause of malignancies related to sex hormones of the breast and endometrium. Intermediate metabolites may also act on both the ovary and the hypothalamopituitary axis reducing feedback effectiveness (Aksel and Jones, 1975; Jones, 1980).

During perimenopause only occasional regular ovulatory cycles are seen leading to estrogen withdrawal with no progesterone. Since estrogen increases its own receptors, and progesterone decreases both the number and effectiveness of estrogen receptors, regular ovulatory menses may be required for estrogen receptor homeostasis (Chan and O'Malley, 1976). The length of the reproductive era differs in individuals; perhaps the receptors have different life spans or responsiveness to aging since it has been seen that estrogen receptors become less efficient as the aging process continues. While animal research has shown this, human studies are still lacking (Roth, 1978).

Postmenopause

When clinical ovarian exhaustion does occur (Fig. 5), a marked rebound elevation of gonadotropin begins with the hypothalamopituitary axis. Gonadotropins are elevated significantly with FSH usually higher than LH due to the slower clearance of FSH from the circulation (Mattingly and Huang, 1969). An excellent review of these changes has been published by Judd (1980).

The androgens normally are secreted from both the ovaries and adrenal during premenopause. In the postmenopause, androstenedione, secreted primarily by the adrenal, has 20% of its secretion from the ovary (Judd et al., 1974). The increased secretion from the ovary may be due to increased gonadotropin. Testosterone is lower, but is higher than that found in young women whose ovaries have been removed (Judd et al., 1974; Judd et al., 1974). Both dihydroepiandrosterone and its sulfate initially are lower, then decelerate to the onset of the adrenopause where a decrease in all adrenal androgens is seen with aging (Abraham and Maroulis, 1975). Thus, the androgens have: (1) a marked reduction in production by the ovary, particularly androstenedione; (2) a continued secretion by the ovary, particularly of testosterone; and (3) a reduced adrenal secretion, particularly dihydroepiandrosterone and its sulfate.

Estrogen is still secreted, but as a result of adrenal androgen secretion with peripheral conversion to estrone and estradiol (Table 1), estrone is favored in the postmenopausal woman (Siiteri and MacDonald, 1973). Evident changes due to reduced estrogen occur in tissues which are most estrogen-responsive such as the vulva, vagina, periurethra, perineum, breasts, hair, and skin. Thus, in this postmenopause period the estrogen deficiency is the result of the decline of the reproductive endocrine system over many years. The clinical findings associated with defective reproductive hormone secretions will be described.

CLINICAL ASPECTS OF REPRODUCTIVE SENESCENCE

During the various stages of reproductive life, aging appears to change steroid secretions and responses quantitatively. Shifts in metabolism by various tissues due to decreasing hormonal stimuli result in clinical symptoms. Some of these are minor and can be adjusted by social or psychological action by the woman. However, at menopause, often the problems become more complex and make coping more difficult.

Certain clinical changes have become associated with reproductive senescence, characterized by estrogen deficiency and related to impaired hormone metabolism (Table 2). It is difficult to decide whether these problems are due to inadequate estrogen or are associated with aging (Eskin, 1980a). Often, in our society, the tactful physician does not directly implicate advancing age, but hints that reproduction is over and that replacement of sex hormones may efficiently replace the losses.

Atrophy of the Perineum, Vagina, and Periurethral Area

While reduced function of all estrogen-responsive tissues occurs, the first symptoms easily recognized by the patient seem to be the loss of elasticity and turgor of the perineum, vagina, and urethral meatus (Fig. 6). When estrogen depletion occurs, end-organ tissue atrophy must eventually result, since these cells are most heavily laden with estrogen receptors. The changes noted in the microphotograph show a thickening of the subdermal tissues; fatty layers are lost and turgor is decreased.

There are many physical problems due to dryness of the vagina and vulva, such as epithelial friability leading to bleeding, infection, or inflammation. Additionally, atrophic vulvovaginitis can bring about discomfort during intercourse since it interferes with lubrication and sexual response.

Dryness near the urethral meatus may cause serious problems of an inflammatory and infectious nature which are localized initially but later escalate into the urinary tract. The loss of turgor of periurethral tissues makes urination difficult, and persistent irritation often causes frequency. Additionally, hyperdystrophy of the periurethral area and urethrovesicle support structures may result in cystic conditions and stress incontinence.

Vasomotor Instability (Hot Flushes)

The presence of vasculomotor flushes due to the senescence of the reproductive system has been described over the centuries. It has been considered as a common

Table 2   Disorders Related to Reproductive Senescence

Directly
  Atrophic vulvovaginitis
  Urethral syndrome
Indirectly
  Hot flushes
  Osteoporosis
  Skin, hair, and breast changes
Possible
  Psychosexual problems
  Psychological conditions and trauma
  Atherosclerotic heart disease

condition occurring in postmenopausal women and is accompanied by disturbing nocturnal sweats and a host of other related changes. Associated with these are perspiration over the chest, decreased peripheral vascular tone, and often intense feeling of heat over the face.

Vasomotor flushes have been established as due to erratic changes in the dilation of microscopic peripheral blood vessels of the skin (Meldrum et al., 1979). The symptom is caused by pulsatile bursts of LH and FSH secretion that occur every 1-2 hr, a frequency similar to that seen in the follicular phase of perimenopausal women (Meldrum et al., 1980). The increased gonadotropin release from the pituitary gland is the result of the lack of estrogen feedback on the hypothalamopituitary system. First, only FSH elevates, but later, in postmenopause, both FSH and LH increase to a level 5-10 times that of the normal reproductive female, although FSH remains higher than LH. As in young women, the levels of FSH-LH are not steady but show random oscillations. Although the frequency is similar, the amplitude is much greater (Fig. 7). This increase in amplitude is thought to be secondary to increased release of the hypothalamic hormone gonadotropin-releasing hormone (GnRH). Postmenopausal women have increased urinary GnRH levels which seem to obviate this increased activity from the hypothalamus.

Studies have also shown that the heat release mechanisms which are responsible for the blood vessel responses are directed within the hypothalamus and affected by GnRH pulses. These hot flushes, as measured by a skin temperature increase, are accompanied by a pulsatile release of LH, showing that these surges of LH may be resultant from central nervous system estrogen action (Meldrum et al., 1979). There is some evidence that nocturnal flushes may be produced by emo-

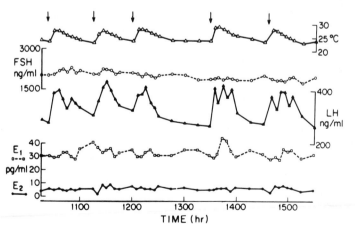

Figure 7 Serial measurements of finger temperature and serum FSH, LH, E_1, and E_2 in an individual subject. Arrows mark the onset of the temperature rise. (From Meldrum et al., 1980.)

tions from rapid eye movement (REM) sleep dreams (Schiff et al., 1979). Stimuli which may provoke these responses include hot weather, exercise, overwork, mental stress, alcohol, caffeine, and spicy foods. The variability of this symptom among women remains somewhat enigmatic. Whether this is a question of receptor function, the action of monoamine effects directly on blood vessels, or a direct central autonomic nervous system response is still unknown.

Osteoporosis

Controversy continues concerning the etiology of osteoporosis. Both reproductive senescence with estrogen depletion and aging of the various organs are involved in bone metabolism (Fig. 8).

There is a long historical relationship for osteoporosis as coincident with the menopause. Osteoporosis is predominantly a disease found in women. Maximum bone mass occurs at approximately 27 years of age, a time in women when both ovarian function and weight and estrogen secretion reach their maximum. Several well-documented studies utilizing photon absorptiometry show the relationship between ovarian function and skeletal homeostasis. From these data sex steroids have been interpolated to have responsibility for prophylaxis of postmenopausal bone loss (Lindsay et al., 1978; Marshall et al., 1977). Recent publications have provided sound evidence of the responsibility of estrogen in this disease (Marshall et al., 1977; Milhaud et al., 1978; Meema and Meema, 1976). These have included prospective data on fractures, estrogen-induced maintenance of bone density, and sex differences in fracture incidence.

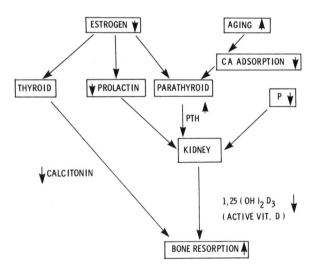

Figure 8 The pathway of osteoporosis in estrogen-deficient women.

Osteoporosis is usually defined as insufficient, but normally calcified bone mass, and is the most common of metabolic bone disease. It results from a number of different processes, the most common of which are: estrogen deficiency due to menopause or bilateral oophorectomy, immobilization, and increased secretion of adrenal steroids. Bone is being remodeled constantly, and bone formation and bone resorption are coupled and homeostatically balanced. In menopause there is a sharp increase in the bone resorption rate that can be prevented by a small dose of estrogen (Meema and Meema, 1976).

The diagnosis of osteoporosis is complex and requires clinical, chemical, and radiological evaluations. Since menopausal osteoporosis mimics a large number of similar conditions, more than radiographic diagnosis is required. Analyses in the laboratory show serum calcium, phosphate, alkaline phosphatase, and electrophoretic protein pattern to be within normal limits. The fact that bone decalcification occurs in untreated gonadal dysgenesis (Turner's syndrome) and in the early and severe osteoporosis seen in women following oophorectomy in the absence of estrogen substitutes has, without a question, placed osteoporosis as one of the evident results of postmenopausal estrogen loss.

The physiological antagonism between parathyroid hormone (PTH) and estrogen was reported as early as 1941. The hypercalcemic action of PTH is opposed by the hypocalcemic action of estrogen. Since that time, research has emphasized this antagonism, both in vivo and in vitro, and has attributed postmenopausal osteoporosis to an increase in bone receptors to PTH, by virtue of the disappearance of the antagonistic hormone. No estrogen receptors have been found in bone. Estrogens may act by virtue of opposing the action of growth hormone (GH) on the bones; hence, the frequent finding of hypophosphatemia in estrogen-deficiency states. It is also possible that estrogens may act by a third mechanism, the stimulatory effect of estrogen on the secretion of thyroid calcitonin (Heaney et al., 1978; Meema et al., 1975).

Several associated factors must be recognized as adding to the problem (Fig. 8). These include inadequate diet, intestinal absorption of calcium or of vitamin D, inadequate physical activity, spontaneous or iatrogenic excess of thyroxin, or drug excess of cortisol. The disease affects most frequently those women who are slight, slender, and have small muscle mass with sedentary lives. Bone formation remains at a normal level, but the rate of bone resorption increases so that the bone density loss renders the skeleton incapable of supporting normal weight and stress. The bone diameter remains the same since the loss is at the endosteal surface of bone and within the cortical and intracortical bone.

It can thus be seen that there are many suggested etiologies for osteoporosis (Fig. 8). All seem to be modified by the presence or absence of estrogen and the action of estrogen in this relatively ubiquitous atmosphere for calcium-phosphorus homeostasis. Because of these results, most authors feel that estrogen therapy is indicated. However, other treatments have been described which are inevitably involved in the series of events that lead to these changes. In all cases, once osteoporosis has developed there is no known therapy for cure, and the bone density remains at the level when therapy was begun (Meema and Meema, 1976; Meema et al., 1975; Gordon and Vaughan, 1980).

Skin, Hair, and Breast Changes

There is relatively sparse literature on integumentary changes due to reproductive senescence, probably due to the general considerations that aging is more likely the primary effector. Nevertheless, the cosmetic industry has for many years maintained that hormonal loss is impressive and countless products for skin and hair improvement have been generated that contain hormonal substances.

Skin and hair follicles contain receptors for both estrogen and androgen steroids. These receptors appear to be most abundant in the perineal area and specific peripheral sites, particularly where secretory activity is abundant. Androgens are seen in hair follicles and, as such, are important to growth, depending on the area of the body. In women, head and pubic hair are under androgen control (Winter and Faiman, 1979). High titers of androgen result in undesirable hair growth on the chest, face, and body. Thus, when unopposed androgen occurs later in the postmenopause, cosmetically unpleasant hair growth may be seen. Increased androgens, especially as testosterone, cause head hair loss or reduction. The critical use of sex steroids for hair control has been questioned.

Breast tissue is activated by estrogen and progesterone causing ductal growth and acinar formation, respectively. In ovulating women biphasic development occurs monthly, often leading to cystic changes. This effect can be produced with moderately large doses of pharmacological hormones, but seems to decrease in effect with aging, which may be a result of receptor insensitivity or modified tissue atrophy. Breast cancer is increased postmenopausally but shows a decrease in mortality.

Psychosexual Problems

Sexual disturbances have been shown to vary individually with aging, although when physical complaints accompany dysfunction, they may be related to reproductive senescence. In the present aging population, which appears to be less tainted with myths, there is a decrease in repression with resultant coital pleasure. While implications of a geriatric sexual revolution are somewhat overstated, sexual activity evidently remains plateaued and adequate.

The loss of turgor in the tissues of the vulvovaginal region is probably the major cause of perimenopausal dyspareunia. This, in turn, can cause sexual dysfunction since intercourse is uncomfortable, adding difficulty to orgasmic response. Specific physiological problems are: increased vaginal diapedesis of lubricating fluid required for sexual intercourse, decreased introital hypertrophy during the plateau and orgasmic stages of sexual responses, and decreased muscular strength and elasticity of the vagina. These changes result in looseness of the vagina which has been described as friction loss by some. Childbirth and aging are generally most responsible for these physical changes.

In the event of a surgical menopause, often the patient is not aware of the psychosexual response that may occur postoperatively. After a bilateral oophorectomy, many physicians feel that if estrogen therapy is given, replacement of ovarian hormones has been effected and no sexual difficulty should be expected afterwards. Actually, these women may have decreased sexual interest and intensity of response. Under most circumstances, most gynecologists attribute this failure to psychological factors, which is part of a mythology which has proliferated over the years. Whereas there is no argument that psychologically disturbed individuals, either before or after reproductive senescence, may have decreased sexual function, specific dysfunctions related to the ovarian deficiencies are seen (Persky et al., 1976).

One of the reasons for the poor sexual response to replacement estrogen is the fact that the normal ovary secretes appreciable amounts of intermediate androgens, such as testosterone and androstenedione, which are converted peripherally to testosterone (Judd, 1980; Judd et al., 1974). It is the normal testosterone that seems to be important in sexual function, probably by sensitizing the clitoris and acting at the hypothalamic area in influencing the sexual drive (Lloyd, 1963; Weisz and Gibbs, 1974). Removal of this androgen causes a decrease in sexual interest and, in general, there is a decreased response to sexual stimulation which is not completely alleviated by the use of pharmacological estrogen products (Eskin and Shah, 1981a).

There is evidence that adrenal outflow of steroids provides a certain amount of intermediate androgens (Judd, 1980; Abraham and Maroulis, 1975). These androgens, however, are primarily androstenedione and dihydroepiandrosterone. The capability of conversion to testosterone is still present, but the amount converted is remarkably reduced. The utilization of androgens with the estrogen substances in patients who have a reduced sexual drive following menopause has been suggested (Greenblatt and Torpin, 1940; Greenblatt et al., 1950). Sexual drive is tied to the feeling of well-being as well. Since the postmenopausal woman may have atrophic changes in her secondary sexual characteristics which may make sexuality difficult, there are peripheral factors that play a role in maintaining a normal sex life (Lloyd, 1980).

Psychological Conditions and Trauma

While much has been written about postmenopausal depression, there have been no mechanisms cited or psychological testing documented. Studies done in geriatric centers primed for individuals in the postmenopausal group showed a marked increase in depression, often defined as involutional (Vanhulle and Demol, 1976; Alyward, 1973). Much of the work has remained anecdotal in nature, and recent evaluations of geriatric psychological testing have begun to show a pattern which may be helped by physical and nutritional treatment.

It has been usual to describe many of the changes noted in geriatric women as being caused by the pathophysiology of the postmenopause rather than as an aging problem, due to involutional trends. This would seem natural since reproductive senescence temporally correlates with aging. On the other hand, several specific organic diseases present in aging individuals are defined as markedly degenerating disease. Only under a few circumstances can the psychological problems of the aged be adequately treated by reproductive hormone replacement (Vanhulle and Demol, 1976).

Attitudinal responses have been studied by several groups as they relate to menopause. There was a great variation in attitudes and experiences in women who were postmenopausal (Winokur, 1973; Campbell, 1976). Most of the findings show the disparity between widely held cultural beliefs and the reality of the menopausal experience. It was through these particular attitudinal issues that the myths of menopause were cultivated, maintained, and promulgated. Most women have ambivalence, uncertainty, and confusion about the menopause, and it is through these attitudes that the psychological trends that have become a part of the mythology are maintained (Thompson, 1977; Wenderlein, 1980).

Atherosclerotic Heart Disease

Literature during the 1950s indicated that estrogen or progesterone were protective for women against atherosclerotic heart disease. In a large series of studies, men were treated with estrogen for several years to evaluate the protective nature of these hormones. Early responses were promising, but later the effect was diminished (Editorial, 1977).

Epidemiological data derived from large female populations confirmed a decreased risk of cardiovascular disease in the premenopausal woman as compared with postmenopause. The Framingham studies showed the probability of developing a cardiovascular problem by age 60 to be 10.1% for women as compared with 27.5% in men, a significant difference. In the age group up to 54 years, menopause, either surgical or natural, increases the risk of coronary heart disease by a factor of 2.7 (Kannel et al., 1976; Gordon et al., 1978).

In terms of generally accepted atherosclerotic risk factors, estrogens seem to do all the things that might worsen the condition. These have been described as elevation of triglycerides, glucose intolerance, increased blood pressure, and increased coagulability of blood. Thus, the beneficial factors have not yet been identified.

INTERVENTIONS IN REPRODUCTIVE SENESCENCE

The earlier sections of this chapter described the physiology and clinical characteristics of reproductive senescence. The prevalent pharmacological interventions into the aging process will be described.

Hormone Replacement Therapies

Considering gestation as the consummate function, the actual length of reproductive life is shorter than menstrual response because ovulation may not occur even though there are bleeding episodes. However, it is apparent that there is a gradual deterioration of the reproductive system and the endocrine backup that controls it. During the stages from reproductive apex to postmenopause, hormonal programs have evolved designed to regulate cycles and even produce ovulation in those individuals who desire it. These interventions are replacement treatment for the depleting endocrine secretions and result in end-organ responses in this curtailed biological system.

Aging appears to affect end-organs through receptor systems as well, for often when replacement is given, the response is not as effective as it was during the temporal reproductive era (Eskin, 1980a). Estrogen replacement given to young women who have had their ovaries surgically removed has a better response than when estrogen therapy is given to women who have gone through physiological menopause.

Estrogen

Replacement estrogen therapy is effective for vascular motor instability, perineal and vaginal atrophism, urethral syndrome, and osteoporosis (Judd et al., 1981; Eskin, 1978). Estrogens, as other steroids, act on the target cell by entering through the cell membrane and combining with a specific protein receptor in the cytoplasm. Through a series of intracellular steps the hormone-receptor complex enters the genome, combines with DNA, and produces messenger RNA (mRNA). Translocated from the nucleus, mRNA returns to the cytosol and enters the ribosome organelles where proteins are synthesized for growth and development (Fig. 9) (Chan and O'Malley, 1976).

The effectiveness of the estrogen depends on the hormone product used, further modified by the specific receptor at the end-organ (Bayward et al., 1978). Estrogens used for treatment differ in specific action on the cells, the efficiency of action varying also according to binding affinity within the cell cytoplasm. The level of response seems to be related to the internal structure responsible for recognition and binding affinity. A prominent consideration appears to be that estrogens respond according to retention time in the nucleus of the estrogen-receptor complex. Potent receptors also promote cytoplasmic resynthesis and replenishment of receptors following the depletion involved in the translocation mechanism to the nucleus (Table 3).

Research evidence accumulated shows that other steroid receptor systems are diminished or modified by aging (Roth and Adelman, 1975; Roth, 1978, 1979; Eskin, 1977). Our studies have shown indirect evidence of aging through modifications of intracellular iodine metabolic pathways in breast tissues (Eskin et al., 1979; Krouse et al., 1979). Iodine pathways are qualitatively associated with estrogen

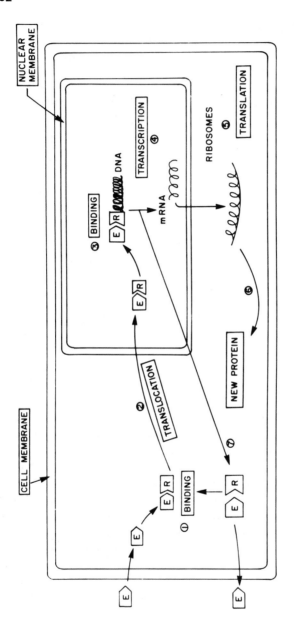

ESTRADIOL RECEPTOR SYSTEM

E = ESTRADIOL
R = RECEPTOR PROTEIN (CYTOSOL)

Figure 9 The mechanism of estradiol receptor activity within the target cell. Description within the text. (From Eskin, 1980a.)

Table 3 Determinants of Estrogen Receptor Response

1. Levels of receptors in target cells
2. Amount of estrogen available
3. Interaction of other steroids
4. How long steroid-receptor complex remains in nucleus
5. Level of dissociation of receptor after nuclear action

protein receptor (Eskin et al., 1977). Roth has indicated a number of mechanisms by which aberrations to the end-organ steroid receptor response could occur (Fig. 10). Pathways are lost and/or distorted in the receptor system causing abnormalities ranging from dysfunction to end-organ deformities to cancer (Roth, 1978, 1979; Nelson et al., 1976).

Estrogen therapy for aging should be used only in relation to those symptoms that are perceived to be the result of reproductive loss. The early changes, which also can be aging-related, should be considered for intervention by hormones. At 27, a woman reaches the peak of reproductive potential and from then on biological aging is a factor and the reproductive system begins its decline. This may be due to the sensitivity of this system and its time-limited status.

Atrophism: The ability of estrogen to improve atrophic changes of the vagina and vulva and to alleviate the urethral syndrome symptoms is limited by the level of receptor function in these tissues. Estrogen therapy depends on the response of the steroid in the target cells themselves (Eskin, 1978). If the receptors are effective, the activity is appropriate; if changes have been made by aging, the clinical result is modified. Thus, estrogens may improve the turgor of such tissues as skin and the quantity of hair follicles as long as the receptor system is active. Generally, the measurement of degree of response is done by cytohormonal diagnosis. The dose required to change the vaginal mitotic index levels to predominantly superficial cells (estrogenic) is low (Sturdec et al., 1978).

Mode of estrogen treatment remains controversial, particularly concerning oral therapy versus direct vulvovaginal application. Whereas consensus has shown that oral treatment is most effective (Jones, 1975), recent studies continue to appear advocating local treatment as an alternative with less potential for endometrial adenocarcinoma (Deutsch et al., 1981). Other techniques such as capsule implantation have gained popularity since they require attention less regularly (2 months to 1 year). Intramuscular injections with both short- and long-acting estrogens are used weekly or monthly depending on the severity of symptoms (Table 4).

Menstrual abnormalities: Manifestations of these changes in early aging are seen by menstrual abnormalities clinically represented by unpredictable or irregular bleeding episodes. This would indicate that the response in the endometrial end-organ is improper, and therefore, the aim of treatment is to provide adequate hormonal replacement to reconstruct tissue framework capable of normal endometrial

Table 4 Commercially Available Ovarian Hormone Therapies in the United States

Generic name	Trade name	Type of preparation
Estrogens		
17-β estradiol	Progynon pellets	Implantation pellets
	Progynon injection	Injectable suspension
	*	Vaginal suppositories
	Estrace	Oral tablets
	*	Percutaneous gel
Estradiol cypionate	E-cypionate	Injectable
Estradiol valerate	Menaval-10	Injectable
Estriol	Hormonin	Oral tablets
Estrogen, conjugated	*	Aqueous and oil injectable
	Premarin	Oral tablets
	Premarin Vaginal Cream	Vaginal cream
Estrogen, conjugated (equine)	*	Oral tablets
Estrogen, esterified	Estratab	Oral tablets
	Evex	Oral tablets
Estrone	Ogen	Oral tablets
Progesterones		
Dydrogesterone	Duphaston	Oral tablets
Progesterone USP	*	Injectable in oil or water
Progesterone caproate	Delalutin	Injectable
Medroxyprogesterone acetate	Amen	Oral tablets
	Provera	Oral tablets
	Depoprovera	Long-acting injectable
Megestrol acetate	Megace	Oral tablets
Norethindrone	Norlutin	Oral tablets
Norethindrone acetate	Norlutate	Oral tablets
	Aygestin	Oral tablets

*Generic only.

growth. Generally, other hormonal factors, such as hypothalamic or pituitary secretions, are overlooked, unless the desired outcome is ovulation.

The most common therapy is estrogen enhancement of the proliferative phase with the assumption that an inadequate secretion of estrogen from an underactive ovary has taken place. The dose of estrogen given is small and sustained from menses to midcycle. Estrogen, as was noted, acts not only on the feedback hypothalamopituitary axis but also directly on the ovary to bring about growth and development of the follicles (Fig. 5). The addition of estrogen in a cyclic fashion in low doses to the woman may bring about normal ovulatory changes. If this is unsuccessful, cyclic treatment with both estrogen and progesterone provide nor-

CONTROL BY HORMONES AND/OR OTHER BIOCHEMICAL AGENTS

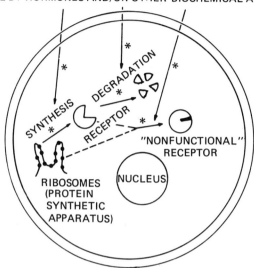

Figure 10 Theoretical positions where hormones or other biochemical agents could control receptor action.* Possible alterations during aging as described in text. (From Roth, 1978.)

mal bleeding episodes and, after several months, may prime regular cyclic responses, usually temporarily, in the individual.

During late reproduction, 36-42, more anovulatory irregular bleeding generally is reported. There are skipped cycles and, because of bleeding episodes, in many cases a series of minor surgical procedures, such as dilatation and curettage (D and C) of the uterus or endometrial biopsies in fear of endometrial cancer are performed. Estrogen therapy is aimed at regulation and is essentially the same as described in the postpeak period. In the late reproductive stage, anatomical diagnoses (i.e., endometrial cancer, myomata, adenomyosis, and so forth) must be ruled out before therapy for irregularity is used. Since 1970, many women have elected bilateral fallopian tubal ligations rather than barrier or steroid contraception, and hence, the various conditions caused by reproductive aging are manifest. Earlier consideration that the sterilization techniques were responsible for menstrual irregularities has been shown to be unfounded.

In the perimenopausal women, the problems seen in the late reproductive phase continue. While reproduction occurs in this age group, it is unusual and the maintenance of a pregnancy is difficult and occasionally hazardous. Most of the medications for dysfunctional vaginal bleeding employed are estrogen and cyclic estrogen and progesterone which are aimed at regulating uterine bleeding and preventing abnormal bleeding. The importance of the support for the functional layers of the endometrium, spongeosa, and compacta continues to be uppermost.

Temperature instability: Vasomotor instability, evident by "hot flashes," first becomes apparent in the perimenopause when the hypothalamopituitary axis starts to compensate by increasing gonadotropin secretions. It is difficult to determine what therapy should be used to treat a women who is having flushes but who has regular menstrual periods. Nevertheless, if the flushes are disturbing to her, small doses of estrogen during the early part of the cycle are given.

The postmenopausal period immediately starts after cessation of bleeding with enhancement of flushes and other symptoms due to the continuation of reproductive aging. Flushes are greatest at the time of menopause, and the pathophysiological cause, described earlier, is further augmented by the response as an autonomic heat dysfunction. Therapy with estrogen is most effective since it reduces the hypothalamic response and output.

Osteoporosis: Estrogen therapy for osteoporosis is required for the normal homeostatic responses of bone metabolism. The dosage required to decrease the calcium:creatinine ratio is 0.3 mg of conjugated estrogens or equivalent doses of estradiol (Table 4). The estrogen receptor system does not appear to be important to the formation of osteoporosis since no estrogen receptors are seen in bone. The mechanism by which estrogen may act is still controversial. It may be directly on the thyroid gland causing calcitonin to be released, or it may be an intermediate in calcium-phosphorus regulation (Fig. 8).

A growing acceptance of treatment for mild hypoestrinism is seen, particularly when vascular changes or reproductive end-organ responses appear. Osteoporosis is more likely to occur in women who show early estrogen-reduction symptoms, and estrogen therapy is more effective as a preventive measure than as a palliative. Since the dose of estrogen required in the perimenopause is less, the side effects appear to be reduced (Meema and Meema, 1976; Lindsay et al., 1976).

Other suggested therapies are less direct, but may be effective. Some believe that vitamin D responds through hydroxylation within the cell binding receptor, acting on intestinal absorption and peripheral bone activity by Ca:P action (Fig. 8). After menopause, estrogen decreases, parathyroid hormone increases, renal conversion to the active form of vitamin D, $1,25(OH)_2D_3$, decreases, calcium absorption from the intestines decreases, and bone resorption dramatically increases (Gordon and Vaughan, 1980).

Additionally, in light of these findings several advocates of calcium therapy have presented the need to maintain the calcium level. Those advocating exercise show that highly active individuals seldom suffer from osteoporosis; nevertheless, obese women, who probably metabolize much of their intermediate steroids to estrogen, are spared.

Progesterone

While progesterone has been described by some investigators as a primary therapy for hot flushes and atrophism, its use for these symptoms remains controversial

(Bullock et al., 1975). Progesterone level in the serum of postmenopausal women is low (Table 1), and there does not appear to be any physiological reason for its presence.

Cyclic progesterone (or progestin) used at least every other month has become accepted therapy for estrogen-treated women. This is particularly true when the uterus is still present. Progesterone treatment in postmenopausal women is advised for more extensive reasons than merely maintaining the endometrial tissue compactness. There is evidence that unopposed estrogen is responsible for changing endometrial progression from cystic hyperplasia to adenomatous hyperplasia (Judd et al., 1981). Progesterone serves both on the endometrium and related hormone-dependent tissues to prevent this overactivity of unopposed estrogen. The various pharmacological progesterone products used are listed in Table 4.

There has been a good deal of discussion concerning the hazards of certain progesterone therapies. Prominent among them is the consideration, as recently described, which shows that certain types, used cyclically, would lower high-density lipoprotein (HDL) cholesterol in postmenopausal women (Hirvonen et al., 1981). These investigators believe that certain 19-nortestosterone derivatives used as progestins have both androgenic and antiestrogenic properties which cause the decrease in HDL. Since an increase in HDL cholesterol presumably decreases the risk of atherosclerosis, consideration of the drug employed is critical. Nevertheless, there are many advocates of progestins (19-nortestosterone derivatives). The latter have been considered more effective since they cause less withdrawal bleeding and have an atrophying effect on the endometrium, a status which may be more desirable in hyperplasia (Gambrell et al., 1979). Employing these steroids, the endometrial support is maintained and breakdown is orderly. Progesterone decreases estrogen receptor proliferation which occurs when estrogen is present and reduces estrogen response to estrogen receptor protein. Cyclic therapy with progesterone may be effective, therefore, in maintaining a normal sequence of sex steroids in the body and may be responsible for a more homeostatic condition in all those tissues that respond to sex steroids in the female.

It is recommended that in conditions where the endometrium is read histologically as nonneoplastic atypical or adenomatous hyperplasia, progesterone or progestin therapy be used for 2-3 months cyclically. At the end of that time reevaluation should be done to determine the results. Genetic carcinomatous growth and development in the endometrium would not be affected by this therapy. Persistent pathohistology requires oncologic evaluation and treatment.

Other Hormonal Therapies

A number of other substances, peptide or steroid in nature, intervene in the reproductive aging process. Where there is inadequate estrogen, anovulation and infertility follow. If infertility is a problem, ovulatory medications, such as clomiphene citrate, human chorionic gonadotropin (hCG), and human menopausal gonadotropins (hMG) with hCG, may be used to try to induce ovulation leading to normal cycles. Clomiphene citrate functions as a weak estrogen signal, acting at the hypothalamopituitary axis and foiling the estrogen receptors, preventing the anticipated negative feedback response. Thus, FSH remains elevated with resultant enhancement of follicular growth, positive estrogen feedback, and often, ovulation.

Gonadotropin therapies (hCG, hMG) act directly on ovarian tissue and provide cyclic activity. They require careful observations and monitoring to prevent hypersensitization of ovarian tissues. In recent years, the number of late pregnancies has increased because women have postponed pregnancy to permit themselves the opportunity to fulfill their professional commitments.

The use of hormones to improve sexuality has been studied (Eskin and Shah, 1981b; Greenblatt et al., 1950; Lloyd, 1980). Androgens are recommended in concert with replacement estrogens. These include the anabolic steroids associated with testosterone products (Eskin, 1980b). Since aging individuals may show an increase in androgens, additional steroids may bring about mild virilization by hirsutism and skin changes. These substances do increase her sexuality by enhancing libido and sexual contacts. In these cases, estrogen must be given as well, since the action of the androgens in increasing sexual appetite without normal vaginal turgor may bring about additional frustration.

Finally, a series of therapeutics becoming available have to do with nonsteroid stimulation of the hypothalamus. Recent studies in sexuality have shown that several neurogenic monoamines as well as catechol estrogens act to increase certain phases of sexuality in women, both in the reproductive and postreproductive periods (Eskin and Shah, 1981a and b). Those available are such substances as dopamine agonists, serotonin stimulators, and norepinephrine mimetics. These drugs, many of which are presently available for the treatment of other problems, have sexual responses as well. The most prominent among these is bromergocriptine, which functions through transmitters to the brain and enhances sexuality, particularly libido, both proceptivity and receptivity (Ambrosi et al., 1980). In the case of tranquilizers, which have both a serotoninlike and serotonin antagonist effect, there are mixed responses causing both enhancement and regression of specific sexual factors depending on the drug used (Eskin and Shah, 1981a and b).

Dopamine agonists, in particularly high doses (such as those used for Parkinsonism), have been known to cause such a stimulation of the hypothalamopituitary axis that the high levels of gonadotropins may renew ovarian activity in postmenopausal women. The use of all of these substances for both postreproductive and aging-related symptoms in women who have a desire for sexuality seems to be a potentially effective intervention (Eskin and Shah, 1981a and b; Ambrosi et al., 1980).

Nonhormonal Therapies

Other drugs not previously mentioned can be used in postmenopausal problems. Again, it is apparent that they would be effective in problems caused by either reproductive loss and/or by aging. Suggested has been the use of vitamin D and the use of calcium therapeutics in osteoporosis (Heaney et al., 1978; Gordon and

Vaughan, 1980). Needless to say, the factors of nutrition and exercise have shown proficiency in all areas. Psychopharmacological therapies, such as tranquilizers and amino acid replacement therapies, have been suggested as they have been for other geriatric symptoms (Clayden et al., 1974).

Risks of Estrogen Therapy

Whenever therapy is employed, regardless of the source, side effects and contra-indications occur. This has become particularly true with estrogen therapy. The absolute contraindications to estrogen therapy are listed in Table 5.

Examining these, it is apparent that estrogen has an effect on liver activity, disturbing normal metabolic function. Oral estrogen therapy is absorbed through the portal circulation and, thus, through the liver, where it is partially metabolized and either detoxified or released systemically. The liver responds to estrogen by increasing renin substrate and clotting factors, leading sequentially to increased estrogen and possible thrombosis. Whereas literature referring to increased renin substrate and clotting factors has been published with contraceptive steroids, little data have been noted for postmenopausal therapy. Cholecystic jaundice occurs two to four times as often during postmenopausal estrogen therapy. Gall bladder disease may increase due to estrogen modifying the bile composition and secondary autoimmune responses (Boston Collaborative Drug Surveillance Program, 1972). Estrogen causes the level of triglycerides to increase through changes in lipid metabolism and fat storage responses within liver depots. The effect of estrogen to increase triglyceride levels (seen more commonly with birth control pills) is due to intracellular lipid transformation in the liver cells.

The hormonal risk of replacement therapy in the premenopausal woman (late reproductive or perimenopausal) has not been clearly determined. However, since

---

Table 5 Contraindications

Estrogens should not be used in women with any of the following conditions:
1. Known or suspected cancer of the breast except in appropriately selected patients with progressing inoperable or radiation-resistant disease
2. Known or suspected estrogen-dependent neoplasia
3. Known or suspected pregnancy
4. Undiagnosed abnormal genital bleeding
5. Active thrombophlebitis or thromboembolic disorders
6. A past history of thrombophlebitis or thromboembolic disorders associated with previous estrogen use (except when used in treatment of breast malignancy)

---

estrogen is an important ingredient of birth control pills, there is likelihood that the risks present or surmised may be similar, although the dose for reproductive aging replacement therapy seems to be much less. The dose of estrogen required for oral birth control has shown a marked increased cardiac risk for women over 35, especially if they smoke. However, little evidence has shown similar heart disease risk in women receiving the low dosage required to treat reproductive senescence (The Coronary Drug Project Research Group, 1978; Jick et al., 1978). A recent study indicates a risk of coronary artery disease with oral contraceptives even if discontinued (Table 6) (Slone et al., 1981).

The effect of estrogen on breast and endometrium remains controversial (Lipsett, 1977), but warrants further discussion (Table 7). Since estrogen is given only by oral or parenteral therapy, the blood level is not stable, and the resulting high doses are not efficient. The use of local estrogen—per vaginum—for atrophic changes is generally ill-advised since the absorption rate is high and the serum estrogen level may be higher than that required orally for comparable local response (Schiff et al., 1977).

Postmenopausal women on estrogen replacement have been described at five to sevenfold risk of endometrial cancer (Geola et al., 1980; Artunes et al., 1979); however, a consideration of quantity and length of therapy is important (Slone et al., 1981). Literature compiled since 1972 has shown that much of the endometrial change seen and considered neoplastic (Lipsett, 1977) may be atypical hyper-

Table 6 Distribution of Cases and Controls According to Duration of Past Use[a] of Oral Contraceptives and Age

Age group	Duration of current use				Never used oral contraceptives
Year	<5 yr	5-9 yr	≥10 yr	unknown	
25-39					
Cases	35	9	3	3	37
Controls	176	46	8	17	153
Rate-ratio estimate[b]	0.8	0.8	1.5	–	1.0[c]
95% confidence limits[d]	0.5-1.4	0.4-1.8	0.4-6.0	–	
40-49					
Cases	93	32	25	6	272
Controls	362	81	40	32	1070
Rate-ratio estimate[b]	1.0	1.6	2.5	–	1.0[c]
95% confidence limits[d]	0.8-1.4	1.1-2.5	1.5-4.1	–	

[a]Last use at least one month before admission. Current users are excluded.
[b]Derived after stratification for half decade of age by the Mantel-Haenszel method.
[c]Reference category.
[d]Computed by Miettinen's test-based method.
Source: Slone et al., 1981.

Table 7 Observed Versus Expected[a] Malignancies for the Uterine Corpus (Adenocarcinoma of the Endometrium), the Breast, and All Sites Listed by the Two Study Groups and by Race. These data are Compared with the Expected Incidences as Documented by the Third National Cancer Survey for the Southeastern Region and Are Also Age-Matched.

Site of malignancy	No E		E	
	White	Nonwhite	White	Nonwhite
Uterine corpus[b]				
Expected	1.85	0.60	1.18	0.02
Observed	2	1	11	0
Risk ratio[c]	1.1	–	9.3	–
95% Confidence interval	0.1-3.9		4.7-16.7	
Breast				
Expected	5.69	1.90	3.77	0.09
Observed	3	1	4	0
Risk ratio[c]	0.5	0.5	1.06	–
95% Confidence interval	0.1-1.5	0.0-2.9	0.3-2.7	
All Sites[b]				
Expected	20.99	8.75	12.5	0.31
Observed	17	9	24	1
Risk ratio	0.8	1.03	1.92	–
95% Confidence interval	0.5-1.3	0.5-2.0	1.2-2.9	

[a]Calculated from age/race incidence data presented in the Third National Cancer Survey.
[b]Carcinoma in situ not included.
[c]Risk ratio = observed/expected.

plasia, which is easily cleared with progesterone therapy (Sturdec et al., 1978; Gambrell et al., 1979). Persistent unopposed estrogen is capable of severe atypical glandular and mitotic change, but in the presence of the physiological stabilizing influence of progesterone, estrogen hypersensitivity is reduced, although not all responses are reduced by this therapy (Judd et al., 1981; Whitehead et al., 1979).

Experimental data on estrogen and endometrial cancer are difficult to assess since there is no tumorigenic model in nonhuman primates. Research programs using rabbits, rodents, and cattle show endometrial changes which do not metastasize or show any characteristics of the human form (Mirriam et al., 1960; Sehya et al., 1972).

Breast tissue has been implicated as affected by excesses of unopposed estrogen, and a risk factor approximately two times for breast cancer has been ascribed

(Hoover et al., 1976). Opposing views consider the long latent period of breast cancer and the many suggested inhibiting factors such as pregnancy, nursing, and family history. Fibrocystic changes have been noted in breasts of women with persistent estrogen therapy with reproductive aging, especially in the perimenopause. Since women with fibrocystic disease have four times the risk for breast carcinoma, the hormonal milieu could be responsible (Ross et al., 1980).

Dosage levels influence complications in hormone replacements (Geola et al., 1980). Low doses of oral estrogen may show liver protein responses (renin substrate and sex-hormone-binding globulin); however, larger oral doses are needed to return fasting calcium excretion and severe vaginal atrophism to normal. In light of possible undesirable responses, several treatment regimens have been suggested (Nachtigall et al., 1979). Low doses of oral estrogen (0.625 mg) daily should be given cyclically with 5-10 days of progesterone (oral Provera 5-10 mg per day) each month. Progesterone can be decreased to every other month, particularly when there is no uterus, since the longer therapy is required only for endometrial protection. The dosage desirable for the breast and liver has not been demonstrated.

From this chapter, it would appear that the main thrusts for estrogen therapy are atrophic changes, hot flushes, and osteoporosis. A recent consensus report on the status of estrogen replacement therapy indicates that hot flushes, atrophy of vaginal epithelium, and prevention of osteoporosis have been established, although the treatment remains under close scrutiny (Judd et al., 1981). Oral estrogen appears to be the preferred route despite misgivings about portal absorption and liver metabolism. The doses required for all of these vary from patient to patient. If a lower dose is started first, determination of optimum therapy can be made by vaginal smears, radiological evaluations of bone, and level of symptomatology. Health control by blood pressure and triglyceride and glucose evaluations may assist in early evidence of other complications.

SUMMARY

The reproductive span is a limited period in a woman's life. Reproductive senescence does not appear to be a serious factor in longevity, but it may play a peripheral role in the quality of life. Because of an aging ovary and the loss of sex hormonal secretions, replacement with estrogen improves the conditions of many sex-dependent tissues. Estrogen interventions are effective for improving atrophic perineal changes, vasomotor dysfunction, and osteoporetic changes.

Side effects to estrogen therapy that have been established are endometrial cancer, hypertension, gall bladder disease, and angina pectoris. No concensus seems to be available for breast cancer, pulmonary embolism, cerebral vascular accident, or myocardial infarction. Progesterone is protective for unopposed estrogen, particularly in the endometrium, and may have desirable responses of its own. Neuroamines are under study for psychosexual and psychiatric problems.

It is impossible to separate most of the conditions postmenopausally into those caused by reproductive senescence and aging phenomena. Thus, therapy must be individualized carefully and its use weighed against the hazards (Eskin, 1978).

REFERENCES

Abraham, G. E., and Maroulis, G. B. (1975). Effect of exogenous estrogen on serum pregnenolone cortisol and androgens in postmenopausal women. *Obstet. Gynecol. 45*: 271.

Aksel, S., and Jones, G. S. (1975). Etiology and treatment of dysfunctional uterine bleeding. *Obstet. Gynecol. 45*: 1.

Alyward, M. (1973). Plasma tryptophan levels and mental depression in post menopausal subjects. *Med. Sci. 1*: 30.

Ambrosi, B., Gaggini, M., Paola, M., and Faglia, G. (1980). Prolactin and sexual function. *JAMA 244*: 2608.

Artunes, C. M. F., Stolley, P. D., Rosenscheim, N. B., Davies, J. L., Tonascia, J. A., Brown, C., Burnett, L., Rutledge, A., Pokempner, M., and Garcia, R. (1979). Endometrial cancer and estrogen use. *N. Engl. J. Med. 300*: 9.

Bayward, F., Damilano, S., Robel, P., and Baulien, E. (1978). Cytoplasmic and nuclear estradiol and progesterone receptors in human endometrium. *J. Clin. Endocrinol. Metab. 46*: 635.

Boston Collaborative Drug Surveillance Program (1972). Gallbladder disease, venous disorders, breast tumors: relationship to estrogen. *N. Engl. J. Med. 287*: 628.

Boyar, R., Finkelstein, J., Roffwarg, H., Kapen, S., Weitzman, E., and Hellman, L. (1972). Synchronization of augmented leutenizing hormone secretion with sleep during puberty. *N. Engl. J. Med. 287*: 582.

Bullock, J. L., Maney, F. M., and Gambrell, R. D. (1975). Use of medroxyprogesterone acetate to prevent menopausal symptoms. *Obstet. Gynecol. 46*: 165.

Campbell, S. (1976). Double blind psychometric studies on the effect of natural estrogens on postmenopausal women. In *The Management of the Menopause and Postmenopausal Years*, S. Campbell (Ed.). University Park Press, Baltimore, p. 152.

Chan, L., and O'Malley, B. W. (1976). Mechanism of action of the sex steroid hormones. *N. Engl. J. Med. 294*: 1322.

Channing, C. P., and Tsafriri, A. (1977). Mechanism of action of leuteinizing hormone and follicle-stimulating hormone on the ovary *in vitro*. *Metabolism 26*: 413.

Clayden, J. R., Bell, J. W., and Pollard, P. (1974). Menopausal bleeding: double-blind trial of a non-hormonal medication. *Br. Med. J. 1*: 409.

Collett, M. E., Werterberger, G. E., and Fiske, V. M. (1954). The effect of age upon the pattern of the menstrual cycle. *Fertil. Steril. 5*: 437.

The Coronary Drug Project Research Group (1978). Findings leading to discontinuation of the 2.5 estrogen group. *JAMA 226*: 652.

Deghenghi, R. (1980). Chemistry and biochemistry of natural estrogens. In *The Menopause and Postmenopause*, N. Pasetto, R. Paoletti, and J. L. Ambrus (Eds.). M. T. P. Press, Lancaster, England, p. 3.

Deutsch, S., Ossowski, R., and Benjamin, I. (1981). Comparison between degree of systemic absorption of vaginally and orally administered estrogens. *Am. J. Obstet. Gynecol. 139*: 967.

Editorial: (1977). Coronary heart disease and the menopause. *Br. Med. J. 1*: 862.

Eisdorfer, C. (1972). Some variables relating to longevity in humans. In *Epidemiology of Aging*, DHEW Publication 75-711, A. M. Ostfeld (Ed.). DHEW, Washington, D.C.

Eskin, B. A. (1977). Intracellular metabolism of iodine in rat breast tissue. In *Inorganic and Nutritional Aspects of Cancer*, G. Schrauzer (Ed.). Plenum Press, New York, p. 293.

Eskin, B. A. (1978). Sex hormones and aging. In *Pharmacologic Interventions in the Aging Process*, J. Roberts, R. C. Adelman, and V. J. Cristofalo (Eds.). Plenum Press, New York, p. 231.

Eskin, B. A. (1980a). Aging and the menopause. In *The Menopause: Comprehensive Management*, B. A. Eskin (Ed.). Masson Publishers, New York, p. 73.

Eskin, B. A. (1980b). Sexuality in athletes using anabolic steroids. *Med. Aspects Human Sexuality 14*: 136.

Eskin, B. A., and Shah, N. M. (1981a). Effects of hormonal steroids and neurotransmitters on sexuality. *Proc. Soc. Sex. Therapy Res. 7*: 8.

Eskin, B. A., and Shah, N. M. (1981b). Non-steroidal sexual therapies in women (in manuscript).

Eskin, B. A., Jacobson, H. I., Bolmarich, V., and Murray, J. A. (1977). Breast atypia in altered thyroid states: Intracellular changes. *Senologia 2*: 67.

Eskin, B. A., Sparks, C. E., and LaMont, B. I. (1979). The intracellular metabolism of iodine in carcinogenesis. *Biol. Trace Element Res. 1*: 101.

Forest, M. G., DePeretti, E., and Bertrand, J. (1976). Hypothalamic-pituitary-gonadal relationships in man from birth to puberty. *Clin. Endocrinol. 5*: 551.

Gambrell, R. D., Many, F. M., and Tristam, A. C. (1979). Reduced incidence of endometrial cancer among postmenopausal women treated with progesterone. *J. Am. Geriatr. 27*: 389.

Geola, F. L., Frumar, A. M., Tataryn, I. V., Lu, K. H., Herhman, J. M., Eggena, P., Sambhi, M. P., and Judd, H. L. (1980). Biological effects of various doses of conjugated equine estrogens in postmenopausal women. *J. Clin. Endocrinol. Metab. 51*: 620.

Goebelsmann, U. (1979). In *Reproductive Endocrinology, Infertility and Contraception*, D. R. Mischell, Jr. and V. Davajan (Eds.). F. A. Davis, Philadelphia, p. 43.

Gordon, G. S., and Vaughan, C. (1980). Prevention and treatment of postmenopausal osteoporosis. In *The Menopause and Postmenopause*, N. Pasetto, R. Paoletti, and J. L. Ambrus (Eds.). M.T.P. Press, Lancaster, England, p. 179.

Gordon, T., Kannel, W. B., Hjortland, M. C., and McNamara, P. M. (1978). Menopause and coronary heart disease. *Ann. Intern. Med. 89*: 157.

Greenblatt, R. B., and Torpin, R. (1940). Some common endocrine disorders in the female: Special references to treatment with male sex hormone. *J. Med. Assoc. Ga. 29*: 68.

Greenblatt, R. B., Barfield, W. E., Gardner, J. F., Calk, G. L., and Harrod, J. P., Jr. (1950). Evaluation of an estrogen, androgen, estrogen-androgen combination and a placebo in the treatment of the menopause. *J. Clin. Endocrinol.* *10*: 1547.

Hammond, C. B., Jelovsek, F. R., and Lee, K. L. (1979). Effects of longterm estrogen replacement therapy. II. Neoplasia. *Am. J. Obstet. Gynecol. 133*: 527.

Heaney, R. P., Recker, R. R., and Saville, P. D. (1978). Menopausal changes in calcium balance performance. *J. Lab. Clin. Med. 92*: 953.

Hemsell, D. L., Grodin, J. M., Brenner, P. F., Siiteri, P. K., and MacDonald, P. C. (1974). Plasma precursors of estrogen. II. Correlation of the extent of conversion of plasma androstenedione to estrone with age. *J. Clin. Endocrinol. Metab. 38*: 476.

Hirvonen, E., Malkonen, M., and Manninen, V. (1981). Effects of different progestogens on lipoproteins during postmenopausal replacement therapy. *N. Engl. J. Med. 304*: 560.

Hoover, R., Gray, L., Cole, P., and MacMahon, B. (1976). Menopausal estrogens and breast cancer. *N. Engl. J. Med. 295*: 401.

Jick, H., Diman, B., and Rothman, K. H. (1978). Noncontraceptive estrogen and nonfatal myocardial infarction. *JAMA 239*: 1407.

Jones, E. C. (1975). The post-reproductive phase in mammals. In *Estrogen in the Post-Menopause. Front. Horm. Res. 3*: 1.

Jones, G. S. (1980). Hormonal changes in perimenopause. In *The Menopause: Comprehensive Management*, B. A. Eskin (Ed.). Masson Publishers, New York, p. 47.

Judd, H. L. (1980). Reproductive hormone metabolism in postmenopausal women. In *The Menopause: Comprehensive Management*, B. A. Eskin (Ed.). Masson Publishers, New York, p. 55.

Judd, H. L., Cleary, R. E., Creasman, W. T., Figge, D. C., Kase, N., Rosenwaks, Z., and Tagatz, G. E. (1981). Estrogen replacement therapy. *Obstet. Gynecol. 58*: 267.

Judd, H. L., Judd, G. E., Lucas, W. E., and Yen, S. S. C. (1974). Endocrine function of the postmenopausal ovary: Concentration of androgens and estrogens in ovarian and peripheral vein blood. *J. Clin. Endocrinol. Metab. 39*: 1020.

Judd, H. L., Lucas, W. E., and Yen, S. S. C. (1974). Effect of oophorectomy on circulating testosterone and androstenedione levels in patients with endometrial cancer. *Am. J. Obstet. Gynecol. 118*: 793.

Kannel, W. B., Hjortland, M. C., and McNamara, P. M. (1976). Menopause and risk of cardiovascular disease: the Framingham study. *Ann. Intern. Med. 85*: 447.

Krouse, T. B. (1980). Pathology of aging. In *The Menopause: Comprehensive Management*, B. A. Eskin (Ed.). Masson Publishers, New York, p. 5.

Krouse, T. B., Eskin, B. A., and Mobini, J. (1979). Age-related changes resembling fibrocystic disease in iodine-blocked rat breasts. *Arch. Pathol. Lab. Med. 103*: 631.

Lindsay, R., Anderson, J. B., Hart, D. M., MacDonald, E. B., and Clarke, A. C. (1976). Long-term prevention of post-menopausal osteoporosis by oestrogen. *Lancet 1*: 1038.

Lindsay, R., MacLean, A., Kraszweski, A., Hart, D. M., Clark, A. C., and Garwood, J. (1978). Bone response to termination of estrogen treatment. *Lancet 1*: 1325.

Lipsett, M. B. (1977). Estrogen use and cancer risk. *JAMA 237*: 1112.

Lloyd, C. W. (1963). Central nervous system regulation of endocrine function in the human. In *Advances in Neuroendocrinology*, A. V. Nalbandov (Ed.). University of Illinois Press, Urbana.

Lloyd, C. W. (1980). Sexuality in the climacteric. In *The Menopause: Comprehensive Management*, B. A. Eskin (Ed.). Masson Publishers, New York, p. 101.

Marshall, D. H., Crilly, R. G., and Nordin, B. E. C. (1977). Plasma androstenedione and estrone levels in normal and osteoporotic postmenopausal women. *Br. Med. J. 2*: 1177.

Mattingly, R. F., and Huang, W. Y. (1969). Steroidogenesis of the menopausal and postmenopausal ovary. *Am. J. Obstet. Gynecol. 103*: 679.

Meema, S., and Meema, H. E. (1976). Menopausal bone loss and estrogen replacement. *Isr. J. Med. Sci. 12*: 601.

Meema, S., Bunker, M. L., and Meema, H. E. (1975). Preventive effect of estrogen on postmenopausal bone loss. *Arch. Int. Med. 135*: 1436.

Meldrum, D. R., Shamonki, I. M., Frumar, A. M., Tataryn, I. V., Chang, R. J., and Judd, H. L. (1979). Elevations in skin temperature of the finger as an objective index of postmenopausal hot flushes. *Am. J. Obstet. Gynecol. 135*: 713.

Meldrum, D. R., Tataryn, I. V., Frumar, A. M., Erlik, Y., Lu, K. H., and Judd, H. L. (1980). Gonadotropins, estrogens and adrenal steroids during the menopause hot flush. *J. Clin. Endocrinol. Metab. 50*: 685.

Milhaud, G., Benezech-Lefevre, M., and Moukhtar, M. S. (1978). Deficiency of calcitonin in age-related osteoporosis. *Biomedicine 29*: 272.

Mirriam, J. C., Jr., Easterdy, C. L., McKay, D. G., and Hertz, A. T. (1960). Experimental production of endometrial carcinoma in the rabbit. *Obstet. Gynecol. 16*: 253.

Nachtigall, L. E., Nachtigall, R. H., Nachtigall, R. D., and Beckman, E. M. (1979). Estrogen replacement therapy. II. A prospective study in the relationship to carcinoma and cardiovascular and metabolic problems. *Obstet. Gynecol. 54*: 74.

Nelson, J. F., Holinka, C. F., and Finch, C. E. (1976). Loss of cytoplasmic estradiol binding capacity during aging in uteri of C57-BL/63 mice. *Proc. Endocr. Soc. 58*: 349.

Persky, H., O'Brian, C. P., and Khan, M. A. (1976). Reproductive hormone levels, sexual activity and moods during the menstrual cycle. *Psychosom. Med. 38*: 62.

Ross, R. K., Paganin, A., Gerkins, V. R., Mack, T. M., Pfeffer, R., Arthur, M., and Henderson, B. E. (1980). A case control study of menopausal estrogen therapy and breast cancer. *JAMA 243*: 1635.

Roth, G. S. (1978). Altered biochemical responsiveness and hormone receptor changes during aging. In *The Biology of Aging*, J. Behnke, G. Finch, and G. Moment (Eds.). Plenum Press, New York, p. 291.

Roth, G. S. (1979). Hormone receptor changes during adulthood and senescence; significance for aging research. *Fed. Proc. 38*: 1910.

Roth, G. S., and Adelman, R. C. (1975). Age related changes in hormone binding by target cells and tissues; possible role in altered adaptive responsiveness. *Exp. Gerontol. 10*: 1.

Schiff, I., Regestein, Q., Tulchinsky, D., and Ryan, K. J. (1979). Effects of estrogens on sleep and psychological state of hypogonadal women. *JAMA 242*: 2405.

Schiff, I., Tulchinsky, D., and Ryan, K. J. (1977). Vaginal absorption of estrone and 17-beta estradiol. *Fertil. Steril. 28*: 1063.

Schneider, J. (1980). Age and the outcome of pregnancy. In *The Menopause: Comprehensive Management*, B. A. Eskin (Ed.). Masson Publishers, New York, p. 93.

Sehya, S., Takamiyawa, H., Wang, F., Takane, T., and Kuwata, T. (1972). *In vivo* and *vitro* studies on uterine adenocarcinoma of the rat induced by 7,12-dimethylbenz(a)anthracene. *Am. J. Obstet. Gynecol. 113*: 691.

Sherman, B. M., and Korenman, S. G. (1975). Hormonal characteristics of the human menstrual cycle through reproductive life. *J. Clin. Invest. 55*: 699.

Siiteri, P. K., and MacDonald, P. C. (1973). Role of extraglandular estrogen in human endocrinology. In *Handbook of Physiology: Endocrinology*, Vol. 2, Part 1, R. O. Greep and E. Astwood (Eds.). American Physiology Society, Washington, D.C., p. 615.

Slone, D., Shapiro, S., Kaufman, D. W., Rosenberg, L., Miettmen, O. S., and Stolley, P. D. (1981). Risk of myocardial infarction in relation to current and discontinued use of oral contraceptives. *N. Engl. J. Med. 305*: 420.

Sturdec, D. W., Wade-Evans, T., Paterson, M. E. L., Thom, M., and Studd, J. W. W. (1978). Relations between bleeding pattern, endometrial histology and oestrogen treatment in menopausal women. *Br. Med. J. 1*: 1575.

Thompson, J. (1977). Double-blind study on the effect of estrogen on sleep, anxiety and depression in perimenopausal women. *Br. Med. J. 6090*: 1317.

Vanhulle, G., and Demol, R. (1976). A double blind study into the influence of estriol on a number of psychological tests in postmenopausal women. In *Consensus on Menopause Research*, P. A. van Keep, R. B. Greenblatt, and M. Albeaux-Fernet (Eds.). M.T.P. Press, Lancaster, England, p. 94.

Weisz, J., and Gibbs, C. (1974). Conversion of testosterone and androstenedione to estrogens *in vitro* in brain of female rats. *Endocrinology 94*: 616.

Wenderlein, J. M. (1980). Psychotherapeutic effects of estrogen substitution during the climacteric period. In *The Menopause and Postmenopause*, N. Pasetto, R. Paoletti, and J. L. Ambrus (Eds.). M.T.P. Press, Lancaster, England, p. 63.

Whitehead, M. I., King, R. J. B., McQueen, J., and Campbell, S. (1979). Endometrial histology and biochemistry in climacteric women during oestrogen and oestrogen/progesterone therapy. *J. Roy. Soc. Med. 72*: 322.

Winokur, G. (1973). Depression in the menopause. *Am. J. Psychiatry 130*: 92.

Winter, J. S. D., and Faiman, C. (1979). The development of cyclic pituitary-gonadal function in adolescent females. *J. Clin. Endocrinol. Metab. 37*: 714.

Part II
Immune Function and Aging

6
Basic Considerations in Immunology

John R. Cohn* / *Veterans Administration and Duke University Medical Centers, Durham, North Carolina*

INTRODUCTION

The latter decades of human life are associated with increasingly well-described alterations in immune function. These changes have profound implications for the study of the biology of aging. Indeed, some research suggests that the aging process itself represents an immunological phenomenon.

This brief discussion will acquaint the reader with the basic concepts of modern immunology. It is hoped that it will prove useful in reading the following chapters, as well as in evaluating developing interventions for correcting immunological dysfunction in the elderly. Detailed monographs, reviews, and books are available to the reader for additional information. Some references are listed at the conclusion of this chapter.

COMPONENTS OF THE IMMUNE SYSTEM

Immune system cells produce numerous humoral substances, including lymphokines, monokines, vasoactive compounds, immunoglobulins, and some complement components. Immunoglobulins and complement often act at sites that are distant from the cells that produced them and are traditionally discussed as humoral im-

---

*Present affiliation: Thomas Jefferson University Hospital, Philadelphia, Pennsylvania.

munity in descriptive chapters such as this. Cells that directly participate in immune responses and their locally active products are customarily considered as cellular immunity. This semantic separation is a useful device for cataloging the individual elements of the immune system. The reader is cautioned that the functional lines separating humoral and cellular immunity are much less distinct.

Cellular Elements

Lymphocytes

Lymphocytes can function as regulatory cells, producers of immunoglobulin, or cytotoxic effector cells. They participate at some point in virtually every type of immune response. Three types of lymphocytes have been described, based on morphological, functional, and surface membrane characteristics.

Thymic-derived or T lymphocytes originate in the fetal hematopoietic tissue, sharing a common stem cell precursor with other immune effector cells. From there, immature T cells migrate to the thymus, where important developmental changes occur before they are released into the circulation. Thymic hormones and epithelium participate in the T-lymphocytes' maturation process. The continued importance of thymic hormones to the function of circulating T lymphocytes is uncertain. Evidence exists for a sustained relationship. It has been proposed that normal aging is the result of T-lymphocyte dysfunction secondary to thymic involution.

Subclasses of T lymphocytes stimulate or inhibit the development of an immune response by many other immune effector cells, including most immunoglobulin production by B lymphocytes and migration and phagocytosis by monocytes and neutrophils. Clinically significant cases of hypogammaglobulinemia have resulted from the excessive action of suppressor lymphocytes on normal immunoglobulin-producing cells. Other subsets of T lymphocytes participate directly in the immune response as cytotoxic effector cells. T lymphocytes produce a variety of lymphokines, including migration-inhibitory factor (MIF), macrophage-activating factor (MAF), leukocyte migration-inhibitory factory (LIF), interleukin II, osteoclast-activating factor (OAF), lymphocyte-derived chemotactic factor (LDCF), lymphotoxin, and interferon. These compounds have a variety of functions. They may activate other effector cells of the immune system, can be directly cytotoxic, may increase the resistance of the host animal's own cells to viral infection, or attract other effector cells to the site of an immune response.

Bursal or B lymphocytes obtain their designation from the chicken's bursa of Fabricius. There, immature chicken lymphocytes acquire immunoglobulin-producing potential. The removal of a chick embryo's bursa will result in an absent immunoglobulin response during adult life. The pathophysiology of this phenomenon is uncertain. The human bursal equivalent is thought to be the bone marrow. In humans, most mature B lymphocytes and plasma cells are found in the bone marrow, spleen, and other lymphoid tissues.

The surface membrane of each B lymphocyte is covered with immunoglobulin molecules which share a single antigen-binding specificity (idiotype). These antibodies serve as the cell's recognition mechanism. When they contact and bind to an appropriate antigen, the membrane-bound immunoglobulin molecules coalesce and are endocytosed into the cell. This process, called "capping," is thought to be part of the antigen recognition-cell activation process. It requires energy and appears to be mediated by the B-cell's cytoskeleton.

In vitro techniques are used to quantitate and characterize B-lymphocyte and T-lymphocyte populations. B cells have strongly adherent surface antibodies, primarily immunoglobulin M (IgM) and immunoglobulin D (IgD), that can be detected with the fluorescein-labeled Fab portion of anti-immunoglobulin. The number of B lymphocytes in a sample capable of producing antibodies against a specific antigen can be determined with a plaque assay. This test is based on the ability of each B-cell's antibody to bind an antigen, forming immune complexes capable of inducing complement-dependent hemolysis. Essentially all T cells bind sheep erythrocytes, forming so-called E rosettes, at 4°C. Activated T lymphocytes bind sheep red blood cells (RBCs) at 37°C, as well. Helper and suppressor T lymphocytes have been differentiated by the immunoglobulin class of their membrane Fc receptors, although recent data suggest this method may not be uniformly reliable. Monoclonal antibodies are also used to identify T-lymphocyte subpopulations. Monoclonal antibodies are raised in vitro from hybridomas that are the result of fusing the spleen cells from immunized animals and permanent myeloma cell lines. By selecting the proper immunoglobulin-producing clone, identical antibodies with the desired binding specificity can be produced. Numerous antibodies have been developed against human and mouse lymphocyte and other cell-surface antigens. Certain monoclonal antibodies appear to distinguish between various types of T lymphocytes, such as helper and suppressor cells. Monoclonal antibody-defined changes in cell-surface antigens have been correlated with stages in the ontogeny of T lymphocytes.

An additional population of lymphocytes has been identified which lacks the membrane markers characteristic of B or T cells. Called null cells, these small lymphocytes are thought to play a major role in antibody-dependent cell-mediated cytotoxicity (ADCC) and in natural killing (NK). Other functions have been postulated for these cells, but their exact nature and role remains to be defined.

Lymphocyte subpopulations, as well as other types of immune system cells, differ in their susceptibility to immunosuppressive drugs and x-irradiation. Low doses of these agents can be used to selectively deplete an animal or in vitro test system of some cell populations (e.g., suppressor cells) while other cells remain functionally intact. Alternatively, the recognition of new antigens may be inhibited, while the secondary response remains intact. There is considerable variability between species in the response to specific immunosuppressive agents.

Systems of gut-associated lymphoid tissue (GALT) and bronchus-associated lymphoid tissue (BALT) have been described. They are both part of a common lymphoid system that connects all mucosal immune responses through circulating lymphocytes. Immunization of the nasal mucosa, for example, results in specific antibody production by immune cells of the gut, genitourinary tract, and mammary tissue.

Immune responsiveness can be transferred between syngeneic animals using sensitized lymphocytes. Called "adoptive transfer," this technique can result in a recall response in a previously unexposed donor. Transfer factor, a small T-lymphocyte-produced protein, may have similar effects. If T lymphocytes are transferred into an immunologically unresponsive, genetically unrelated recipient, graft-versus-host (GVH) disease results from the transfused donor lymphocytes attacking the host's cells.

Phagocytes

The two major populations of phagocytic cells that participate in the immune response are the monocytes and polymorphonuclear leukocytes. Both cell types originate in the bone marrow from a common precursor stem cell. Monocytes circulate briefly in the blood before migrating into tissues. In tissue, monocytes transform into macrophages. Macrophages are important in phagocytosis in the lung, skin, liver as Kupffer cells, spleen, and other locations. Macrophages process antigens for presentation to lymphocytes in the development of an immune response. Mononuclear phagocytes may also function as tissue effector cells, often at the direction of lymphocytes via lymphokines. Liver and spleen macrophages filter from the circulation-opsonized bacteria, senescent red blood cells, and other debris. Monocytes discharge a variety of enzymes and prostaglandins that have direct end-organ effects, and inactivate mast cell products released in immediate hypersensitivity reactions. The epitheliloid or giant cells found in granulomatous lesions are derived from macrophage precursors.

Macrophages produce monokines that further modulate the immune response. Examples are lymphocyte-activating factor (LAF), a neutrophil chemotactic factor, and some complement components. Mononuclear phagocytes are suppressor cells in some circumstances, a function that may be particularly important in the elderly. Laboratory evidence suggests that suppressor macrophages are responsible for the immunological dysfunction of multiple myeloma.

Polymorphonuclear leukocytes are produced in quantity in the bone marrow. They phagocytize and destroy bacteria and fungal organisms. They are also important in the development of an inflammatory response due to their content of enzymes, peroxide, and similar compounds. Neutrophils are important effector cells in diseases such as rheumatoid arthritis, where abnormal release of enzymes is responsible for tissue damage.

Mast Cells and Basophils

Basophils are produced in the bone marrow. They circulate in the blood in limited quantities and settle in the tissues where they become mast cells. Minor functional differences exist between mast cells and basophils. The surface of each mast cell is covered with up to 100,000 molecules of IgE in equilibrium with reagenic antibodies in surrounding fluids.

Mast cells are important in the development of an allergic response. They may also play a role in other immunological processes, such as the facilitation of immune complex disposition at blood vessel basement membranes. Mast cells contain and produce a variety of vasoactive compounds including histamine, platelet-activating factor (PAF), and eosinophil chemotactic factor of anaphylaxis (ECF-A). Slow-reacting substance of anaphylaxis (SRS-A) is also thought to be a mast cell product, but this viewpoint has been questioned.

Platelets

Platelets are more important in the development of immune responses in certain animal species than in humans. In some animal serum sickness models, they serve a role similar to that of the mast cell, and release vasoactive mediators that are important in immune complex deposition.

Eosinophils

Eosinophils are being actively studied to determine their function as immune effector cells. Eosinophils are associated with allergic processes. Blood eosinophilia is commonly found in patients with a variety of allergic diseases, and eosinophils may be found in nasal secretions or sputum of patients with allergic rhinitis or asthma. It is now thought that eosinophils inactivate many of the mediators released by mast cells and also participate in the defense against infection by certain parasites.

Humoral Elements

Immunoglobulins

The basic immunoglobulin molecule consists of two long peptide chains, designated as heavy chains, and two shorter chains, called light chains. Each light chain is attached to a heavy chain, and the heavy chains are joined together. The shared end of a heavy chain and a single light chain is called an Fab region. This region binds to antigens. Variations in the amino acid sequence of the light chain and the corresponding portion of the heavy chain in the Fab region determine the antibody's specificity. The heavy chains are joined together in the Fc region. This region participates in the binding of complement, interactions with cell membranes, and other biological activities of antibodies. A monomeric antibody molecule consists of two Fab portions and a single Fc portion in a Y-shaped configuration. Isolated Fab regions from the enzymatic cleavage of an antibody molecule retain their antigen-binding capacity.

There are two types of light chains, kappa and lambda, shared by all immunoglobulin classes. Heavy chains vary between the different immunoglobulin classes, and there are important functional differences based on heavy chain composition.

Subclasses of immunoglobulin have been described for IgG and IgA. Functional differences have been associated with these subclasses as well. Genetically determined immunoglobulin allotypes have been described, but they are of uncertain significance.

The most abundant immunoglobulin in serum is IgG. This protein circulates in the monomeric form and participates actively in many immunological processes. Under normal circumstances, it appears in the circulation 10-14 days after the start of an acute infection. It is the primary circulating immunoglobulin produced on second exposure to an infecting organism. Most of the antibodies produced in autoimmune illness, such as antinuclear antibodies, are in this class.

The second major immunoglobulin with a well-defined role in immune defense mechanisms is IgM. The intact IgM molecule consists of five immunoglobulin monomers joined together. IgM is the first antibody produced as part of the primary immune response. Most rheumatoid factor is in this class, and IgM is a major constituent of most cryoglobulins.

IgA is important in secretory immunity. Isolated acquired IgA deficiencies are observed in asymptomatic patients, and in persons with frequent respiratory or gastrointestinal infections. This immunoglobulin is produced by plasma cells located in areas adjacent to mucosal surfaces. Usually, two IgA molecules are joined together by a J chain. Epithelial cells attach an additional secretory component, which facilitates the secretion of IgA into fluids such as saliva and breast milk.

IgE is synthesized in plasma cells. It is found in serum as well as attached to mast cells and circulating basophils. IgE molecules are freely mobile on the cell membrane, and many different antigen specificities are represented on each cell.

The role of IgD is not yet defined. This immunoglobulin is found in the serum as well as on the surface of mature B lymphocytes. It has been postulated that the absence of surface IgD on immature lymphocytes allows for the development of tolerance to "self" antigens during fetal development.

Complement System

The complement system is a collection of circulating proteins that differ in size and other physical characteristics. The primary components of this system are nine peptide chains numbered C1-C9. There are two pathways to complement activation. The classical pathway is activated by the interaction of C1q and a molecule of IgM or two molecules of IgG that are bound to specific antigen. Aggregates of IgG will also activate the classic pathway. The alternative pathway requires additional factors, primarily properdin and factors B and D, to activate the complement cascade beginning with C3. This pathway can be triggered by an expanding list of substances, including IgA and endotoxin.

Complement factors have a variety of biological activities. These include chemotaxis, immune adherence, stimulation of histamine release, and cytotoxicity. Labeled anticomplement antibodies are used to identify complement components in tissue sections from patients and laboratory animals with a variety of disease states. This provides presumptive evidence of complement involvement in the condition under study.

Inactivators of the complement cascade have been described. C1 esterase inhibitor binds to C1 esterase blocking the activation of C4. With the help of beta-1-H, C3 inactivator cleaves C3b into two biologically inert compounds, C3c and C3d. The inactivation of C3b inhibits both the classic and alternative complement pathways.

MECHANISMS OF IMMUNOLOGICAL RESPONSE

Recognition

Immune recognition proceeds through a well-defined sequence of events. An immunogen is first recognized by macrophages, processed, and then presented to T lymphocytes. Lymphokines may then direct the mobilization of additional lymphocytes, macrophages, and other effector cells. If an immunoglobulin response is called for, B lymphocytes will be recruited. B cells proliferate and produce plasma cells developing first IgM and then IgG antibodies. Some less complex antigens, such as bacterial polysaccharide, are capable of provoking an antibody response without the involvement of T lymphocytes. These antigens are called T-independent antigens.

The anamnestic immune response requires less elaborate interaction. Certain drugs and aging itself may be associated with an impaired primary immune response but an intact secondary response.

The genetically determined histocompatibility antigen system plays a major role in this process. This is the means by which immune response cells recognize normal host cells from foreign antigens. It is also important in the cell-to-cell interaction that occurs as part of the immune response. The histocompatibility complex is termed HLA in humans and H-2 in the mouse. In humans, four loci have been defined. They are given the letter designations A-D. Some of the HLA-defined surface antigens provoke a serological response. Others are detected by the proliferation of lymphocytes cocultured with allogenic cells in the mixed lymphocyte reaction (MLR). The major histocompatibility complex also participates in regulating the vigor of the immune response.

Response

Immune responses take several forms. In health, each begins with a series of directed and specific cellular and humoral events that may terminate in nonspecific activity, such as the release of mast cell mediators or the activation of macrophages. Protective mechanisms function as part of this system to limit responses and prevent inadvertent damage to host tissues. These mechanisms include suppression of immunoglobulin production and cell-mediated cytotoxicity by lymphocytes, inactivation of mast cell products by macrophages and eosinophils, and proteins that inactivate components of the complement cascade. Disease results from improper regulation of the immune response.

Congenital defects of most of the components of the immune response have been described, and acquired abnormalities have also been reported. These may result from or be associated with drug therapy, infection, neoplasm, or aging. At a cellular level, dysfunction may be caused by abnormal helper or suppressor cell activity, blocking antibodies, circulating immune complexes, or primary effector cell abnormalities. All of these mechanisms may play a role in the immunological dysfunction of the elderly.

Human and laboratory models of illness caused by immunological processes are protean in their manifestations. Examples are autoimmune diseases, lymphoproliferative disorders, allergies, and plasma cell dyscrasias. In most cases, the mechanism by which these immunological disorders occurs is unknown. Loss of tolerance plays a part in some conditions. Whether this occurs at the recognition or the response level is unknown.

Coombs and Gell (1963) have divided immune responses into four types. Although in vivo there is frequent overlap between these groups, they provide a useful means of understanding the diversity of the immune response.

Immediate Hypersensitivity

Immediate hypersensitivity reactions are caused by homocytotropic antibody-induced mast cell activation. The most common mechanism for this is the interaction of cell surface IgE and a specific antigen. Studies with anti-IgE and anti-IgE receptor antibodies have demonstrated that the initiation of the mast cell response requires two cell membrane IgE receptors to be brought together by the reaction of two IgE molecules with an antigen. There is some evidence to suggest that certain immunoglobulins of the IgG class, termed "short-termed sensitizing antibody," may also activate mast cells. Radiographic contrast media, opiates, and other drugs may directly induce the release of mast cell mediators in susceptible individuals. This can result in an anaphylactoid reaction. Aspirin and other cyclooxygenase inhibitors can produce bronchospasm and related symptoms in susceptible individuals. Since these drugs block the synthesis of prostaglandins, it is thought that they may direct the common precursor arachidonic acid into the lipoxygenase pathway, resulting in increased symptoms due to production of slow-reacting substance of anaphylaxis (SRS-A). Alternatively, a decrease in bronchodilating prostaglandins may account for this interesting disorder.

All of these mechanisms result in reactions beginning as soon as a few minutes after exposure. The rapidity of the response will be determined by the route of challenge. The extent of the reaction is in large part related to host factors. Particularly important may be the status of the autonomic nervous system and the distribution of autonomic receptors on target cells.

The atopic predisposition of an individual can be assessed by immediate hypersensitivity skin tests, as well as serum measurements of total and antigen-specific IgE. The latter is measured by means of the radioallergosorbent test (RAST).

Direct Cytotoxicity

Direct cytotoxicity is mediated by antigen-specific antibody. Once bound to a cell membrane, additional mechanisms of inflammation are recruited. This may include activation of the classic complement pathway or mobilization of cytotoxic effector cells, such as lymphocytes and neutrophils. Macrophages in the liver and spleen remove antibody and complement-coated cells from the circulation. Some drug reactions and a variety of hematological disorders are associated with cytotoxic antibody damage. In some cases, such as Graves' disease, autoimmune antibodies may provoke hypersecretion from endocrine glands.

Immune Complexes

An immune complex is formed when a specific antibody reacts with its soluble antigen. Immune complexes can bind complement as well as other serum proteins. Disease is thought to occur when immune complexes are trapped and activate complement in locations such as the renal glomerulus, joints, or lungs. Serum sickness is a diffuse vasculitis resulting from the deposition of immune complexes. When heterologous serum was used for treating infection, serum sickness was a common occurrence. Since antibiotics and immunization have made the use of heterologous serum less common, the study of immune complexes is now focused on the collagen vascular diseases, neoplasms, infectious diseases, and unexplained inflammatory disorders.

The postulated mechanism for immune complex disease is that circulating immune complexes are deposited in tissues based on their size and charge characteristics. Deposited complexes activate complement, resulting in organ damage. Animal models of immune complex-induced glomerulonephritis support this theory. This model does not explain the heterogeneity of presentation, from asymptomatic to fulminant disease, of patients with apparently similar immune complexes. An alternative hypothesis is that some immune complex diseases are the result of antigen-antibody interactions originating in the target organ.

Circulating immune complexes may be detected by the Raji cell assay, several C1q-based binding assays, cryoprecipitation, polyethylene glycol precipitation, nephelometry, and other techniques. All of these methods have limitations and no two methods are in consistent agreement. Immune complexes in tissue are detected by staining histology sections with labeled antibodies against complement and immunoglobulin. The detection of abnormal quantities of these proteins in an irregular (lumpy-bumpy) pattern is presumptive evidence of immune complex deposition.

Cryoglobulins are a type of immune complex with marked temperature-dependent solubility. They may contain only one class of immunoglobulin or may be of the mixed type. Frequently, cryoglobulin molecules contain an anti-immunoglobulin.

There is evidence that mast cell mediators participate in human immune complex disease. In some animal systems, platelets play a similar role. Vasoactive mediators facilitate the deposition of immune complexes at blood vessel basement membranes. Antihistamines have inhibited the development of serum sickness in clinical settings.

Cell-Mediated Immunity

Lymphocytes and macrophages are the principle effectors of cell-mediated immunity. This response is important in the defense against organisms such as mycobacteria and fungi, in eradicating neoplastic cells, and in contact hypersensitivity.

Cell-mediated immunity can be assessed in vivo and in vitro. The principle in vivo test is the intradermal injection of 0.1 ml of a specially treated and prepared form of a microbiological antigen such as purified protein derivative of *Mycobacterium* (PPD), tetanus toxoid, *Candida albicans*, streptokinase-streptodornase, or tricophyton. There is no single antigen to which all patients respond, so a selected panel is required to define responsiveness. After 48 hr, the development of an appropriate area of induration at the site of the injection provides presumptive evidence that cell-mediated immunity is intact. Patients may not respond to a specific antigen because they have not been exposed to that organism previously, because of a specific or generalized loss of immunological memory (anergy), or because of effector cell failure. In some instances of impaired cellular immunity, the response may be abnormally delayed rather than absent. The development of anergy can be due to the infection itself, and responsiveness may be restored after the disease is treated.

In vitro tests of cell-mediated immunity are most often based on the induction of lymphocyte proliferation when exposed to mitogens. Mitogens are compounds that nonspecifically stimulate large numbers of lymphocytes. Specific antigens, such as PPD, have a similar effect on sensitized cells. Common mitogens for T cells include phytohemagglutinin, concanavalin A, and pokeweed mitogen. Pokeweed mitogen will also nonspecifically stimulate B lymphocytes. Newer tests have been or are being developed to further assess cellular immunity. These tests measure functions such as chemotaxis, migration inhibition, and cytotoxicity.

ACKNOWLEDGMENTS

I want to thank C. E. Buckley and Hillel Koren for their thoughtful comments and Elsie Morris and Julie Farr for their able secretarial assistance.

REFERENCES

Adkinson, N. F. (1980). The radioallergosorbent test: uses and abuses. *J. Allergy Clin. Immunol. 65*: 1-4.

Aisenberg, A. C. (1981). Cell surface markers in lymphoproliferative disease. *N. Engl. J. Med. 304*: 331-336.

Ammann, A. J., and Hong, R. (1971). Selective IgA deficiency: presentation of 30 cases and a review of the literature. *Medicine 50*: 223-236.

Amos, D. B., and Kostyu, D. D. (1980). HLA—a central immunological agency of man. *Adv. Hum. Genet. 10*: 137-208.

Askenase, P. W. (1980). Effector cells in late and delayed cutaneous hypersensitivity reactions that are dependent on antibodies or T-cells. In *Progress in Immunology IV*, J. Pausset (Ed.). Academic Press, New York, pp. 829-845.

Austen, K. F., and Orange, R. P. (1975). Bronchial asthma: the possible role of the chemical mediators of immediate hypersensitivity in the pathogenesis of subacute chronic disease. *Am. Rev. Resp. Dis. 112*: 423-436.

Butterworth, A. E., and David, J. R. (1981). Eosinophil function. *N. Engl. J. Med. 304*: 154-156.

Chess, L., and Schlossman, S. F. (1977). Human lymphocyte subpopulations. *Adv. Immunol. 25*: 213-241.

Coombs, R. R. A., and Gell, P. G. H. (1963). The Classification of Allergic Reactions Underlying Disease. In *Clinical Aspects of Immunology*, P. G. H. Gell and R. R. A. Coombs (Eds.). F. A. Davis, Philadelphia, pp. 317-337.

Fearon, D. T., and Austen, K. F. (1980). The alternative pathway of complement —a system for host resistance to microbial infection. *N. Engl. J. Med. 303*: 259-263.

Fey, G., and Colten, H. R. (1981). Biosynthesis of complement components. *Fed. Proc. 40*: 2099-2104.

Fudenberg, H. H., Strites, D. P., Caldwell, J. L., and Wells, J. V. (1980). *Basic and Clinical Immunology*. Lange Medical Publications, Los Altos, Calif.

Grey, H. M., and Kohler, P. F. (1973). Cryoimmunoglobulins. *Sem. Hematol. 10*: 87-112.

Lambert, P. H., Dixon, F. J., Zubler, R. H., Agnello, V., Cambiaso, C., Casali, P., Clarke, J., Cowdery, J. S., McDuffie, F. C., Hay, F. C., MacLennan, I. C. M., Masson, P., Muller-Eberhard, H. J., Penttinen, K., Smith, M., Tappeiner, G., Theofilopoulos, A. N., and Verroust, P. (1978). A WHO collaborative study for the evaluation of eighteen methods for detecting immune complexes in serum. *J. Clin. Lab. Immunol. 1*: 1-15.

McDevitt, H. O. (1980). Regulation of the immune response by the major histocompatibility system. *N. Engl. J. Med. 303*: 1514-1517.

Middleton, E., Jr., Reed, C. E., and Ellis, E. F. (1978). *Allergy Principles and Practice*. C. V. Mosby, St. Louis.

Nathan, C. F., Murray, H. W., and Cohn, Z. N. (1980). The macrophage as an effector cell. *N. Engl. J. Med. 303*: 622-626.

Parker, C. W. (1980). *Clinical Immunology*. Saunders, Philadelphia.

Patterson, R. (1979). *Allergic Diseases: Diagnosis and Management*. Lippincott, Philadelphia.

Reinherz, E., and Schlossman, S. F. (1980). Regulation of the immune response— induce and suppressor T-lymphocyte subsets in human beings. *N. Engl. J. Med. 303*: 370-373.

Rose, N. R., and Friedman, H. (1980). *Manual of Clinical Immunology*. 2nd ed. American Society for Microbiology, Washington, D.C.

Sirois, P., and Borgeat, P. (1980). From slow reacting substance of anaphylaxis (SRS-A) to leukotriene D4 (LTD4). *Int. J. Immunophasmac. 2*: 281-293.

Theofilopoulos, A. N., and Dixon, F. J. (1979). The biology and detection of immune complexes. *Adv. Immunol. 28*: 89-220.

Unanue, E. R. (1980). Cooperation between mononuclear phagocytes and lymphycytes in immunity. *N. Engl. J. Med. 303*: 977-985.

Waldmann, T. A., Blaese, R. M., Broder, S., and Krakauer, R. S. (1978). Disorders of suppressor immunoregulatory cells in the pathogenesis of immunodeficiency and autoimmunity. *Ann. Intern. Med. 88*: 226-238.

7

Treatments that Retard or Reverse Immunological Losses Due to Aging

Joy Cavagnaro* / *Duke University Medical Center, Durham, North Carolina*

EFFECTS OF AGE ON THE IMMUNE SYSTEM

The immune system is important in controlling the age-determined evolution of physiological changes. The effectiveness of this control may be influenced by the age-related decline in the immune system (Hirokowa, 1972; Roberts-Thomson et al., 1974; Makinodan et al., 1977; Kay, 1979). This decline, manifested by a decrease in the number and function of immune cells or alteration of the environment in which they function, may be responsible for the diseases which are associated with increasing age.

Experiments using in vivo cell transfer techniques have shown that the immune system's control is influenced by both intrinsic and extrinsic factors (Price and Makinodan, 1972a, b; Singhal et al., 1978; Kay, 1979). Intrinsically, the selectivity and the extent of this process is genetically determined by the major histocompatibility complex (MHC) in mice and the HLA system in man (Greenberg and Yunis, 1978; Smith and Walford, 1978; Yunis and Lane, 1979; Amos and Yunis, in press; Williams and Yunis, in press). Extrinsically, environmental factors including chronic antigen stimulation and virus infection may be involved.

Changes in the T-cell populations in the lymphoid organs and the peripheral blood probably account for most of the functional decline that accompanies aging (Kishimoto et al., 1978; Yunis and Lane, 1979). Such changes, represented as an

*Present affiliation: Hazleton Laboratories America, Inc., Vienna, Virginia

133

age-related decrease in T-cell function, are reflected in the normal age-dependent involution of the thymus (Kay and Makinodan, 1976; Yunis and Lane, 1979; Weksler, 1980). Most studies of age-associated immune changes have concentrated on cellular function (e.g., cell-mediated immunity) as related to the involution of the thymus gland, the decline in thymus hormone levels with age (Yunis and Lane, 1979; Weksler, 1980), and qualitative defects in both T cells and B cells (Callard et al. 1979; Weksler, 1980). It is also interesting to consider some biochemical factors which may be involved.

Callard et al. (1979) proposed that metabolic or structural abnormalities affecting the cell membrane may prevent the aged immune cells from responding normally to extrinsic signals. Following analysis of spleen cell populations from old Lewis rats and from young Lewis rats, Woda and Feldman (1979) suggested that changes in capping (cell surface polarization of membrane components) in old rats were due, in part, to alterations in membrane fluidity and cytoskeleton function. Age-related biochemical changes have further been attributed to the appearance of a unique class of cytoplasmic filaments in lymphoid cells (Phillips and Koppenheffer, 1978).

A pituitary factor might also promote immune senescence, via direct interference with cyclic nucleotide metabolism (Denckla, 1974, 1978) by blocking the action of thyroid hormone in adenyl cyclase synthesis (Parker et al., 1974; Tam and Walford, 1978). Watson (1975) suggested that alterations in the ratio of cyclic adenosine monophosphate (cAMP) to cyclic guanosine monophosphate (cGMP) might have a controlling effect on cell proliferation. Later, Tam et al. (1979) reported an age-related decrease in splenic cAMP and an increase in cGMP.

Other biochemical factors which may contribute to the immunodeficient state of the aged are the levels and activities of certain enzymes. Scholar et al. (1980) showed that a decrease in purine nucleoside phosphorylase (PNP), an enzyme involved in purine metabolism, is related to depressed T-cell function. There is also evidence which suggests that an endogenous chromosomal protease may be involved with the thymus gland and the aging process (Cavagnaro et al., 1978).

A common diisopropylfluorophosphate- (DFP) binding protease shown to migrate at 25,000 daltons on SDS polyacrylamide gel electrophoresis has been found in a variety of rat and mouse tissues (Furlan et al., 1968; Kurecki et al., 1975; Heinrich et al., 1976; Cavagnaro et al., 1980). This 25,000-dalton serine protease associated with chromatin can be cross-linked to the DNA in chromatin by formaldehyde under conditions which favor selective cross-linking of DNA-bound protein to DNA (Brutlag et al., 1969; Bartley and Chalkley, 1970; Jackson and Chalkley, 1974; Chalkley and Hunter, 1975; Doenecke and McCarthy, 1975a, b; Jackson, 1978) (Fig. 1) (Cavagnaro, 1979).

When the chromatin from aging tissue is labeled with (^{3}H)-DFP, there is a sharp increase in binding of DFP exclusive to the thymus gland, while the level of the chromosomal protease(s) in the other tissues remains constant (Fig. 2) (Cavagnaro, 1979). This sharp increase in the level of the thymus chromosomal protease

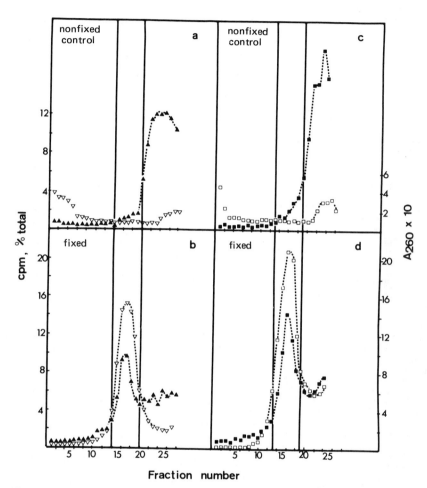

Figure 1 Equilibrium density-banding patterns of (^{3}H)-DFP-labeled chromatin in cesium chloride after treatment with formaldehyde. (a) Thymus chromatin, non-fixed control; (b) thymus chromatin, fixed; (c) spleen chromatin, nonfixed control; and (d) spleen chromatin, fixed. The absorbance was monitored at 260 nm and an aliquot was assayed for percent total radioactivity. Fractions were collected from the bottom of the tube. Open symbols, A_{260}; closed symbols, percent total radioactivity in counts per minute.

of the aged animal may be due to the activation of the protease in the residual T cells in aged animals or to the proportionate increase in the nonlymphoid mass, which may have a higher level of the chromosomal protease than the T cells. It is assumed that the protease is involved in the continuous turnover of chromosomal proteins throughout the cell cycle and in the limited turnover of histone H1 in the

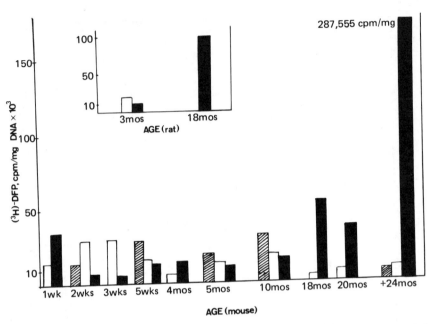

Figure 2 Level of chromosomal protease during aging. Chromatin was labeled with (^{3}H)-DFP (50 μCi/mg/ml DNA at 4°C for 36 hr and dialyzed against 0.01 M sodium phosphate buffer, pH 7.0 containing 1% sodiumdodecylsulfate and 0.1% 2-mercaptoethanol). Aliquots were counted for radioactivity in a scintillation counter and counts per minute per milligram DNA were determined. Chromatin: kidney (□), liver (□), and thymus (■).

G1 phase of the cell cycle (Hale, 1978). Further studies on the nuclear protease of the thymus may help to explain the biochemical influence of the thymus on the immunology of aging.

Immune Cells

Lymphocytes and macrophages, both derived from bone marrow stem cells, are involved in most types of immune responses. The lymphocytes are further classified as T cells and B cells, and differ morphologically, functionally, and ontogenetically during maturation and senescence (Leech, 1980). The age-dependent efficiency to mount an immune response depends on the interaction and collaboration of T cells, B cells, and macrophages. The age-related decline in responsiveness may be attributed to an alteration(s) in the qualitative or functional property of any or all of these cell populations (Fig. 3).

Macrophages from old mice are abnormal in their ability to function as stimulator cells in the allogeneic mixed lymphocyte reaction (MLR) (Callard, 1978), although their ability to collaborate with T and B cells in antibody production is

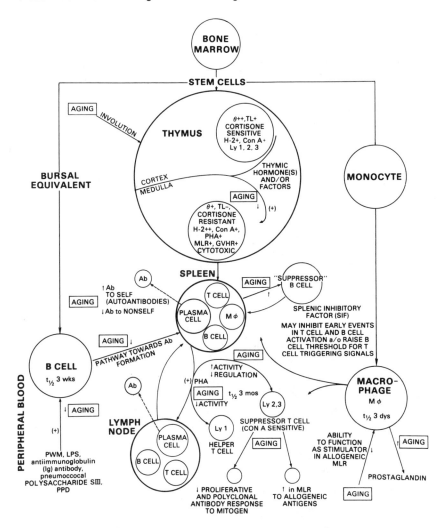

Figure 3 Model outlining the developmental stages and interrelationships of immune cells. (↑) Increase, (↓) decrease.

not impaired with age (Price and Makinodan, 1972a, b; Teller, 1972a, b; Heidrick and Makinodan, 1973; Konen et al., 1973).

Aging promotes a decline in maturation and immune reactivity of T cells (Makinodan and Adler, 1975; Han and Johnson, 1976; Kay, 1978; Rosenstein and Strausser, 1980), but the relative percent of peripheral T cells remains normal (Yunis and Lane, 1979). There is an age-associated increase in the number of suppressor T cells, suggested by the increase in the number of I-J bearing cells (Callard et al., 1979) and an increase in the number of T cells possessing receptors for immunoglobulin-G-containing immune complexes (Moretta et al., 1977; Kishimoto et al., 1978). Concomitant with the suppressor cell changes with age, which include a failure in the mechanism of regulation of these cells (Naor et al., 1976), is the decline of the helper function of T cells with age (Price and Makinodan, 1972a, b; Hardin et al., 1973; Heidrick and Makinodan, 1973).

In addition to the age-related changes in suppressor and helper T cells, there is a significant defect in the effectiveness of the B-cell population which accompanies age (Makinodan and Adler, 1975; Kishimoto et al., 1976). It appears as though aging causes some type of deregulation which permits an increased expression of autoreactive B-cell clones (Meredith and Walford, 1979). B cells from aged mice also respond to, and are poorly inhibited by, anti-immunoglobulin (Scribner et al., 1978). This response appears to occur as a result of decreased receptor-mediated immunoregulation of the responding B cells. The recent experiments of Nariuchi and Adler (1979) further support the idea that age-associated B-cell changes are qualitative changes. They proposed that B cells from aged mice have a defect in their metabolic pathway which is essential for antibody formation but is not necessary for proliferation.

In addition to the above studies, Singhal et al., (1978) have demonstrated an age-related increase in suppressor B cells, as well as increased release of low molecular weight soluble factors capable of suppressing in vitro plaque-forming cell (PFC) response. They concluded that the deficient immune response in aging animals is not the result of an intrinsic deficit in B-cell responsiveness or lack of progenitor cells, but rather results from an active block in some late maturation stage, such as T- or B-cell activation by antigen or mitogen.

Regardless of the qualitative or quantitative affects on the immune cells, the integrity and efficiency of the immune system depends upon the effective interaction of both the cellular (T cell) and humoral (antibody-mediated) subsystems (Meredith and Walford, 1979) (Table 1).

Cell-Mediated Immunological Responses

Age-related effects have been investigated in many areas of the cellular immune system. These investigations have included the actions of cytotoxic T cells, natural killer cells (NK), and suppressor T cells. Konen et al. (1973) showed a decrease in stimulation in the MLR with age. More recently, Schulof et al. (1980) reported that aged subjects exhibited intact autologous concanavalin A- (Con-A) induced suppressor cell activity, but a depressed allogeneic activity when compared with young subjects. Kyewski and Wekerle (1978) also found a decrease in the allogeneic and mitogen responsiveness in aged rats (20 months) when compared with young controls (3 months).

In 1980, Kruisbeck and Steinmeir reported on the biological relevance of high-frequency alloreactive T cells. These cells, which specifically lyse autologous cells

Table 1 Effects of Age on the Immune System

Immune cells	References
Decrease in T-cell immune reactivity	Rosenstein and Strausser, 1979; Antel et al., 1980
Shift in relative proportions of T-cell progenitors	Antel et al., 1980
Age-related decrease in mouse T-cell progenitors	Tyan, 1977
Cessation of stem cell movement into the thymus	Kay, 1978
Decrease in proportion of lymphocytes bearing the theta antigen	Brennan and Jaraslow, 1975
Decline in Ly-1, 2, 3 cells, increase in Ly-1 and Ly-2, 3 cells	Cantor et al., 1978
Decline in helper function T cells	Price and Makinodan, 1972a,b; Hardin et al., 1973; Heidrick and Makinodan, 1973; Krogsrud and Perkins, 1977; Callard and Basten, 1978; Greenberg and Yunis, 1978; Leech, 1980
Decrease in ease of induction of tolerance in helper T cells	DeKruyff et al., 1980
Increase in I-J-bearing T cells corresponding to the presence of T-cell suppressors	Callard et al., 1978; Perry et al., 1978
Increase in suppressor T-cell activities in long-lived mice	Price and Makinodan, 1972a,b; Goidl et al., 1976; Segre and Segre, 1976; Callard et al., 1980
Decrease in regulatory function by suppressor T cells	Naor et al., 1976
Decrease in effectiveness of the B-cell population	Makinodan and Adler, 1975; Kishimoto et al., 1976
Reduced capacity of B cells to respond to T-dependent antigens	DeKruyff et al., 1980
Increase of suppressor B cells	Singhal et al., 1978
Impaired ability of the macrophages to collaborate with T and B cells in antibody production (antigen handling during both induction of immune response and phagocytosis)	Price and Makinodan, 1972a,b; Teller, 1972a,b; Heidrick and Makinodan, 1973; Konen et al., 1973
Abnormal ability of macrophages to function as stimulator cells in allogeneic MLR	Callard, 1978

Table 1 (continued)

Cell-mediated immunological responses	References
Decrease in stimulation in MLR (indicator system for cellular immunity)	Adler et al., 1971; Hori et al., 1973; Konen et al., 1973; Gerbase-DeLima et al., 1975; Meredith et al., 1975; Gershon et al., 1979

Decrease in allo and mitogen responsiveness
   Supression of PHA, PWM, PPD, and pneumococcal polysaccharide III
   Depressed allogeneic Con-A-induced suppressor cell activity
	Heidrick and Makinodan, 1972; Konen et al., 1973; Adler, 1975; Hallgren et al., 1975; Pisciotta et al., 1976; Gershon et al., 1979; Kyewski and Wekerle, 1980; Schulof et al., 1980

Decline in cell-mediated lymphocytotoxic reaction (CML) (involves the killer lymphocytes and is important in the response to viruses; moderate against allogeneic tumor cells and not readily apparent against certain syngeneic tumor cells)	Teller, 1972a,b; Goodman and Makinodan, 1975
Increase in antibody-dependent lymphocyte-mediated cytotoxicity (ADLMC)	Haffer et al., 1979
Resistance to challenge with syngeneic and allogeneic tumor cells in vivo	Stjernsward, 1966
Decreased ability to mount GVH (increased retention of allografts)	Teller et al., 1964; Heidrick and Makinodan, 1972; Walters and Claman, 1975
Deficiency in production of cytotoxic cells following appropriate stimulation in vitro	Goodman and Makinodan, 1975; Shigemoto et al., 1975
Decline in natural killer-cell-(NK) mediated cytotoxicity	Herberman et al., 1975; Kiessling et al., 1975; Nunn et al., 1976

Humoral immunological responses	References
Defect in metabolic pathway which is for antibody formation but is not necessary for proliferation	Callard and Basten, 1978; Nariuchi and Adler, 1979
Decrease in antibody production	Friedman and Globerson, 1978
Decline in antibody response in vivo to foreign antigens	Makinodan and Peterson, 1966; Cheney and Walford, 1974; Makinodan et al., 1976; Leech, 1980
Reduction of primary and secondary antibody responses to T-dependent antigens and the IgM response to T-independent antigens	Callard et al., 1977; Callard and Basten, 1978

Table 1   (continued)

Humoral immunological responses	References
Decline in responses to T-dependent antigens and a concomitant decrease in autoantibody production against DNA in NZB mice	Talal and Steinberg, 1974; Roder et al., 1977
Decline in plaque-forming cell response (accompanied by the appearance of suppressor B cells in the spleen and increase in the ability of cells from bone marrow to suppress anti-SRBC response to young syngeneic spleen cells in vitro)	Singhal et al., 1978
Increase in proliferative response to anti-Ig	Scribner et al., 1978
Decrease of suppressor activity of antigen-primed spleen cells	Butenko and Adrianova, 1979
Increase in nonspecific B-cell suppression as cells migrate from bone marrow to peripheral lymphoid organs	Leech, 1980
Decrease of avidity of antibody produced by mice (restriction in magnitude and heterogeneity)	Goidl et al., 1976; Doria et al., 1978; Leech, 1980
Increase in B-cell activity in producing autoantibodies	Leech, 1980

coupled to trinitrobenzene sulfonate, represent the consequence of the T-cell response against self, modified by various agents (e.g., chemical modification, viral antigens, or malignant transformation). They hypothesized from their results that either a decline in suppressor cells or a prolonged exposure to autologous major histocompatibility (MHC) determinants modified by natural pathogens might be involved in the generation of the increased spectrum of age-dependent cross-reactivities observed (Kruisbeck and Steinmeir, 1980).

There is a deficiency in aged animals in the production of cytotoxic cells following appropriate stimulation in vivo (Shigemoto et al., 1975; Goodman and Makinodan, 1975). There is also an age-dependent affect on the expression of natural killer-cell- (NK) mediated cytotoxicity in mice (Herberman et al., 1975; Kiessling et al., 1975) and rats (Nunn et al., 1976; Shellam and Hogg, 1977). Although exceptions have been noted, activity is generally higher in younger animals and starts to decline with age (Altman and Rapp, 1978).

The graft-vs.-host (GVH) assay has also been used in studies relating immune function and age. The syngeneic GVH response between old donors and young host cells represents an immunological attack that is due to the antigenic differences between the two. The differences that exist between old and young animals have been attributed to the former's loss of regulatory function (perhaps regulated by suppressor cells or suppressor humoral factors), thus permitting reactive clones to express themselves (Gozes et al., 1978; Kay, 1979).

Humoral Immunological Responses

Many reports indicate that there is a decreased antibody (Ab) response in vivo coincident with increasing age (Makinodan and Peterson, 1966; Cheney and Walford, 1974; Makinodan et al., 1976), as well as a decrease of antigen-binding capacity of the antibody that is produced (Goidl et al., 1976). Greenberg and Yunis (1978) and Friedman and Globerson (1978) concluded that the decline in Ab-forming capacity was due primarily to a decrease in T-helper-cell activity. The humoral response to T-dependent antigens appeared to decline faster and at an earlier age than the ability to respond to T-independent antigens (Greenberg and Yunis, 1978).

Data obtained by Butenko and Adrianova (1979) showed a decreased suppressor activity of the antigen-primed spleen cells from animals of increasing age. The adoptive transfer of spleen cells of primed young-adult mice suppressed antibody production in immunized recipients, whereas that of primed spleen cells from aged mice produced no reaction.

Roder et al. (1978a) studied suppressed humoral immunity using NZB strain mice which exhibit a progressive age-dependent decline in response to T-dependent antigens and mitogens, as well as a concomitant decline in autoantibody production against DNA (Talal and Steinberg, 1974; Roder et al., 1977). Results indicated that the suppression of immunity could be attributed to the presence of soluble mediators released from spontaneously appearing splenic suppressor cells (Roder et al., 1978b).

The studies of Callard and Basten (1978) supported the idea that a defect exists in B cells which is independent of T-cell help. Their experimental system involved the adoptive transfer of purified lymphocyte populations derived from the spleens of old and young mice into young irradiated recipients. A dramatic decline in B-cell function with age was demonstrated in both primary and secondary antibody responses. The authors attributed the defect to a loss in the potential of old B cells to enter the differential pathway towards antibody-forming cells. The kinetics of the primary response of both young and old animals, as well as the number of antibody cell precursors between each group, were comparable. More recently, Callard et al. (1980) have suggested that the age-related decline in T-cell-dependent antibody responses is probably best explained in terms of a qualitative defect at the level of both the B cell and the helper T cell.

Finally, Delpierre et al. (1980) have shown that aged lymphoid cells, either in vitro or in vivo, during natural senescence, synthesize or activate specific protein(s) capable of interfering with the differentiation of stimulated lymphocytes into antibody-producing cells. The exact mechanism has not been determined.

FACTORS CONTROLLING GROWTH AND AGE INVOLUTION OF THE THYMUS

It appears that the immune system is unique in attempts to intervene in the age-associated physical deterioration processes. More importantly, it is a system that interacts with, protects, and affects activities of all other systems (Kay, 1979). In this section, a decline in the rate of deterioration of the immune system will be discussed with respect to in vivo macroenvironmental manipulation, (e.g., dietary restriction and lowering of body temperature, as well as surgical and chemical interventions). An excellent review of this topic has been reported earlier by Makinodan (1978).

Regulation of Diet

Dietary restriction early in life reportedly prolongs proper immunological responsiveness (Ross, 1972; Walford et al., 1974; Young, 1978). Dietary restrictions appear to alter the age-dependent changes in the growth and structure of the thymus (Weindruch and Suffin, 1980). When 6-month-old mice maintained on a restricted diet were compared with unrestricted-diet controls, the thymuses of the former appeared histologically younger than those of controls. Furthermore, they showed a more vigorous spleen cell proliferative response to the T-cell mitogens PHA and Con-A.

Dietary restriction also appears to influence the life span of the short-lived, autoimmune-prone NZB-NZW (B/W) mouse. Early studies by Fernandes et al. (1976, 1977a,b, and 1978) showed that dietary manipulation inhibited thymic involution and the age-related decline in certain immunological functions in B/W mice. In later experiments, Safai-Kutti et al. (1980) suggested that restricted diets may inhibit the formation and deposition of immune complexes in vital organs. Other investigations utilizing NZB mice showed that diets relatively high in fat and low in protein and fiber accelerated the development of autoimmune disease and shortened life span; diets high in protein and fiber and low in fat, however, delayed the development of autoimmunity, thereby prolonging the life span in these animals (Fernandes et al., 1972, 1973, and 1978; Fernandes, 1979; Fernandes et al., 1979).

A relationship between dietary protein and carbohydrate intake has also been reported concerning the metabolism of serotonin and catecholamines. These substances ultimately influence the control of pituitary hormone output (Wurtman et al., 1974). This will be of interest in the final section of this chapter where the interrelationships between the neuroendocrine and immune systems will be discussed.

The effect of selective nutrient deficiencies has also been explored with respect to prolongation of life span (Schloen et al., 1979). Experiments by Chandra et al. (1980) showed that deficiencies of calories, zinc, and pyridoxine resulted in significant lowering of serum thymic hormonal activity, whereas deficiency in vitamin A had no effect. Specific nutrients may thus modulate different steps in cell-mediated immunity.

Lowering of Body Temperature

The immune response in animals is influenced by environmental temperature (Tait, 1969; Jaraslow, 1971; Cone and Marcholonis, 1972; Liu and Walford, 1972, 1975; Egami, 1980). Both humoral antibody production and cell-mediated immunity are suppressed when immunized animals are maintained at low environmental temperatures. Evidence from Cone and Marcholonis (1972) suggests that the different phases of the immune response can be dissociated and certain steps in the maturation of immunocompetent cells can be influenced by environmental temperature changes. The experiments of Liu and Walford (1972, 1975) and a recent review by Egami (1980) demonstrate that mild hypothermia can prolong the life span of poikilothermic vertebrates.

Surgical Manipulation

Selective surgery at a well-defined time in development can extend the life span. In 1944, McEndy et al. reported that the thymus is a key organ in determining the time of death in short-lived AKR mice, since thymectomy of very young animals prolonged their life span. Later, Furth also showed that AKR mice would live longer if they were thymectomized before they manifested the tumors characteristic of their strain (Furth, 1946). The temporal importance of thymectomy was stressed in studies by Nakakuki et al. (1967) who reported that the incidence of leukemia in AKR mice was reduced; hence, their mean survival time was enhanced, but only when thymectomy was performed on animals between 35 and 150 days of age.

In 1969, Albright et al. reported that the life expectancy of $(C57Bl \times C3H)F_1$, a long-lived mouse strain, could be doubled if spleens were removed at 2 years of age. Like thymectomy, there is a critical time period linked with increasing life expectancy (Peter et al., 1975). More recently, Meyer and Meyer (1978) have reported that splenectomy retards thymic involution. Their hypothesis focuses on polypeptides designated as immunoregulatory globulins (IRA) or IRA-like substances causing progressive thymic involution. They suggested that the long-continued presence of such factors in control animals may be responsible for the process of "normal" thymic involution.

Szewczuk and Campbell (1980) proposed that the age-dependent loss of immune competence in the spleen B-cell population was caused by the presence of auto-anti-idiotypic antibody production. Schrater et al. (1979) have suggested that this antibody produced during the aging response combines with B-cell surface antigen receptors and, thus, inhibits antibody secretion. Ablation of the spleen succeeded in depressing this response.

There has also been much evidence suggesting that the immune system is influenced directly or indirectly by the sexual endocrine system. The findings have indicated that sex steroids inhibit thymus growth, either by inhibiting cellular proliferation or by accelerating cellular loss. As early as 1940, Chiodi demonstrated that gonadectomy leads to thymic hypertrophy. Depending on the strain of the animal and the age, gonadectomy may result in either an increase in thymic growth rate or a continuation of the initial growth rate for a longer period of time (Bellamy et al., 1976). In 1974, Castro reported that the orchidectomy, but not ovariectomy, causes hypertrophy of the thymus and, hence, a delay in its involution. Experimentally, although orchidectomy has its primary effects upon thymus tissues (by delaying the rate of normal involution and augmenting cell-mediated immune responses), it also caused enlargement of lymph nodes, as well as an increase in spleen size (Castro, 1974a,b).

It is not unreasonable to suggest that the normal time of age involution in the thymus may be set by the gonads. Growth of the thymus may be initiated by gonadectomy during the early stages of age involution, at a rate equal to the preinvolution rate. However, there also appears to be an upper limit to the thymic cell population that is set independently by the gonads (Bellamy et al., 1976).

In 1937, Schacher et al. demonstrated thymus atrophy in rats following administration of adrenocortical extracts. It is, therefore, not surprising that in later studies, Ishidate and Metcalf demonstrated that adrenalectomy as a surgical intervention may lead to thymic hypertrophy (Ishidate and Metcalf, 1963).

Cell Grafts

Transplantation of aged immune tissue into healthy young recipients should determine if the age-related defect is caused by factors intrinsic or extrinsic to the immune tissue. Based on transplantation experiments, Harrison (1975) suggested that loss with age in erythrocyte production was not directly related to the age of the bone marrow cell lines. In almost all cases, bone marrow cells from old donors, which have a normal rate of proliferation, function as well as the cells from young donors, after transplantation into normal irradiated recipients. From these results, it was suggested that senescence of the organism is caused by intrinsically "timed" functional declines in only a few vital cell types. Hirokowa later showed that immune function of long-lived mice can be restored to levels approaching those of adult mice by grafting young-adult bone marrow cells and newborn thymus (Hirokowa et al., 1976).

Bone marrow cells have a substantially normal rate of proliferation which should act to select out defective cells. Thus, a conceivable method of intervention, suggested by Callard, to rejuvenate the immune system might be achieved by using existing normal stem cells to replace the defective long-lived peripheral lymphocyte pool (Callard, 1978).

Another form of intervention aimed at extending life expectancy is T-cell graft treatment. Kysela and Steinberg (1973) showed that such replacement may extend life expectancy of old NZB mice, although it did not prevent pathological changes (Yunis et al., 1971). Other experimenters showed that grafting of T cells (Ebbesen et al., 1971) or of the whole thymus (Gershwin et al., 1976) from young syngeneic donors to intact recipients did not influence the development of leukemia or the time of death in AKR or other mice (Albright and Makinodan, 1966).

Millan et al. (1980) have described their observations following transplantation of cultured thymic epithelial cells. Replacement with these cells and the suspected hormone release of thymic factors resulting from the transplant were not able to act upon the recipient's thymus to confer a capacity for cellular attraction and differentiation. Perkins et al. (1972) also attempted to restore immune function in aged mice by replacing the immune cells with those from young syngeneic mice. Experimentally, this was achieved by exposing aged mice to x-rays to destroy most of the radiosensitive immune cells, and then injecting spleen cells from young donors which had been previously immunized with *Salmonella typhimurium*. After such treatment, the aged mice were able to resist lethal doses of the virus for an extended period of time.

Although immunorestoration may be achieved by spleen grafts, it is not obvious that the life expectancy can be prolonged. This has been demonstrated by Teague et al. (1972), Yunis et al. (1971), and Yunis and Greenberg (1974), who have shown that when young spleen cells are injected into old mice, the appearance of certain types of autoantibodies is delayed or prevented, without appreciably prolonging life.

Lymph node cells, on the other hand, have been demonstrated as effective life-prolonging agents. The life span of short-lived hypopituitary dwarf mice, which suffer from a thymic immunodeficiency due to an inherited endocrine imbalance (Fabris et al., 1971), could be extended by injecting large doses of lymph node cells (Fabris et al., 1972).

Chemical Therapy

Immunological capacity has been restored in both young and aged immunologically insufficient animals using polynucleotide adjuvants (e.g., poly A:U) (Han and Johnson, 1976). In the aged mice, the poly A:U may have induced the release of soluble factors from the thymocytes. Improvement of impaired immune responses also has been observed following the joint administration of antigen and double-stranded synthetic polynucleotides (Braun et al., 1970; Halsall and Perkins, 1974). Cyclophosphamide has been used clinically to control autoimmune activity and extend foreign graft survival (Makinodan, 1978). However, later studies (Mitsuoka et al., 1979) have shown that delayed hypersensitivity (DTH) to methylated human serum albumin could be enhanced with cyclophosphamide in young mice but not in aged mice. They suggested that the enhancement with cyclophosphamide may have been the result of an elimination of suppressor T cells involved in DTH. Effector T cells were also sensitive to cyclophosphamide; however, the damaging effect was only transient.

Administration of immunostimulatory agents has also been used extensively in attempts to correct age-dependent immunodepression. Levamisole, an antihelmintic drug and immunostimulatory agent (Renoux and Renoux, 1972, 1977) has been shown to restore the impaired immunological system of aged mice (Goldstein, 1978). Studies of the in vivo effect of levamisole on antibody production in aged mice by Morimoto et al. (1979) showed that long-term administration can restore helper and suppressor T-cell function. Furthermore, they suggested that levamisole probably was not the active effector in vitro, but rather executed its effects through metabolites in vivo. Bruley-Rosset et al. (1979) showed that when bestatin, a more suitable chemical for immunorestoration than levamisole because of its absence of toxicity, was injected into young mice, it was able to activate macrophages, to potentiate humoral responses to thymus-dependent and thymus-independent antigens, and to increase the antibody-dependent cellular cytotoxicity of spleen cells. Munthe et al. (1979) have found a similar kind of therapeutic effect with penicillamine, a dimethylcysteine formed by the hydrolysis of penicillin. Some of the more specific effects of penicillamine include: reduction of the concentration of pathological immune complexes, both in the circulation and in the tissue; inhibition of PHA-induced activation of lymphocytes; enhancement of the modulation effect of macrophages on Con-A-stimulated lymph nodes; and inhibition of granulocyte migration.

In 1959, Hohn demonstrated that daily injections of thyroxine for 4 weeks into laying hens increased thymic weights and histological development of the thymic cortex. Adrenocortical steroids have been shown to increase the life span of hypophysectomized rats (Everitt, 1976) and a strain of short-lived mice (Bellamy, 1968), thereby relating adrenocortical function to life duration. As noted before, there is evidence which suggests that an excess of corticosteroids may also accelerate the aging phenomenon (Schacher et al., 1937).

Another means of chemical intervention investigated has been chalone therapy. Lymphoid tissues contain a macromolecule or macromolecules which specifically inhibit the proliferation of lymphocytes in vitro (chalones). The in vivo effects of lymphocyte chalone have been shown to include inhibition of the GVH reaction (Garcia-Giralt et al., 1972) and skin allograft rejection (Houck et al., 1973). In addition, Attallah et al. (1979) have shown that adult NZB and B/W mice are responsive to lymphocyte chalone. The loss of chalone activity with age may thus play a role in the disturbance of the negative feedback control system which contributes to NZB autoimmune disease.

Beta-aminoproprionitril (BAPN) added to the drinking water of 2-month-old male LAF/J mice significantly increased the survival time of the mice (LaBella and

Vivian, 1978). BAPN prevents the formation of stable cross-links between peptide chains in collagen and elastin (LaBella, 1971, 1972). The rationale for using this therapy as a possible inhibition of the aging process was based on the hypothesis that the drug might delay the age-related, deleterious cross-linking processes which continue with age.

The sulfhydryl compound mercaptoethanol has proved to be effective in enhancing various responses of young and old lymphocytes. Although the exact mechanism has not been defined, a variety of mechanisms have been suggested, for example, mercaptoethanol acts by replacing a macrophage factor (Chen and Hirsch, 1972; Hewlett et al., 1977); and by activating a component of fetal calf serum and/or by stabilizing cell membranes (Forsdyke and David, 1978). Makinodan and Albright (1979a,b) showed that mercaptoethanol enhanced the time of peak antibody response in certain strains of mice. Of particular interest are the studies by Heidrick et al. (1980), which showed that mercaptoethanol had a significantly greater enhancing effect on old cells when compared with young. These data suggest that mercaptoethanol, in addition to enhancing the response of functioning old cells, may partially restore function to age-defective cells.

By far, the most encouraging results of immunorestoration by chemical intervention have been the use of various thymic hormones. Thymosin restores the cellular immunity of immunodeficient animals (Asanuma et al., 1970; Dauphinee and Talal, 1975; Dauphinee et al., 1978; Goldstein et al., 1976; Goldstein et al., 1978). Further, the evidence that thymosin induces suppressor T cells makes it clinically attractive for use in certain autoimmune diseases such as systemic lupus erythematosis (SLE) (Horowitz et al., 1977). Aged spleen cells incubated with thymic humoral factor regain their in vitro GVH reactivity (Friedman and Globerson, 1978). A practical but significant reactivation of the age-related impaired immune response in aged mice can also be achieved from subcutaneous administration of thymopoietin II, the nonapeptide facteur thymique serique (FTS), or a dodecapeptide analogue of FTS (Bliznakov et al., 1978). Age-dependent immunodeficiencies were reversed, either by treating old mice with thymopoietin in vivo or by incubating their spleen cells with thymopoietin before adoptive transfer to young irradiated thymectomized syngeneic mice (Weksler et al., 1978). When young and old C_3H mice were immunized with cross-reacting rat erythrocytes, they produced erythrocyte autoantibodies that usually persisted for more than 10 weeks. Injection of thymopoietin pentapeptide (TP5), the biologically active fragment, accelerated the loss of erythrocyte autoantibodies 7 weeks after immunization (Lau et al., 1980).

THE PITUITARY-THYMUS-OVARIAN AXIS: ASSOCIATION OF NEURO-ENDOCRINE HOMEOSTATIC MECHANISMS WITH THE AGE-RELATED DETERMINATION OF CELLULAR AND HUMORAL IMMUNOLOGICAL FUNCTIONS

The growth and development of the immune system is regulated partly by the thymus and elaboration of its humoral factors. Although normal aging is probably under genetic control (i.e., MHC), part of this effect may be influenced through a regulatory center in the brain which directs the programmed events of aging. There is increasing evidence which indicates that vasoactive substances, such as catecholamines, histamines, and prostaglandins, may influence the immune response, when studied in vitro (Braun et al., 1970). In vivo, the physiological regulation of the immune system may be controlled by endocrine organs.

To date, not one of the hormones known to modulate lymphocytic organs is solely responsible for age involution. At present, it is not clear if hormonal administration produces acute involution or merely enhances the rate of normal thymic involution. Since the nervous system and endocrine system have been implicated in influencing, as well as integrating with the immune system, it was interesting to consider how changes in age, as well as experimental intervention of these systems, may influence the immune response (Fig. 4).

There appear to be significant changes with increasing age in the production of releasing hormones from the hypothalamus. Reductions have been reported for the contents of growth hormone-releasing factor (GRF), luteinizing hormone-releasing factor (LRF), and prolactin-inhibitory factor (PIF), whereas increases have been observed in follicle-stimulating hormone releasing factor (FRF) (Everitt, 1980). LRF is increased in the plasma of postmenopausal females. The level of plasma thyroxine (T_4) does not change with age, but the level of triiodothyronine (T_3) shows a significant age-related decrease (Snyder and Utiger, 1972). There is also an age-dependent decrease in the level of a pituitary factor believed responsible for influencing peripheral tissue responsiveness to thyroid hormone (Denckla, 1974). Both follicle-stimulating hormone (FSH) and luteinizing hormone (LH) increase with age, whereas the level of plasma prolactin remains constant (Yamaiji et al., 1976). The basal plasma growth hormone (GH) levels show little or no change with age (Blichert-Toft, 1975). The level of plasma glucocorticoids does not change with increasing age (Tang and Phillips, 1978). Through the counterbalancing effects of all these hormonal secretions, the immune system is maintained within the range characteristic to its particular age.

Acute thymic involution is produced by enhanced and endogenous secretion or administration of a wide variety of androgenic, estrogenic, and adrenocortical steroid hormones (Dougherty, 1952). More specifically, a study of local hormone production by various tissues, and the local effects of steroid hormones implanted into the rat thymus, revealed that cortisone, cortisol, and testosterone produce zonal involution, whereas estradiol, estriol, and estrone cause diffuse involution of the thymus (Friedman et al., 1964).

Isakovic and Jankovic (1973) have demonstrated acute involution of the thymus 32 days after electrolytic lesioning to the brain. The thymuses of rats with lesions in the hypothalamus, reticular formation, and superior colliculus, exhibited the most dramatic changes (e.g., a profound depletion of lymphocytes, drastic reduction of the thymic cortex, and disappearance of the cortical-medulla junction). Only hypothalamic lesioned rats exhibited any significant alteration in the spleen and lymph nodes.

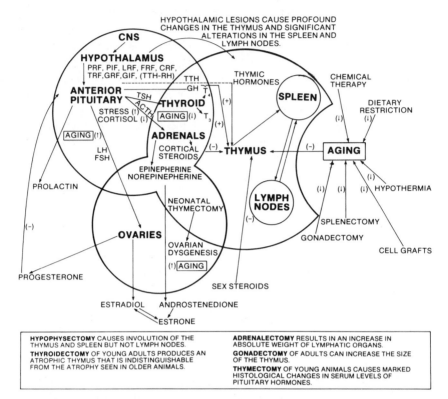

Figure 4 Influence of age on the neuroendocrine, ovarian, and immune systems. Prolactin-releasing factor (PRF), prolactin-inhibitory factor (PIF), luteinizing hormone-releasing factor (LRF), follicle-stimulating hormone-releasing factor (FRF), thyrotropin-releasing factor (TRF), growth hormone-releasing factor (GRF), somatotropin-releasing-inhibitory factor (GIF), thymotropin hormone-releasing factor (TTH-RH), thymotropin hormone (TTH), thyroid-stimulating hormone (TSH), adrenocorticotropic hormone (ACTH), growth hormone (GH), luteinizing hormone (LH), follicle-stimulating hormone (FSH), thyroxine (T_4), triiodothyronine (T_3); ($\uparrow$) increase, ($\downarrow$) decrease, (−) inhibits, (+) stimulates.

Tyrey and Nalbandov (1978) showed that rats with midline bilateral lesions in the anterior hypothalamus developed circulating antibodies with significantly lower precipitin titers than those obtained from sham-operated controls. Furthermore, neither hypophysectomy nor adrenalectomy alone altered antibody precipitin titers, but the depression of precipitin titers in lesioned animals was prevented when either operation was performed concomitant with lesioning. Cross et al. (1980) also presented data implying that the neuroendocrine pathway is capable of modulating immune function. Rats with electrolytic anterior hypothalamic lesions showed changes in lymphoid tissue cellularity and a decrease in the Con-A response, which were not seen by release of corticosteroids alone.

The following scheme has been proposed by Isakovic and Jankovic (1973) to correlate their results with the interaction of the neuroendocrine system and the immune response. These authors suggested that the anterior hypothalamus, perhaps through the elaboration of an hypothetical thymotropin hormone-releasing factor (TTH-RF), affects the secretion of thymotropin hormone (TTH) by the pituitary, which acts on the release of thymic hormones as a consequence to lymphocyte proliferation. Changes in the anterior hypothalamus caused by electrolytic lesions may result in a diminished release or inhibition of the release of TTH-RF, and thus hyposecretion of TTH. The low levels of TTH may be responsible for the changes observed in the lymphocyte populations (Isakovic and Jankovic, 1973).

The experiments of Pierpaoli and Maestroni (1977) demonstrate further an appreciation for the interrelationships among the neuroendocrine, immune, and ovarian systems. They showed that antigen injected into mice induces a rapid increase in FSH and LH. Suppression of these hormonal changes by a combination of drugs acting on neuroendocrine regulation as well as on cell membrane receptors resulted in a blockade of antibody synthesis and specific tolerance.

In summary, the pituitary appears to secrete substances which exert positive (i.e., LH, FSH, and ACTH) influences on the immune system (Denckla, 1978). In addition, the thymus may also secrete substances that both potentiate the beneficial effects of the pituitary hormones and antagonize some of the pituitary-dependent hormones (Denckla, 1978). A consideration of the exquisite relationship among the neuroendocrine, immune, and ovarian systems is warranted when designing future treatments to retard or reverse the immunological losses of age.

ACKNOWLEDGMENT

To Sara Lewis for her "untimely" association and A. J. Lewis, who made it "just in time."

REFERENCES

Adler, W. H. (1975). Aging and immune function. *Bioscience 25*:652-657.
Adler, W. H., Takiguchi, T., and Smith, R. T. (1971). Effect of age upon primary alloantigen recognition by mouse spleen cells. *J. Immunol. 107*: 1357-1362.
Albright, J. F., and Makinodan, T. (1966). Growth and senescence of antibody-forming cells. *J. Cell Physiol. 67*: 185-206.
Albright, J. F., Makinodan, T., and Deitchman, J. W. (1969). Presence of life-shortening factors in spleens of aged mice of long life span and extension of life expectancy by splenectomy. *Exp. Gerontol. 4*: 267-276.
Altman, A., and Rapp, H. J. (1978). Natural cell-mediated cytotoxicity in guinea pigs: properties and specificity of natural killer cells. *J. Immunol. 121*: 2244-2252.

Amos, D. B., and Yunis, E. J. (in press). An introduction to HLA and disease. In *Interfaces Between Immune Mechanisms*, D. B. Amos (Ed.). Academic Press, New York.

Antel, J. P., Oger, J. J. F., Dropcho, E., Richman, D. P., Kuo, H. H., and Arnason, B. G. W. (1980). Reduced T-lymphocyte cell reactivity as a function of human aging. *Cell Immunol. 54*: 184-192.

Asanuma, Y., Goldstein, A. L., and White, A. (1970). Reduction in the incidence of wasting disease in neonatally thymectomized CBA-W mice by the injection of thymosin. *Endocrinology 86*: 600-610.

Attallah, M. M., Steinberg, A. D., Ahmed, A., and Sell, K. W. (1979). Loss of lymphocyte chalone activity in mice with autoimmune disease. *Int. Arch. Allergy Appl. Immunol. 59*: 186-191.

Bartley, J., and Chalkley, R. (1970). Further studies of a thymus nucleohistone-associated protease. *J. Biol. Chem. 245*: 4286-4292.

Bellamy, D. (1968). Long-term action of predisolone phosphate on a strain of short-lived mice. *Exp. Gerontol. 3*: 327-333.

Bellamy, D., Hinsull, S. M., and Phillips, J. G. (1976). Factors controlling growth and age involution of the rat thymus. *Age and Aging 5*: 12-19.

Blichert-Toft, M. (1975). Secretion of corticotrophin and somatotrophin by the senescent adenohypophysis in man. *Acta Endocrinol. (Kbh.) 78, Suppl. 195*: 15-154.

Bliznakov, E. G., Wan, Y. P., Chang, D., and Folkers, K. (1978). Partial reactivation of impaired immune competence in aged mice by synthetic thymus factors. *Biochem. Biophys. Res. Commun. 80*: 631-636.

Braun, W., Yajima, Y., and Ishizuka, M. (1970). Synthetic polynucleotides as restorers of antibody formation capacities in aged mice. *J. Reticuloendothel. Soc. 7*: 418-425.

Brennan, P. C., and Jaroslow, B. N. (1975). Age-associated decline in theta antigen on spleen thymus-derived lymphocytes of B6CF1 mice. *Cell Immunol. 15*: 51-56.

Bruley-Rosset, M., Florentin, I., Kiger, N., Schulz, J., and Mathe, G. (1979). Restoration of impaired immune function of aged animals by chronic bestatin treatment. *Immunology 38*: 75-83.

Brutlag, D., Schlehuber, C., and Bonner, J. (1969). Properties of formaldehyde-treated nucleohistone. *Biochemistry 8*: 3214-3218.

Butenko, G. M., and Adrianova, F. (1979). The effect of antigen priming on immunological response regulation in aging. *Exp. Gerontol. 14*: 87-93.

Callard, R. E. (1978). Immune function in aged mice. III. Role of macrophages and effect of 2-mercaptoethanol in the response of spleen cells from old mice to phytohemagglutinin, lipopolysaccharide and allogeneic cells. *Eur. J. Immunol. 8*: 697-705.

Callard, R. E., and Basten, A. (1978). Immune function in aged mice. IV. Loss of T cell and B cell function in thymus-dependent antibody responses. *Eur. J. Immunol. 8*: 552-558.

Callard, R. E., Basten, A., and Blanden, R. V. (1979). Loss of immune competence with age may be due to a qualitative abnormality in lymphocyte membranes. *Nature 281*:218-220.

Callard, R. E., Basten, A., and Waters, L. K. (1977). Immune function in aged mice. II. B cell function. *Cell Immunol. 31*: 26-36.

Callard, R. E., De St. Groth, B. F., Basten, A., and McKenzie, I. F. (1980). Immune function in aged mice. V. Role of suppressor cells. *J. Immunol. 124*: 52-58.

Cantor, H., McVay-Boudreau, L., Hugenberger, J., Naidorf, K., Shen, S. W., and Gershon, R. K. (1978). Immunoregulatory circuits among T-cell sets. II. Physiologic role of feedback inhibition *in vitro*: absence in NZB mice. *J. Exp. Med. 147*: 1116-1125.

Castro, J. E. (1974a). Orchidectomy and the immune response. I. Effect of orchidectomy on lymphoid tissues of mice. *Proc. R. Soc. Lond. B. 185*: 425-436.

Castro, J. E. (1974b). Orchidectomy and the immune response. II. Response of orchidectomized mice to antigens. *Proc. R. Soc. Lond. B. 185*: 437-451.

Cavagnaro, J. A. (1979). *Localization and Further Characterization of an Endogenous Chromosomal Protease*. Ph.D. thesis, University of North Carolina at Chapel Hill. (supported in part by National Institute on Aging grant AG00103).

Cavagnaro, J. A., Pierce, D. A., Lucchesi, J. C., and Chae, C. B. (1980). Association of a protease with polytene chromosomes of *Drosophila melanogaster*. *J. Cell. Biol. 87*: 415-419.

Chalkley, R., and Hunter, C. (1975). Histone-histone propinquity by aldehyde fixation of chromatin. *Proc. Natl. Acad. Sci. USA 72*: 1304-1308.

Chandra, R. K., Heresi, G., and Au, B. (1980). Serum thymic factor activity in deficiencies of calories, zinc, vitamin A and pyridoxine. *Clin. Exp. Immunol. 42*: 332-335.

Chen, C., and Hirsch, J. G. (1972). The effects of mercaptoethanol and of peritoneal macrophages on the antibody forming capacity of nonadherent mouse spleen cells *in vitro*. *J. Exp. Med. 136*: 604-617.

Cheney, K. E., and Walford, R. L. (1974). Immune function and dysfunction in relation to aging. *Life Sci. 14*: 2075-2084.

Chiodi, H. (1940). The relationship between the thymus and the sexual organs. *Endocrinology 26*: 107-116.

Cone, R. E., and Marcholonis, J. J. (1972). Cellular and humoral aspects of the influence of environmental temperature on the immune response of poikilothermic vertebrates. *J. Immunol. 108*: 952-957.

Cross, R. J., Markesbery, W. R., Brooks, W. H., and Roszman, T. L. (1980). Hypothalamic-immune interactions. I. The acute effect of anterior hypothalamic lesions on the immune response. *Brain Res. 196*: 79-87.

Dauphinee, M. J., and Talal, N. (1975). Reversible restoration by thymosin of antigen-induced depression of spleen DNA synthesis in NZB mice. *J. Immunol. 114*: 1713-1716.

Dauphinee, M. J., Talal, N., Goldstein, A. L., and White, A. (1978). Thymosin corrects the abnormal DNA synthetic response of NZB mouse thymocytes. *Proc. Natl. Acad. Sci. USA 71*: 2637-2641.

De Kruyff, R. H., Rinooy-Kan, E. A., Weksler, M. E., and Siskind, G. W. (1980). Effect of aging on T-cell tolerance induction. *Cell Immunol. 56*: 58-67.

Delpierre, M. A., Panijel, J., and Terquem, M. (1980). Lymphoid cells from senescent animals contain specific inhibitors of immune response. *Cell Immunol. 52*: 204-210.

Denckla, W. D. (1974). Role of the pituitary and thyroid glands in the decline of minimal O_2 consumption with age. *J. Clin. Invest.* *53*: 572-581.

Denckla, W. D. (1978). Interactions between age and the neuroendocrine and immune systems. *Fed. Proc. 37*: 1263-1267.

Doenecke, D., and McCarthy, B. J. (1975a). Protein content of chromatin fractions separated by sucrose gradient centrifugation. *Biochemistry 14*: 1366-1372.

Doenecke, D., and McCarthy, B. J. (1975b). The nature of protein associated with chromatin. *Biochemistry 14*: 1373-1378.

Doria, G., D'Agostaro, G., and Poretti, A. (1978). Age-dependent variations in antibody avidity. *Immunology 35*: 601-611.

Dougherty, T. F. (1952). Effects of hormones on lymphatic tissue. *Physiol. Rev. 32*: 379-401.

Ebbesen, P., Doenhoff, M. J., and Thorn, N. A. (1971). Abrogated thymoma development in estrogenized mice grafted spleen and bone marrow cells. *Proc. Soc. Exp. Biol. Med. 133*: 850-855.

Egami, N. (1980). Environment and aging: an approach to the analysis of aging mechanisms using poikilothermic vertebrates. *Adv. Exp. Med. Biol. 129*: 249-259.

Everitt, A. V. (1976). Hypophysectomy in aging in the rat. In *Hypothalamus, Pituitary and Aging*, A. V. Everitt and J. A. Burgess (Eds.). Charles C Thomas, Springfield, Ill., pp. 68-75.

Everitt, A. V. (1980). The neuroendocrine system and aging. *Gerontology 26*: 108-119.

Fabris, N., Pierpaoli, W., and Sorkin, E. (1971). Hormones and the immunological capacity. III. The immunodeficiency disease of the hypopituitary Snell-Bagg dwarf mouse. *Clin. Exp. Immunol. 9*: 209-225.

Fabris, N., Pierpaoli, W., and Sorkin, E. (1972). Lymphocytes, hormones and aging. *Nature 240*: 557-559.

Fernandes, G. (1979). Nutrition, immunity and cancer. *Clin. Bull. 9*: 91-106.

Fernandes, G., Friend, P., and Yunis, E. J. (1977a). Influence of calorie restriction on autoimmune disease. *Fed. Proc. Fed. Am. Soc. Exp. Biol. 36*: 1313a.

Fernandes, G., Friend, P., Yunis, E. J., and Good, R. A. (1978). Influence of dietary restriction on immunological functions and renal disease in (NZB x NZW)F1 mice. *Proc. Natl. Acad. Sci. USA 75*: 1500-1504.

Fernandes, G., Good, R. A., and Yunis, E. J. (1977b). Attempts to correct age-related immunodeficiency and autoimmunity by cellular and dietary manipulation in inbred mice. In *Immunology and Aging*, T. Makinodan and E. Yunis (Eds.). Plenum Press, New York, pp. 111-133.

Fernandes, G., West, A., and Good, R. A. (1979). Nutrition, immunity and cancer. A review: Part III: Effects of diet on the diseases of aging. *Clin. Bull. 9*: 91-106.

Fernandes, G., Yunis, E. J., and Good, R. A. (1976). Influence of diet on survival of mice. *Proc. Natl. Acad. Sci. USA 73*: 1279-1283.

Fernandes, G., Yunis, E. J., Jose, D. G., and Good, R. A. (1973). Dietary influence on antinuclear antibodies and cell-mediated immunity in NZB mice. *Int. Arch. Allergy Appl. Immunol. 44*: 770-782.

Fernandes, G., Yunis, E. J., Smith, J., and Good, R. A. (1972). Dietary influence on breeding behavior, hemolytic anemia and longevity in NZB mice. *Proc. Soc. Exp. Biol. Med. 139*: 1189-1196.

Forsdyke, D. R., and David, C. M. (1978). Comparison of enhancement by heated serum and 2-mercaptoethanol of lymphocyte transformation induced by high concentrations of concanavalin A. *Cell. Immunol. 36*: 86-96.

Friedman, D., and Globerson, A. (1978). Immune reactivity during aging. I. T-helper dependent and independent antibody responses to different antigens, *in vivo* and *in vitro*. *Mech. Ageing Dev. 7*: 289-298.

Friedman, N. B., Bonze, E. J., Rothman, S., and Drutz, E. (1964). The effects of local hormonal organ transplants and steroid hormone implants upon the thymus gland. *Ann. N. Y. Acad. Sci. 113*: 916-932.

Furlan, M., Jericijo, M., and Suhar, A. (1968). Purification and properties of a neutral protease from calf thymus nuclei. *Biochem. Biophys. Acta. 167*: 154-160.

Furth, J. (1946). Prolongation of life with prevention of leukemia by thymectomy in mice. *J. Gerontol. 1*: 46-52.

Garcia-Giralt, E., Morales, H., Lasalvia, E., and Mathe, G. (1972). Suppression of graft-versus-host reaction by spleen extract. *J. Immunol. 109*: 878-880.

Gerbase-De Lima, M., Meredith, P., and Walford, R. (1975). Age-related changes, including synergy and suppression, in the mixed lymphocyte reaction in long-lived mice. *Fed. Proc. 34*: 159-161.

Gershon, H., Merhav, S., and Abraham, C. (1979). T-cell division and aging. *Mech. Ageing Dev. 9*: 27-38.

Gershwin, R. J., Gershwin, M. E., Steinberg, A. D., Ahmed, A., and Ochiai, T. (1976). Relationship between age and thymic function in the development of leukemia in AKR mice. *Proc. Soc. Exp. Biol. Med. 152*: 403-407.

Goidl, E. A., Innes, J. B., and Weksler, M. E. (1976). Immunological studies of aging. II. Loss of IgG and high avidity plaque-forming cells and increased suppressor cell activity in aging mice. *J. Exp. Med. 144*: 1037-1048.

Goldstein, A. L., Thurman, G. B., Cohen, G. H., and Rossio, J. L. (1976). The endocrine thymus: potential role for thymosin in the treatment of autoimmune disease. *Ann. N. Y. Acad. Sci. 174*: 390-401.

Goldstein, A. L., Thurman, G. B., Low, T. L. K., Rossio, J. L., and Trivers, G. E. (1978). Hormonal influences on the reticuloendothelial system: current status of the role of thymosin in the regulation and modulation of immunity. *J. Reticuloendothel. Soc. 23*: 253-266.

Goldstein, G. (1978). Mode of action of levamisole. *J. Rheum. 5, Suppl. 4*: 143-148.

Goodman, S. A., and Makinodan, T. (1975). Effect of age on cell-mediated immunity in long-lived mice. *Clin. Exp. Immunol. 19*: 533-547.

Gozes, Y., Umiel, T., Meshorer, A., and Trainin, N. (1978). Syngeneic GVH induced in popliteal lymph nodes by spleen cells of old C57 BL/6 mice. *J. Immunol. 121*: 2199-2204.

Greenberg, L. J., and Yunis, E. J. (1975). Immunopathology of aging. *Hum. Pathol. 5*: 122-124.

Greenberg, L. J., and Yunis, E. J. (1978). Genetic control of autoimmune disease and immune responsiveness and the relationship to aging. *Birth Defects 14*: 249-260.

Haffer, K., Freeman, M. J., and Watson, R. R. (1979). Effects of age on cellular immune responses in BALB/CJ mice: increase in antibody-dependent T lymphocyte mediated cytotoxicity. *Mech. Ageing Dev. 11*: 279-285.

Hale, P. M. (1978). *Endogenous Chromosomal Proteolysis of Histones*. Ph.D. thesis, University of North Carolina at Chapel Hill.

Hallgren, H. M., and Yunis, E. J. (1977). Supressor lymphocytes in young and aged humans. *J. Immunol. 118*: 2004-2008.

Hallgren, H. M., Buckley, E. C., III, Gilbertson, V. A., and Yunis, E. J. (1975). Lymphocyte phytohemagglutinin responsiveness, immunoglobulins and auto-antibodies in aging humans. *J. Immunol. 111*: 1101-1107.

Halsall, M. H., and Perkins, E. H. (1974). The restoration of phytohemagglutinin responsiveness of spleen cells from aged mice. *Fed. Proc. 33*: 736.

Han, I. H., and Johnson, A. G. (1976). Regulation of the immune system by synthetic polynucleotides. VI. Amplification of the immune response in young and aging mice. *J. Immunol. 117*: 423-427.

Hardin, J. A., Chuseo, T. M., and Steinberg, A. D. (1973). Suppressor cells in the graft versus host reaction. *J. Immunol. 111*: 650-651.

Harrison, D. E. (1975). Normal function of transplanted marrow cell lines from aged mice. *J. Gerontol. 30*: 279-285.

Heidrick, M. L., and Makinodan, T. (1972). Nature of cellular deficiencies in age-related decline of the immune system. *Gerontologia 18*: 305-320.

Heidrick, M. L., and Makinodan, T. (1973). Presenescence of impairment of humoral immunity in nonadherent spleen cells of old mice. *J. Immunol. 111*: 1502-1506.

Heidrick, M. L., Albright, J. W., and Makinodan, T. (1980). Restoration of impaired immune functions in aging animals. IV. Action of 2-mercaptoethanol in enhancing age-reduced immune responsiveness. *Mech. Ageing Dev. 13*: 367-378.

Heinrich, P. C. Raydt, G., Puschendorf, B., and Jusic, M. (1976). Subcellular distribution of histone-degrading enzyme activities from rat liver. *Eur. J. Biochem. 62*: 37-43.

Herberman, R. B., Nunn, M. E., and Lavrin, D. H. (1975). Natural cytotoxic reactivity of mouse lymphoid cells against syngeneic and allogeneic tumors. I. Distribution of reactivity and specificity. *Int. J. Can. 16*: 216-229.

Hewlett, G., Opitz, H. G., Schlumberger, H. D., and Lemke, H. (1977). Growth regulation of a murine lymphoma cell line by a 2-mercaptoethanol or macrophage-activated serum factor. *Eur. J. Immunol. 7*: 781-785.

Hirokowa, K. (1972). The thymus and aging. In *Immunology and Aging*, T. Makinodan and E. J. Yunis (Eds.). Plenum Press, New York, pp. 51-72.

Hirokowa, K., Albright, J. W., and Makinodan, T. (1976). Restoration of impaired immune functions in aging animals. I. Effect of syngeneic thymus and bone marrow cells. *Clin. Immunol. Immunopathol. 5*: 371-376.

Hohn, E. D. (1959). Action of certain hormones on the thymus of the domestic hen. *J. Endocrinol. 19*: 282-287.

Hori, Y., Perkins, E. H., and Halsall, M. K. (1973). Decline in phytohemagglutinin responsiveness of spleen cells from aging mice. *Proc. Soc. Exp. Biol. Med.* *144*: 48-55.

Horwitz, S., Borcherding, W., Moorthy, A. V., Chesney, R., Shulte-Wissermann, H., and Hong, R. (1977). Induction of supressor T cells in systemic lupus erythematosus by thymosin and cultured thymic epithelium. *Science 197*: 999-1001.

Houck, J. C., Attallah, A. M., and Lilly, J. R. (1973). Some immunosuppressive properties of lymphocyte chalone. *Nature (Lond.) 245*: 148-150.

Isakovic, K., and Jankovic, B. D. (1973). Neuroendocrine correlates of immune response. II. Changes in the lymphatic organs of brain-lesioned rats. *Int. Arch. Allergy 45*: 373-384.

Ishidate, M., and Metcalf, D. (1963). The pattern of lymphopoiesis in the mouse after cortisone administration or adrenalectomy. *Aust. J. Exp. Biol. Med. Sci. 41*: 637-649.

Jackson, V. (1978). Studies on histone organization in the nucleosome using formaldehyde as a reversible crosslinking agent. *Cell 15*: 945-954.

Jackson, V., and Chalkley, R. (1974). Separation of newly synthesized nucleohistone by equilibrium centrifugation in cesium chloride. *Biochemistry 13*: 3952-3956.

Jaroslow, B. N. (1971). Hibernation and different stages in the sequence of immune responsiveness. *Cryobiology 8*: 306-307.

Kay, M. M. B. (1978). Effect of age on T cell differentiation. *Fed. Proc. 37*: 1241-1244.

Kay, M. M. B. (1979). The thymus: clock for immunologic aging? *J. Invest. Dermatol. 73*: 29-38.

Kay, M. M. B., and Makinodan, T. (1976). Immunobiology of aging: evaluation of current status. *Clin. Immunol. Immunopathol. 6*: 394-413.

Kiessling, R., Klein, E., and Wigzell, H. (1975). "Natural" killer cells in the mouse. I. Cytotoxic cells with specificity for mouse Moloney leukemia cells. Specificity and distribution according to genotype. *Eur. J. Immunol. 5*: 112-117.

Kishimoto, S., Takahama, T., and Mizumachi, H. (1976). *In vitro* immune response to the 2, 4, 6-trinitrophenyl determinant in aged C57BL/6J mice: changes in the humoral response to avidity for the TNP determinant and responsiveness to LPS effect with aging. *J. Immunol. 116*: 294-300.

Kishimoto, S., Tomino, S., Inomata, K., Kotegawa, S., Saito, T., Kuroki, M., Mitsuye, H., and Hisamitsu, S. (1978). Age-related changes in the subsets and functions of human T lymphocytes. *J. Immunol. 121*: 1773-1780.

Konen, T. G., Smith, G. S., and Walford, R. L. (1973). Decline in mixed lymphocyte reactivity of spleen cells from aged mice of a long-lived strain. *J. Immunol. 110*: 1216-1221.

Krogsrud, R. L., and Perkins, E. H. (1977). Age-related changes in T cell function. *J. Immunol. 118*: 1607-1611.

Kruisbeek, A. M., and Steinmeir, F. A. (1980). Alloreactive cytotoxic T lymphocytes from aged mice express increased lysis of autologous and third-party target cells. *J. Immunol. 125*: 858-864.

Kurecki, T., Kowalska-Loth, B., Toczko, K., and Chmielewska, I. (1975). Evidence that neutral protease from calf thymus chromatin is a serine type enzyme. *FEBS Letts.* *53*: 313-315.

Kyewski, B., and Wekerle, H. (1978). Increase of T lymphocyte self-reactivity in aging inbred rats: *in vitro* studies with a model of experimental autoimmune orchitis. *J. Immunol. 120*: 1249-1255.

Kysela, S., and Steinberg, A. D. (1973). Increase survival of NZB/W mice given multiple syngeneic young thymus grafts. *Clin. Immunol. Immunopathol. 2*: 133-136.

LaBella, F. S. (1971). Cross-links in elastin and collagen. In *Biophysical Properties of the Skin*, H. R. Elden (Ed.). Wiley-Interscience, New York, pp. 243-301.

LaBella, F. S. (1972). Pharmacolongevity: control of aging by drugs. In *Search for New Drugs*, A. A. Rubin (Ed.). Marcel Dekker, New York, pp. 347-383.

LaBella, F., and Vivian, S. (1978). Beta-aminoproprionitrile promotes longevity in mice. *Exp. Gerontol. 13*: 251-254.

Lau, C. Y., Freestone, J. A., and Goldstein, G. (1980). Effect of thymopoietin pentapeptide (TP5) on autoimmunity. I. TP5 suppression of induced erythrocyte autoantibodies to C_3H mice. *J. Immunol. 125*: 1634-1638.

Leech, S. H. (1980). Cellular immunosenescence. *Gerontologia 26*: 330-345.

Liu, R. K., and Walford, R. L. (1972). The effect of lowered body temperature and life span on immune and non-immune processes. *Gerontologia 18*: 363-388.

Liu, R. K., and Walford, R. L. (1975). Mid-life temperature transfer effects on life span of annual fish. *J. Gerontol. 30*: 121-131.

Makinodan, T. (1978). Mechanism, prevention and restoration of immunologic aging. *Birth Defects 14*: 197-212.

Makinodan, T., and Adler, W. (1975). The effects of aging on the differentiation and proliferation potentials of cells in the immune system. *Fed. Proc. 34*: 153-158.

Makinodan, T., and Albright, J. W. (1979a). Restoration of impaired immune functions in aging animals. II. Effect of mercaptoethanol in enhancing the reduced primary antibody responsiveness *in vitro*. *Mech. Ageing Dev. 10*: 325-340.

Makinodan, T., and Albright, J. W. (1979b). Restoration of impaired immune function in aging animals. III. Effect of mercaptoethanol in enhancing the reduced primary antibody responsiveness *in vivo*. *Mech. Ageing Dev. 11*: 1-8.

Makinodan, T., and Peterson, W. J. (1966). Secondary antibody-forming potential of mice in relation to age—its significance to senescence. *Dev. Biol. 13*: 96-111.

Makinodan, T., Albright, J. W., Good, P. I., Peter, C. P., and Heidrick, M. L. (1976). Reduced humoral immune activity in long-lived mice: an approach to elucidating its mechanism. *Immunology 31*: 903-911.

Makinodan, T., Good, R. A., and Kay, M. M. B. (1977). In *Comprehensive Immunology I. Immunology and Aging*, T. Makinodan, R. A. Good, and M. M. B. Kay (Eds.). Plenum Press, New York.

McEndy, D. P., Boon, M. C., and Furth, J. (1944). On the role of the thymus, spleen and gonads in the development of leukemia in a high leukemia stock of mice. *Can. Res. 4*: 377-383.

Meyer, J. A., and Meyer, J. D. (1978). Splenectomy and the thymic involution of increasing age. *Arch. Surg. 113*: 972-975.

Meredith, P. J., and Walford, R. L. (1979). Autoimmunity, histocompatability, and aging. *Mech. Ageing Dev. 9*: 61-77.

Meredith, P. J., Kristie, J. A., and Walford, R. L. (1979). Aging increases expression of LPS-induced autoantibody-secreting B cells. *J. Immunol. 123*: 87-91.

Meredith, P., Tittor, W., Gerbase-De Lima, M., and Walford, R. (1975). Age-related changes in the cellular immune response of lymph node and thymus cells in long-lived mice. *Cell. Immunol. 18*: 324-330.

Millan, J. C., Santosham, M., Khaneja, S., Winkelstein, J. A., Schulte-Wisserman, H., Horowitz, S., and Hong, R. (1980). Long-term observations in a patient with severe combined immunodeficiency after transplantation with cultured epithelium. *Clin. Immunol. Immunopathol. 17*: 382-388.

Mitsuoka, A., Morikawa, S., Baba, M., and Harada, T. (1979). Cyclophosphamide eliminates suppressor T cells in age-associated central regulation of delayed hypersensitivity in mice. *J. Exp. Med. 149*: 1018-1028.

Moretta, L., Webb, S. R., Grossi, C. E., Lydyard, P. M., and Cooper, M. D. (1977). Functional analysis of two human T-cell subpopulations: help and suppression of B-cell responses by T cells bearing receptors for IgM or IgG. *J. Exp. Med. 146*: 184-200.

Morimoto, C., Abe, T., and Homma, M. (1979). Restoration of T-cell function in aged mice with long-term administration of levamisole. *Clin. Immunol. Immunopathol. 12*: 316-322.

Munthe, E., Jellum, E., and Aageth, J. (1979). Some aspects of the mechanism of action of penicillamine in rheumatoid arthritis. *Scand. J. Rheum., Suppl. 28*: 6-12.

Nakakuki, K., Shisa, H., and Nishizuka, Y. (1967). Prevention of AKR leukemia by thymectomy at varying ages. *Acta Haematol. Jap. 38*: 317-323.

Naor, D., Bonavida, B., and Walford, R. L. (1976). Autoimmunity and aging: the age-related response of mice of a long-lived strain to trinitrophenylated syngeneic mouse red blood cells. *J. Immunol. 117*: 2204-2208.

Nariuchi, H., and Adler, W. H. (1979). Dissociation between proliferation and antibody formation by old mouse spleen cells in response to LPS stimulation. *Cell Immunol. 45*: 295-302.

Nunn, M. E., Djeu, J. Y., Glaser, M., Lavrin, D. H., and Herberman, R. B. (1976). Natural cytotoxic reactivity of rat lymphocytes against syngeneic Gross virus-induced lymphoma. *J. Natl. Can. Inst. 56*: 393-399.

Parker, C. W., Sullivan, T. J., and Wedner, H. J. (1974). Cyclic AMP and the immune response. *Adv. Cycl. Nucl. Res. 4*: 1-79.

Perkins, E. H., Makinodan, T., and Seibert, C. (1972). Model approach to immunological rejuvenation of the aged. *Infect. Immun. 6*: 518-524.

Perry, L. L., Benacerraf, B., and Greene, M. I. (1978). Regulation of the immune response to tumor antigen. IV. Tumor antigen-specific suppressor factor(s) bearing I-J determinants and induce suppressor cells *in vivo. J. Immunol. 121*: 2144-2147.

Peter, C. P., Perkins, E. H., Peterson, W. J., Walburg, H. E., and Makinodan, T. (1975). The late effects of selected immune suppressants and immunocompetence, disease incidence and mean life span. III. Disease incidence and life expectancy. *Mech. Ageing Dev. 4*: 251-261.

Phillips, J. H., Jr., and Koppenheffer, T. L. (1978). Age-related appearance of a unique class of cytoplasmic filaments in murine lymphoid cells. *Dev. Comp. Immunol.* 2: 741-746.

Pierpaoli, W., and Maestroni, J. M. (1977). Pharmacological control of the immune response by blockade of the early hormonal changes following antigen injection. *Cell. Immunol.* 31: 355-363.

Pisciotti, A. V., Westring, D. W., De Prey, C., and Walsh, B. (1976). Mitogenic effect of phytohemagglutinin at different ages. *Nature (Lond.)* 215: 193-194.

Price, G. B., and Makinodan, T. (1972a). Immunologic deficiencies in senescence. I. Characterization of intrinsic deficiencies. *J. Immunol.* 108: 403-412.

Price, G. B., and Makinodan, T. (1972b). Immunologic deficiencies in senescence. II. Characterization of extrinsic deficiencies. *J. Immunol.* 108: 413-417.

Renoux, G., and Renoux, M. (1972). Restauration par le phenylimidothiazole de la response immunologique des souri àgreés. *Acad. Sci. (Paris)* 274: 3034-3035.

Renoux, G., and Renoux, M. (1977). Roles of the imidazole and thiol moiety on the immunostimulant action of levamisole. In *Control of Neoplasia by Modulation of the Immune System*, M. A. Chirigos (Ed.). Raven Press, New York, pp. 67-80.

Roberts-Thomson, I., Whittingham, J., Youngchaiyud, U., and MacKay, I. R. (1974). Aging, immune response and mortality. *Lancet 2*: 368-370.

Roder, J. C., Bell, D. A., and Singhal, S. K. (1977). Regulation of the immune response in autoimmune NZB/NZW F_1 mice. I. Spontaneous generation of splenic suppressor cells. *Cell Immunol.* 29: 272-284.

Roder, J. C., Bell, D. A., and Singhal, S. K. (1978a). Regulation of the immune response in autoimmune NZB/NZW F_1 mice II. Age-dependent release of suppressive factors from spleen cells. *Immunology 34*: 1017-1026.

Roder, J. C., Duwe, A. K., Bell, D. A., and Singhal, S. K. (1978b). Immunological senescence. I. The role of suppressor cells. *Immunology 35*: 837-847.

Rosenstein, M. M., and Strausser, H. R. (1980). Macrophage-induced T cell mitogen suppression with age. *J. Reticuloendothel. Soc.* 27: 159-166.

Ross, M. H. (1972). Length of life and caloric intake. *Am. J. Clin. Nutr. 25*: 834-838.

Safai-Kutti, S., Fernandes, G., Wang, Y., Safai, B., Good, R. A., and Day, N. K. (1980). Reduction of circulating immune complexes by calorie restriction in (NZB x NZW) F_1 mice. *Clin. Immunol. Immunopathol. 15*: 293-300.

Schacher, J., Brown, J. S. L., and Selye, H. (1937). Effect of various steroids on thymus in the adrenalectomized rat. *Proc. Soc. Exp. Biol. Med. 36*: 488-491.

Schloen, L. H., Fernandes, G., Garafalo, J. A., and Good, R. A. (1979). Nutrition, immunity and cancer—a review. Part II. Zinc, immune function and cancer. *Clin. Bull. 9*: 63-75.

Scholar, E. M., Rashidian, M., and Heidrick, M. L. (1980). Adenosine, deaminase and purine nucleoside phosphorylase activity in spleen cells of aged mice. *Mech. Ageing Dev. 12*: 323-329.

Schrater, A. F., Goidl, E. A., Thorbecke, G. J., and Siskind, G. W. (1979). Production of auto-anti-idiotypic antibody during the normal immune response to

TNP-ficoll. I. Occurrence in AKR/J and Balb/c mice of hapten-augmentable, anti-TNP plaque-forming cells and their accelerated appearance in recipients of immune spleen cells. *J. Exp. Med. 150*: 138-153.

Schulof, R. S., Garafalo, J. A., Good, R. A., and Gupta, S. (1980). Concanavalin A induced suppressor cell activity for T-cell proliferative response: autologous and allogeneic suppression in aging humans. *Cell Immunol. 56*: 80-88.

Scribner, D. J., Weiner, H. L., and Moorehead, J. W. (1978). Anti-immunoglobulin stimulation of murine lymphocytes. V. Age-related decline in Fc receptor-mediated immunoregulation. *J. Immunol. 121*: 377-382.

Segre, D., and Segre, M. (1976). Humoral immunity in aged mice. II. Increased suppressor T cell activity in immunologically deficient old mice. *J. Immunol. 116*: 735-758.

Shellam, G. R., and Hogg, N. (1977). Cross virus-induced lymphoma in the rat. IV. Cytotoxic cells in normal rats. *Int. J. Can. 19*: 212-224.

Shigemoto, S., Kishimoto, S., and Yamamura, Y. (1975). Change in cell-mediated cytotoxicity with aging. *J. Immunol. 115*: 307-309.

Singhal, S. K., Roder, J. C., and Duwe, A. K. (1978). Suppressor cells in immunosenescence. *Fed. Proc. 37*: 1245-1252.

Smith, G. S., and Walford, R. L. (1978). Influence of the H2 and H1 histocompatability systems upon life span and spontaneous cancer incidences in congenic mice. *Birth Defects 14*: 281-312.

Snyder, P. J., and Utiger, R. D. (1972). Response to thyrotropin releasing hormone (TRH) in normal man. *J. Clin. Endocrinol. 34*: 380-385.

Stjernsward, J. (1966). Age-dependent tumor-host barrier and effect of carcinogen initiated immune depression of rejection of isografted methylcholanthrene induced sarcoma cells. *J. Natl. Can. Inst. 37*: 505-512.

Szewczuk, M. R., and Campbell, R. J. (1980). Loss of immune competence with age may be due to auto-anti-idiotypic antibody regulation. *Nature 286*: 164-166.

Tait, N. N. (1969). The effect of temperature on the immune response in cold-blooded vertebrates. *Physiol. Zool. 42*: 29-35.

Talal, N., and Steinberg, A. D. (1974). The pathogenesis of autoimmunity in New Zealand black mice. *Curr. Top. Microbiol. Immunol. 64*: 79-103.

Tam, C. F., and Walford, R. L. (1978). Cyclic nucleotide levels in resting and mitogen-stimulated spleen cell suspensions from young and old mice. *Mech. Ageing Dev. 7*: 309-320.

Tam, C. F., Smith, G. S., and Walford, R. L. (1979). Resting and concanavalin-A stimulated levels of cyclic nucleotides in splenic cells of aging mice with spontaneous cancers. *Life Sci. 24*: 311-322.

Tang, F., and Phillips, J. G. (1978). Some age-related changes in pituitary-adrenal function in the male laboratory rat. *J. Gerontol. 33*: 377-382.

Teague, P. O., Friou, G. Y., Yunis, E. J., and Good, R. A. (1972). Spontaneous autoimmunity in aging mice. In *Tolerance, Autoimmunity and Aging*, M. M. Siegel and R. A. Good (Eds.). Charles C Thomas, Springfield, Ill., pp. 33-61.

Teller, M. N. (1972a). Age changes and immune resistance to cancer. *Adv. Gerontol. Res. 4*: 25-43.

Teller, M. N. (1972b). Interrelationships among aging, autoimmunity, and cancer. In *Tolerance, Autoimmunity and Aging*, M. M. Siegel and R. A. Good (Eds.). Charles C Thomas, Springfield, Ill., pp. 18-22.

Teller, M. N., Stohr, G., Curlett, W., Kubisek, M. L., and Curtis, D. (1964). Aging and cancerogenesis. I. Immunity to tumor and skin grafts. *J. Natl. Can. Inst. 33*: 649-656.

Tyan, M. L. (1977). Age-related decrease in mouse T cell progenitors. *J. Immunol. 118*: 846-851.

Tyrey, L., and Nalbandov, A. V. (1978). Influence of anterior hypothalamic lesions on circulating antibody titers in the rat. *Am. J. Physiol. 222*: 179-185.

Walford, R. L., Liu, R. K., Mathies, M., Gerbase-De Lima, M., and Lipps, L. (1974). Long-term dietary restriction and immune function in mice, response to sheep red blood cells and to mitogens. *Mech. Ageing Dev. 2*: 443-451.

Walters, C. S., and Claman, H. N. (1975). Age-related changes in cell mediated immunity of Balb/c mouse. *J. Immunol. 115*: 1438-1443.

Watson, J. (1975). The influence of intracellular levels of cyclic nucleotides on cell proliferation and the induction of antibody synthesis. *J. Exp. Med. 141*: 97-111.

Weindruch, R. H., and Suffin, S. C. (1980). Quantitative histological effects on mouse thymus of controlled dietary restriction. *J. Gerontol. 35*: 525-531.

Weksler, M. E. (1980). The immune system and the aging process in man. *Proc. Soc. Exp. Biol. Med. 165*: 200-205.

Weksler, M. E., Innes, J. D., and Goldstein, G. (1978). Immunological studies of aging. IV. The contribution of thymic involution to the immune deficiencies of aging mice and reversal with thymopoietin 32-36. *J. Exp. Med. 148*: 996-1006.

Williams, R. M., and Yunis, E. J. (in press). Genetics of immunity and its relation to disease. In *Genetics, Infection and Immunity*, H. Friedman and T. J. Linna (Eds.). University Park Press, Baltimore.

Woda, B. A., and Feldman, J. D. (1979). Density of surface immunoglobulin and capping on rat B lymphocytes. I. Changes with aging. *J. Exp. Med. 149*: 416-423.

Woda, B. A., Yguerabide, J., and Feldman, J. D. (1979). Mobility and density of age. IA and Fc receptors on the surface of lymphocytes from young and old rats. *J. Immunol. 123*: 2161-2167.

Wurtman, R. J., Larin, F., Mostafapour, J., and Fernstrom, J. D. (1974). Brain catechol synthesis: control by brain tyrosine concentrations. *Science 185*: 183-184.

Yamaiji, T., Shimamoto, K., Ishibashi, M., Kosaka, K., and Orimo, H. (1976). Effect of age and sex on circulating and pituitary prolactin in humans. *Acta Endocrinol. (Kbh.) 83*: 711-719.

Young, V. R. (1978). Nutrition and aging. *Adv. Exp. Med. Biol. 97*: 85-110.

Yunis, E. J., and Greenberg, L. J. (1974). Immunopathology of aging. *Fed. Proc. 33*: 2017-2019.

Yunis, E. J., and Lane, M. A. (1979). Cellular immunity in aging. *J. Invest. Dermatol. 73*: 24-28.

Yunis, E. J., Fernandes, G., and Stutman, O. (1971). Susceptibility to involution of the thymus-dependent lymphoid system and autoimmunity. *Am. J. Clin. Pathol. 56*: 280-292.

8

Neuroimmunomodulation and Senescence

Thomas L. Roszman, Richard J. Cross, William H. Brooks, and William R. Markesbery / *University of Kentucky Medical Center, Lexington, Kentucky*

INTRODUCTION

Although aging is a predictable and natural sequence of biological events, precise understanding and correlation of the multiple factors associated with this process remain elusive. Of the numerous theories proposed to explain the cellular mechanisms of aging, those suggesting that (1) the pacemakers of aging are intrinsic and subject to genetic instability and thus, cells are programmed to lose their ability to divide (Hayflick, 1975, 1979); and/or (2) groups of cells or organs regulate aging via hormonal, neural, or other systemic controls (Finch, 1979) come closest to a unifying concept of senescence. In addition to these cellular mechanisms, survival and individual longevity also are determined at a higher level by integrated performances of different organ systems of the host. It is clear, therefore, that attempts to unify those mechanisms associated with control of aging must consider a single system which is capable of modulating biological events at the cellular level as well as pivotal in control and integration of different organ systems.

The organ system that potentially best fulfills this requirement is the central nervous system (CNS). In proposing a network theory of immunological responsiveness, Jerne (1974) concluded that the immune and nervous systems are phenotypically quite similar. Each is capable of responding to an infinite variety of external and internal stimuli by displaying dichotomous and dualistic enhancing and suppressor modulation to maintain homeostatic immunological and neurological competence. Adaptive behaviors of both systems are based upon experience and memory which are sustained by reinforcement and plasticity of network modifications. Continual internal modulation of these networks, therefore represents the organism's attempt to appropriately respond to the external environment. The data demonstrating that more than a conceptual link exists between the brain and immune system are reviewed in this chapter. More specifically, it is concluded that age-related changes in the hypothalamus occur concomitant with decline in immune function. Thus, a unified concept of neuroimmunomodulation is conceived as operating during development, maturation, and senescence.

IMMUNE-ENDOCRINE INTERDEPENDENCE DURING DEVELOPMENT

Interactions between one effector of the nervous system, the neuroendocrine system, and the immune system begin during development. Congenitally athymic mice are severely compromised with regard to the development of the neuroendocrine system (Pierpaoli and Besedovsky, 1975). These animals display depressed serum levels of both thyroxine and gonadotropic hormones which, present neonatally, persist throughout life. An attempt to restore neuroendocrine function by implanting thymus tissue results in a return of estrogen concentration to normal levels; however, the concentrations of other hormones do not increase. Supplemental therapy with luteinizing hormone (LH), thyroid-stimulating hormone (TSH), and adrenocorticotropin (ACTH) restores endocrine function, indicating no abnormality exists in the target gland or its hormone receptors. These data indicate a functional thymus, a primary lymphoid organ, must be present prior to birth for the development of the hypothalamopituitary axis. Additional thymic-hypothalamic interactions also have been detected. Thus, thymosin, a thymic-derived hormone, has been shown to interact with hypothalamic tissue to induce the release of LH-releasing factor from adjacently cultured, membrane-separated, pituitary glands (Rebar et al., 1981). This study provides further evidence of a direct effect of thymic hormone on the hypothalamus.

Arrenbrecht and Sorkin (1973) showed growth hormone promotes the differentiation of thymus-derived lymphocyte precursors to mature T cells. More recently, Snow et al. (1981) have demonstrated that growth hormone and insulin must be added to serum-free spleen cell cultures to promote the development of cytotoxic T lymphocytes. Thus, these data support the theory of the interdependence of the neuroendocrine and immune systems during development.

EFFECTS OF HORMONES ON THE IMMUNE RESPONSE

In addition to the role hormones play during immunological development, endocrine factors also are implicated in many immunopotentiating and immunosuppressive events. Many of these events may be manifest through the specific binding of these hormones through specific hormone receptors. Arrenbrecht (1974) has shown that specific growth hormone receptors are present on the lymphocyte membrane as are insulin receptors (Harrison et al., 1979).

The results of Pandian and Talwar (1971) demonstrate that treatment of rats with antigrowth hormone serum diminishes the humoral immune response to sheep red blood cells (SRBC). Subsequent treatment with growth hormone restores the antibody response. The cell-mediated component of the immune response also can be influenced by hormones. Thus, as previously mentioned, insulin and growth hormone are required for the generation of cytotoxic T lymphocytes (Snow et al., 1981).

Adrenocortical hormones, primarily glucocorticoids, have marked effects on lymphocyte function, number, and migration. Ambrose (1970) has shown an absolute requirement for cortisone for the initiation of a humoral immune response in lymphoid organ cultures. In contrast to these effects, high doses of corticosteroids markedly alter both lymphoid cell function (Blomgren and Svedmyr, 1971; Doughery et al., 1964; Mansour and Nelson, 1978) and migratory patterns (Fauci, 1975). Vischer (1972) reports mice injected with hydrocortisone exhibit marked splenic involution with a similar decrease in splenic lymphocyte responsiveness to mitogens and allogeneic cells. Likewise, the number of cells in the thymus decreased; however, responsiveness to phytohemagglutinin and allogeneic cells is increased. This enhanced response is interpreted as a condition in which a subpopulation of thymocytes that do not respond well to mitogens or alloantigens is selectively depleted by cortisone, thereby effectively enriching a population of cells that respond well to mitogens or alloantigens (Anderson et al., 1972). Blomgren and Anderson (1971) also reported that the cortisone effect on lymphocytes is acute, with complete recovery from the effects 14 days after treatment.

Besedovsky et al. (1975) have measured serum hormone levels during the humoral immune response to foreign erythrocytes and found that the concentration of ACTH increases while the level of thyroxine decreases after the injection of antigen. Autologous erythrocytes do not affect hormone levels. Similarly, Pierpaoli and Maestroni (1977) have reported that the injection of allogeneic lymph node cells into mice induces a rapid increase in the serum levels of both LH and FSH. These data taken together suggest that fluctuations in hormone levels may serve as mediators within an integrated, communicating network between the endocrine and immune systems to modulate immune responsiveness.

NEUROTRANSMITTERS AND IMMUNOREGULATION

In addition to the influence of the neuroendocrine system on immune parameters, evidence also exists implicating the autonomic nervous system and autonomic neurotransmitters in immunoregulation. A number of studies demonstrate that rats injected with reserpine display prolonged skin graft survival, decreased intensity of delayed-type hypersensitivity reactions to bovine serum albumin, and involution of the thymus (Draskoci and Jankovic, 1964; Draskoci et al., 1966; Jankovic et al., 1965). In addition, Devoino et al. (1970) showed that reserpine, serotonin, or 5-hydroxytryptophan (5-HTP) treatment increases the latent period of the primary and secondary antibody responses. Therefore, they suggested that increases in free serotonin inhibit the antibody response. In a subsequent report (Devoino et al., 1975), they extended these observations by demonstrating that an intact pituitary gland is required for these effects to occur.

Reports indicating that the neurotransmitter norepinephine affects immune responsiveness are conflicting. Kasahara et al. (1977) have shown that chemical ablation of the sympathetic nervous system with 6-hydroxydopamine (6-OHDA), a drug known to deplete norepinephrine, decreases both the hemagglutinin titer and the plaque-forming cell response to SRBC. Conversely, Besedovsky et al. (1979), using rats surgically sympathectomized by denervating the spleen of animals or that were chemically sympathectomized by injection of 6-OHDA in combination with adrenalectomy, reported that depletion of norepinephrine enhances the plaque-forming cell response to SRBC. Assays of norepinephrine showed that the concentration of the neurotransmitter decreases immediately prior to the detection of plaque-forming cells. Thoenen and Tranzer (1968) have reported that 6-OHDA does not decrease the concentration of norepinephrine in the adrenal glands. Thus, the discrepancies between the data of Kasahara et al. (1977) and Besedovsky et al. (1979) may result from norepinephine remaining in the adrenal following 6-OHDA sympathectomy. These data do indicate, however, that norepinephrine may be a potential immunomodulator. Williams et al. (1981) in a similar experiment ablated the sympathetic nervous system by injecting 6-OHDA at birth followed by injection of 6-OHDA or alpha-methytyrosine 24 hr prior to antigenic challenge. Their data confirm the previous report of Besedovsky et al. (1979) indicating that an enhanced plaque-forming cell response occurs following chemical sympathectomy.

An accumulation of experiments performed over the last several decades has led to the formulation of a pathway outlining neurotransmitter control of pituitary hormone secretion. Experiments show that neurotransmitter binding to a receptor in the hypothalamus controls the release of specific pituitary hormones (Schally et al., 1977). Pierpaoli and Maestroni (1978) built on these theories to integrate neurotransmitters and neurohormones with immune response regulation. Previously, they reported that stimulation of the immune system with antigen invokes a rapid change in serum gonadotropin levels (Pierpaoli and Maestroni, 1977). They postulate that this change in hormone levels is required to initiate an immune response. In subsequent experiments, an attempt was made to block immune responsiveness by inhibiting the shift in hormone levels by injection of a combination of drugs which modify neurotransmitter function (Pierpaoli and Maestroni, 1978). They found that by injecting 5-HTP (which increases serotonin synthesis), phentolamine (an a-adrenergic receptor antagonist), and haloperidol (a dopamine receptor blocker), lymphoid cells become unresponsive to SRBC. Replacement of LH, FSH, and ACTH results in the abrogation of the effects of these neuroleptic drugs.

Thus, LH, FSH, and ACTH are required to initiate an immune response, and the release of these hormones is regulated by the synthesis, release, and binding of neurotransmitters.

Additional support for this concept is provided by Besedovsky et al. (1977) who showed that an immune response to SRBC induces changes in the electrical activity within the hypothalamus. Recording electrodes, placed in the ventromedial hypothalamic nucleus, detected an increase in neuronal firing rate 5-8 days following antigen injection. Thus, these findings suggest the presence of a neurotransmitter-neurohormone network in regulating immune responsiveness.

EFFECTS OF EXPERIMENTAL CNS ABLATION ON IMMUNE RESPONSIVENESS

Recently we have demonstrated that a more than hypothetical correlation exists between anatomical changes in the hypothalamus, endocrine function, and immunity. Thus, bilateral electrolyte lesions were placed in the anterior hypothalamic area (AHT) of Fischer 344 rats, and at various intervals the spleen cell responsiveness to the mitogen concanavalin A (Con-A) was determined (Cross et al., 1980). The results demonstrated that AHT lesions but not frontal cortex (FC) lesions induced an acute change in splenocyte and thymocyte numbers and diminished splenocyte mitogenic reactivity. The maximum effect was noted 4 days after lesioning, with a return to normal by day 14 postlesioning. Quantitation of serum corticosterone levels in lesioned animals revealed a similar increase in AHT- and FC-lesioned animals, but quantitative and qualitative immunological changes were confined to rats with AHT lesions. This indicates that the results observed were not due to increased levels of corticosterone but to other neural effectors. The decreased spleen cell responsiveness observed in AHT-lesioned animals was further investigated. It was ascertained that this impaired lymphocyte reactivity could be restored to normal by removal of a subpopulation of spleen cells with macrophage-like properties (Roszman et al., 1982). Although naturally occurring suppressor macrophages are detectable in normal and FC-lesioned rats, substantially more activity was present after AHT destruction. This increased suppressor activity observed in AHT-lesioned animals was not due to an increase in the number of splenic macrophages but rather a neurally induced qualitative change in suppressor macrophage function. Thus, one way in which the immune response can react to alterations in brain function is to activate a suppressor cell circuit.

As previously discussed, not all perturbations of the brain by electrolytic lesioning result in decreased immune responsiveness. We have studied immune parameters in rats with bilateral electrolytic lesions in specific limbic nuclei (Brooks et al., 1982). Employing splenic and thymic reactivity to Con-A as an in vitro correlate of cell-mediated immunity, we observed that, dependent on the location of the lesion, lymphocyte reactivity increased, decreased, or evidenced no change. Thus, spleen cell responsiveness to Con-A decreased subsequent to AHT lesioning, whereas enhanced reactivity occurred after lesion placement in the mamillary bodies, hippocampus (HC), and amygdaloid complex (AM) with no change observed with lesions in the ventral medial hypothalamus or fornix. Alterations in thymocyte mitogenic reactivity were limited to increases noted only after lesions in the hippocampus and amygdaloid complex. These effects manifested themselves maximally 4 days after lesioning, with a return to normal by day 14. These data suggest that one facet of enhanced or suppressed lymphocyte activation emanates from specific areas of the brain. Moreover, the variable modulations of blastogenic reactiveness produced by isolated lesions in the richly interconnecting lymbic system indicate that a single nucleus acting as a central immunoregulatory center probably does not exist.

The primary effectors of neuroimmunomodulation remain conjectural, yet study of the kinetics of the observed immunological effects suggests that one mediator may be the neuroendocrine system. The alterations in lymphocyte number and function are short-lived and completely reversed by 14 days, and thereby are consistent with the endocrine effects of hormonal release and metabolism. Furthermore, specific hormonal receptors are present on the lymphocyte plasma membrane (Arrenbrecht, 1974; Harrison et al., 1979) and would provide a means for lymphocytes to perceive changes in hormone levels. To test this hypothesis, neural-induced changes in lymphocyte responsiveness were assessed before and after hypophysectomy (Cross et al., 1982). As previously discussed, lesions in the AHT result in a decreased spleen cell response to Con-A, whereas lesions in the HC and AM result in increased mitogenic reactivity. If the animals are hypophysectomized, the inhibitory and facilitary lymphocyte blastogenic effects of lesioning of the AHT and HC or AM lesions, respectively, are abrogated. Hypophysectomy has no effect on Con-A responsiveness of splenocytes obtained from normal and FC-lesioned rats. Similar types of observations were made with the responsiveness of thymocytes from hypophysectomized animals with one major exception. Although hypophysectomy does not alter the Con-A responsiveness of thymocytes obtained from normal or FC-lesioned animals, it completely reverses the enhancement observed after HC or AM lesions. Interestingly, lesions in the AHT in intact animals have no effect on the Con-A reactivity of thymocytes, but in hypophysectomized animals, AHT lesions induce a decreased responsiveness. These results suggest that the neuroendocrine system can have an influential regulatory role in the immune response and are consistent with the observation that a variety of hormones are capable of influencing and maintaining mitogen-induced lymphocyte activation and antibody production (Beling and Weksler, 1974; Pierpaoli and Maestroni, 1977, 1978; Snow et al., 1981).

Other work using experimental animal models and ablation techniques supports the hypothesis that the hypothalamus plays a role in the immune response. Besedovsky et al. (1977) have shown a significant increase in the firing rate of ventromedial hypothalamic neurons during the first 5 days following antigen administration. Thymic involution has been observed following lesions of the hypothalamus (Isakovic and Jankovic, 1973). Decreased antibody titers have been correlated with lesions in the AHT of rats (Tyrey and Nalbandov, 1972), whereas decreased intensity of anaphylactic shock (Stein et al., 1976) and lymphocyte mitogenic responsiveness (Keller et al., 1980) was found in guinea pigs with AHT lesions.

The mechanisms by which brain lesions modulate the immune response involve complex interactions between neuroendocrine influences and the autonomic nervous system as previously discussed. Receptors for both mediators, that is, hormones (Arrenbrecht, 1974) and neurotransmittors (Pochet et al., 1979), are present on the lymphocyte surface. Thus, it may be hypothesized that changes in AHT or limbic nuclei function result in alterations in sympathetic or parasympathetic activity or hormonal secretion which in turn affect changes in lymphocyte function by interaction with specific surface receptors. More recently, direct innervation of thymus and lymph nodes has been demonstrated which lends further support to a functioning link between the CNS and immune system (Bulloch and Moore, 1981; Giron et al., 1980). Changes in thymic innervative patterns associated with immunity and aging remain to be defined.

AGE-RELATED NEUROIMMUNOMODULATION

Several independent avenues of investigation lend support to an age-related neuro-immunomodulation hypothesis. Fabris and co-workers (Fabris et al., 1971a,b) have studied endocrine control of the immune response in the hypopituitary dwarf mouse. These mice exhibit marked retardation in growth, sterility, and an underdeveloped endocrine system. More interestingly, these animals are affected by an immunodeficiency syndrome characterized by hypotrophy of the thymus, spleen, and lymph nodes, impairment of humoral and cellular immunity, and a decreased life span. These immunodeficiencies can be corrected by treatment with bovine growth hormone or thyroxine for 30 days beginning immediately after weaning. If the mice are thymectomized, these hormones have no effect. Further studies indicate that the life span of these mice can be prolonged from 4 months to 15-18 months if growth hormone is administered during the first 30 days after weaning. Treatment begun after 90 days of life was not effective.

It appears, therefore, that a particular hormonal balance may be important during a critical period of development which is essential for maturation of the immune response, beginning with neonatal life and extending through adulthood and senescence. This hormonal balance, or perhaps alteration, may account for the cellular environment that is responsible for age-related immunological decline. That such a decline in immune responsiveness occurs with age is extensively documented (Walford, 1974; Kay and Makinodan, 1976; Hirokawa, 1977; MacKay et al., 1977; Makinodan et al., 1977; Kay and Baker, 1979). What is less obvious is the explanation of the biological event.

In conclusion, it may be hypothesized that morphological alterations in the hypothalamus, such as occur with aging (Machado-Salas et al., 1977), alter immune responsiveness by affecting changes in endocrine, biochemical, or anatomic milieu. Thus, anatomic changes in the central nervous system may be correlated with fluctuations in neurosecretory activity and lymphoid innervative activity which, in turn, influence the cellular mediators of immune responsiveness. Exploration and elucidation of this hypothalamic-immune network will greatly contribute to explaining the age-related decline of immunological function.

ACKNOWLEDGMENTS

This work was supported in part by N.I.H. grants CA-18234, CA-23891, NS-1742, and AG-02759.

REFERENCES

Ambrose, C. T. (1970). Hormones and the immune response. In *Ciba Foundation Study Group #36*, G. E. W. Wolstenholme and J. Knight (Eds.). Churchill, London, pp. 100-135.

Anderson, J., Moller, G., and Sjoberg, O. (1972). Selective induction of DNA synthesis in T and B lymphocytes. *Cell. Immunol. 4*: 381-393.

Arrenbrecht, S. (1974). Specific binding of growth hormone to thymocytes. *Nature 252*: 255-257.

Arrenbrecht, S. and Sorkin, E. (1973). Growth hormone-induced T-cell differentiation. *Eur. J. Immunol. 3*: 601-604.

Bartrop, R. W., Lazarus, E., and Luckhurst, L. G. (1977). Depressed lymphocyte function after bereavement. *Lancet 1*: 834-836.

Beling, C. G., and Weksler, M. E. (1974). Suppression of mixed lymphocyte reactivity by human chorionic gonadotrophin. *Clin. Exp. Immunol. 18*: 537-541.

Besedovsky, H. D., Del Rey, A., Sorkin, E., DaPrada, M., and Keller, H. H. (1979). Immunoregulation mediated by the sympathetic nervous system. *Cell Immunol. 48*: 346-355.

Besedovsky, H. W., Sorkin, E., Felix, D., and Haas, H. (1977). Hypothalamic changes during the immune response. *Eur. J. Immunol. 7*: 323-325.

Besedovsky, H. O., Sorkin, E., Keller, M., and Muller, J. (1975). Changes in blood hormone levels during the immune response. *Proc. Soc. Exp. Biol. Med. 150*: 466-470.

Blomgren, H. and Anderson, B. (1971). Characteristics of the immunocompetent cells in the mouse thymus: Cell population changes during cortisone-induced atrophy and regeneration. *Cell. Immunol. 1*: 545-560.

Blomgren, H., and Svedmyr, E. (1971). *In vitro* stimulation of mouse thymus cells by PHA and allogeneic cells. *Cell. Immunol. 2*: 285-299.

Brooks, W. H., Cross, R. J., Roszman, T. L., and Markesbery, W. R. (1982). Neuroimmunomodulation: Neural anatomical basis for impairment and facilitation. *Ann. Neurol. 12*:56-61.

Bulloch, K., and Moore, R. Y. (1981). Innervation of the thymus gland by brain stem and spinal cord in mouse and rat. *Am. J. Anat. 162*: 157-166.

Cross, R. J., Brooks, W. H., Roszman, T. L., and Markesbery, W. R. (1982). Hypothalamic-immune intereactions. III. Effect of hypothalamic lesions on neuroimmunomodulation. *J. Neurol. Sci. 53*:557-566.

Cross, R. J., Markesbery, W. R., Brooks, W. H., and Roszman, T. L. (1980). Hypothalamic-immune interactions. I. The acute effect of anterior hypothalamic lesions on the immune response. *Brain Res. 196*: 79-87.

Devoino, L., Eliseeva, L., Eremina, O., Idova, G., and Cheido, M. (1975). 5-Hydroxytryptophan effect on the development of the immune response: IgM and IgG antibodies and rosette formation in the primary and secondary responses. *Eur. J. Immunol. 5*: 394-399.

Devoino, L. V., Eremina, O. F., and Yu Illyutchenok, R. (1970). The role of the hypothalamic-pituitary system in the mechanism of action of reserpine and 5-hydroxytryptophan on antibody production. *Neuropharmacology 9*: 67-72.

Doughery, T. F., Berliner, M. L., Schneebeli, G. L., and Berliner, D. L. (1964). Hormonal control of lymphatic structure and function. *N.Y. Acad. Sci. 113*: 825-843.

Draskoci, M., and Jankovic, B. D. (1964). Involution of thymus and suppression of immune response in rats treated with reserpine. *Nature 202*: 408-409.

Draskoci, M., Janjic, M., and Jankovic, B. D. (1966). Immunological capacity of rats treated with reserpine. *Ingosl. Physiol. Pharmacol. Acta 2*: 79-81.

Fabris, N., Pierpaoli, W., and Sorkin, E. (1971a). Hormones and the immunological capacity. III. The immunodeficiency disease of the hypopituitary Snell-Bagg dwarf mouse. *Clin. Exp. Immunol. 9*: 209-225.

Fabris, N., Pierpaoli, W., and Sorkin, E. (1971b). Hormones and the immunological capacity. IV. Restorative effects of developmental hormones or of lymphocytes on the immunodeficiency syndrome of the dwarf mouse. *Clin. Exp. Immunol. 9*: 227-240.

Fauci, A. S. (1975). Mechanisms of corticosteriod action on lymphocyte subpopulations. I. Redistribution of circulating T- and B-lymphocytes to the bone marrow. *Immunology 28*: 669-680.

Finch, C. E. (1979). Neuroendocrine mechanisms and aging. *Fed. Proc. 38*: 178-183.

Giron, L. T., Crutcher, K. A., and Davis, J. N. (1980). Lymph nodes—A possible site for sympathetic neuronal regulation of immune responses. *Ann. Neurol. 8*: 520-525.

Harrison, L. C., Flier, J., and Itin, A. (1979). Radioimmunoassay of the insulin receptor: A new probe of receptor structure and function. *Science 203*: 544-547.

Hayflick, L. (1975). Current theories of biological aging. *Fed. Proc. 34*: 9-12.

Hayflick, L. (1979). Cell aging. In *Physiology and Cell Biology of Aging*, A. Cherkin, C. E. Finch, N. Kharasch, T. Makinodan, F. L. Scott, and B. Strehler (Eds.). Raven Press, New York, pp. 3-19.

Hirokawa, K. (1977). The thymus and aging. In *Immunology and Aging*, T. Makinodan and E. Yunis (Eds.). Plenum, New York, pp. 51-70.

Isakovic, K., and Jankovic, B. D. (1973). Neuroendocrine correlates of immune response. II. Changes in the lymphatic organs of brain-lesioned rats. *Int. Arch. Allergy 45*: 373-384.

Jankovic, B. D., Draskoci, M., Janjic, M., and Isvaneski, M. (1965). Immunosuppressive effect of reserpine on delayed hypersensitivity reactions. *Int. Arch. Allergy Appl. Immunol. 27*: 376.

Jerne, N. K. (1974). Towards a theory of the immune system. *Ann. Immunol. (Inst. Pasteur) 125C*: 373-389.

Kasahara, K., Tanaka, S., Ito, T., and Hamashima, Y. (1977). Suppression of the primary immune response by chemical sympathectomy. *Res. Comm. Chem. Pathol. Pharmacol. 16*: 687-694.

Kay, M. M. D., and Baker, L. S. (1979). Cell changes associated with declining immune function. In *Physiology and Cell Biology of Aging*, A. Cherkin, C. E. Finch, N. Karasch, T. Makinodan, F. L. Scott, and B. Strehler (Eds.). Raven Press, New York, pp. 27-49.

Kay, M. M. D., and Makinodan, T. (1976). Immunobiology of aging: Evaluation of current status. *Clin. Immunol. Immunopathol. 6*: 394-413.

Keller, S. E., Stein, M., Camerino, M. S., Schleifer, S. J., and Sherman, T. (1980). Suppression of lymphocyte stimulation by anterior hypothalamic lesions in the guinea pig. *Cell. Immunol. 52*: 334-340.

Machado-Salas, J., Scheibel, M., and Scheibel, A. B. (1977). Morphologic changes in the hypothalamus of the old mouse. *Exp. Neurol. 57*: 102-111.

Mac Kay, I. R., Whittingham, S. F., and Matthews, J. D. (1977). The immunoepidemiology of aging. In *Immunology and Aging*, T. Makinodan and E. Yunis (Eds.). Plenum, New York, pp. 35-48.

Makinodan, T., Good, R. A., and Kay, M. M. D. (1977). Cellular basis of immunosenescence. In *Immunology and Aging*, T. Makinodan and E. Yunis (Eds.). Plenum, New York, pp. 9-19.

Mansour, A., and Nelson, D. S. (1978). Effect of hydrocortisone on the response of rat lymphocytes to phytohemagglutinin. *AJEBAK 5C*: 301-311.

Panadian, M. R., and Talwar, G. P. (1971). Effect of growth hormone on the metabolism of thymus and on the immune response against SRBC. *J. Exp. Med. 134*: 1095-1113.

Pierpaoli, W., and Besedovsky, H. O. (1975). Role of the thymus in programming of neuroendocrine functions. *Clin. Exp. Immunol. 20*: 323-338.

Pierpaoli, W., and Maestroni, G. J. M. (1977). Pharmacological control of the immune response by blockade of the early hormonal changes following antigen injection. *Cell. Immunol. 31*: 355-363.

Pierpaoli, W., and Maestroni, G. J. M. (1978). Pharmacological control of the hormonally-modulated immune response. II. Blockade of antibody production by a combination of drugs acting on neuroendocrine functions: Its prevention by gonadotropins and corticotropin. *Immunology 34*: 419-430.

Pochet, R., Delesperse, G., Gauseet, P. W., and Collet, H. (1979). Distribution of beta-adrenergic receptors on human lymphocyte subpopulations. *Clin. Exp. Immunol. 38*: 578-584.

Rebar, R. W., Miyake, A., Low, T. L. K., and Goldstein, A. (1981). Thymosin stimulates secretion of luteinizing hormone-releasing factor. *Science 214*: 669-671.

Roszman, T. L., Cross, R. J., Brooks, W. H., and Markesbery, W. R. (1982). Hypothalamic-Immune interactions. II. The effect of hypothalamic lesions on the ability of adherent spleen cells to limit lymphocyte blastogenesis. *Immunology 45*:737-742.

Schally, A., Kastin, A., and Arimura, A. (1977). Hypothalamic hormones: The link between brain and body. *Am. Sci. 65*: 712-719.

Schiavi, R. C., Adams, J., and Stein, M. (1966). Effect of hypothalamic lesions on histamine toxicity in the guinea pig. *Am. J. Physiol. 211*: 1269-1273.

Snow, E. C., Feldbush, T. L., Oaks, J. A. (1981). The effect of growth hormone and insulin upon MLC responses and the generation of cytotoxic lymphocytes. *J. Immunol. 126*: 161-164.

Stein, M., Schiavi, R. C., and Camerino, M. S. (1976). Influence of brain and behavior on the immune system. *Science 191*: 435-440.

Thoenen, H., and Tranzer, J. P. (1968). Chemical sympathectomy by selective destruction of adrenergic nerve endings with 6-hydroxydopomine. *Naunyn Schmiedebergs Arch. Pharmakol. Exp. Pathol. 261*: 271-278.

Tyrey, L., and Nalbandov, A. V. (1972). Influence of anterior hypothalamic lesions on circulating antibody titers in the rat. *Am. J. Physiol. 222*: 179-185.

Vischer, T. L. (1972). Effect of hydrocortisone on the reactivity of thymus and spleen cells of mice to *in vitro* stimulation. *Immunology 23*: 777-784.

Walford, R. L. (1974). Immunologic theory of aging: Current status. *Fed. Proc. 33*: 2020-2027.

Williams, J. M., Peterson, R. G., Shea, P. A., Schmedtje, J. F., Bauer, D. C., and Felten, D. L. (1981). Sympathetic innervation of murine thymus and spleen: Evidence for a functional link between the nervous and immune systems. *Brain Res. Bull. 6*: 83-94.

9

Clinical Interventions in Immunological Dysfunction

John R. Cohn* / *Veterans Administration and Duke University Medical Centers. Durham, North Carolina*

C. Edward Buckley, III / *Duke University Medical Center, Durham, North Carolina*

INTRODUCTION

Immune dysfunction is a common problem encountered by physicians caring for the elderly. Clinical disease may result from a deficient immune response, such as the increased susceptibility of geriatric patients to soft tissue neoplasms and infections; or paradoxically, it may be a direct result of an inappropriate augmentation of immune processes. Rheumatoid arthritis and multiple myeloma represent extremely different examples of this last group of illnesses. Walford (1974) has suggested that the aging process itself is a manifestation of immune dysfunction, noting the similarities that exist between the graft-vs.-host reaction and normal aging. Burnett (1970) has hypothesized that the immune system may translate the genetic clock controlling longevity into the somatic events which limit life. Yunis and Greenberg (1974) have theorized that "optimal functional longevity" is regulated by the individual's immune response genes. The possibility exists that genetic manipulation of the immune system could ultimately permit intervention in the physiological decline associated with aging. This type of immunological intervention could hold the key to prolonging healthy function in our increasing population of older persons.

---

*Present affiliation: Thomas Jefferson University Hospital, Philadelphia, Pennsylvania.

Certain limited forms of immunological intervention are currently feasible in caring for the elderly. An understanding of the changes in immunity characteristic of older patients is important in understanding the ways in which these primitive modalities are used. After briefly reviewing the immunological changes that occur with aging, this chapter will focus on those interventions which have unique or important clinical applications in the geriatric population.

AGING HUMAN IMMUNE SYSTEM

The alterations that occur in the aging human immune system closely parallel changes described in experimental animals. A comprehensive review of this topic was presented by Makinodan and Kay (1980).

Immunoglobulin (Ig) Production

The ease and safety with which small samples of serum can be obtained have provided many opportunities to describe and quantify age-related changes in serum antibody levels. Buckley and Dorsey (1970, 1971) measured serum concentrations of IgG, IgA, and IgM in 811 healthy persons aged from birth to 92 years. Maximum serum immunoglobulin concentrations occurred near the third decade of life, followed by a gradual decline in IgG and IgM in postmature adults. Increased levels of IgG and IgA were detected near the end of life. In a study of paired observations in elderly persons (Buckley et al., 1974), serum IgG and IgA appeared to increase slightly with advanced age in healthy subjects, while IgG concentrations measured in those near to death were decreased. Extension of these studies to up to five sequential observations has revealed very little change in serum IgG and IgA, a gradual decline in IgM, and evidence of a profound preterminal decrease in IgG and IgM which appears independent of chronological age (unpublished observation). Radl and his associates (Radl et al., 1975) reported a cross-sectional study of immunoglobulin levels in individuals aged 95 years and older who were compared with younger controls. A significant increase in IgG and IgA was detected in their particularly aged population, while serum IgM and IgD concentrations were decreased. Buckley and Trayer (1972) also demonstrated a significant decrease in serum IgD in elderly patients.

The reason for the reported increase in serum IgG and IgA levels in cross-sectional studies is unknown. Possibly, it results from a beneficial effect of relatively higher serum concentrations of these immunoglobulin classes on the survival of older persons (Buckley and Roseman, 1976). The reduced serum levels of IgM and IgD, also characteristic of the elderly, are of special interest. Infection with novel organisms generates IgM antibodies. Other evidence suggests IgD is important in the generation of antibodies to novel antigens, and the absence of IgD on the B-cell surface appears related to the development of tolerance (Vitetta and Uhr, 1977). Makinodan and Kay (1980) reviewed a number of animal studies which demonstrated a decline in the primary but not the secondary antibody response with increasing age, a finding consistent with similar observations in humans. It is tempting to speculate that a common basis exists for the decreased primary immune response, increased susceptibility to infection, and low serum concentrations of IgD and IgM found in the aged.

Cell-Mediated Immunity

Cell-mediated immunity, or delayed hypersensitivity, can be assessed in vivo either by provoking contact dermatitis or by measuring the response to intradermal injections of antigens. Study of the primary immune response generally employs the contact hypersensitivity model. This requires an antigen that is safe, reliably induces sensitization in normals, and to which the subject is unlikely to have been previously exposed. Dinitrochlorobenzene (DNCB) is most often used for this purpose. After this compound is applied to the skin of normal individuals, a typical cell-mediated contact hypersensitivity response will occur on reexposure. The ability to be sensitized to DNCB, and presumably the primary cell-mediated immune response, is decreased in the elderly (Baer and Bowser, 1963; Gross, 1965; Girard et al., 1977).

The secondary or recall immune response is most often studied using the intradermal injection of antigen. Since it is frequently impossible to be certain of prior exposure, multiple antigens must be used, or patients with known infection, particularly with *Mycobacterium tuberculosis*, must be selected. The latter technique is easiest to employ, but has the disadvantage that age- and infection-related effects often cannot be separated.

Grossman and his associates (Grossman et al., 1975) determined in healthy volunteers tested with seven antigens the number of positive delayed hypersensitivity responses. The number of positive tests per subject increased with age until the fifth decade. After that age, a gradual decline in the number of positive tests was noted. The actual average number of positive responses in the 40 to 49-year age range was 3.2. This decreased to 1.7 in subjects aged 80-99 years. The absolute percentage of subjects who exhibited one or more positive skin test reactions declined from 100% during the fifth decade to 85% during the ninth to tenth decades, although this change was not statistically significant. We found similar results in nursing home patients tested with eight delayed-type hypersensitivity recall antigens (Cohn et al., 1982). This suggests that elderly persons, even with chronic illness, retain the potential for a cutaneous cell-mediated response. Multiple antigens may be required to elicit this reactivity, however. Evidence also suggests that the size of the response is decreased, although this may not be true for tuberculin in the face of acute mycobacterial infection.

Buckley and White (1978) examined the diameters of the cutaneous hypersensitivity responses to a standard panel of recall antigens in responders among 1350 patients aged 15-85 years. Maximum responsiveness after 48 hr was detected in subjects in the third decade of life to streptokinase, mumps, and *Candida albicans* skin test antigens. A fivefold decline in responsiveness to streptokinase was detected between the fourth and eighth decades, whereas the age-associated decline in the size of the reactions to mumps and *C. albicans* was gradual through the sixth decade, becoming more pronounced near the end of life. Age-dependent trends in delayed hypersensitivity could be distinguished from those attributed to neoplasia and other chronic diseases common in older persons. Of interest, the magnitude of age-adjusted responses in patients with neoplasia appeared related to survival time.

Battershill (1980) examined the skin test response to 5 U of purified protein derivative of tuberculin (PPD) in 776 patients with tuberculosis. The percentage of patients with anergy (no response to PPD) increased with advancing age. However, no age-related difference was detected in the mean reaction size of responders. A portion of the anergic patients were retested with PPD after their infection had resolved and exhibited typical cutaneous delayed hypersensitivity.

Girard and his associates (Girard et al., 1977) evaluated 880 elderly persons hospitalized in a geriatric hospital. Sixty-seven patients failed to respond to a 100-TU PPD. Of this group, 54 also failed to respond to three control antigens. This represented a much higher prevalence of unresponsiveness than that found in younger controls.

Previously, tuberculin responses 10 mm or greater in size were thought to identify patients sensitized to *M. tuberculosis*. Responses between 5 and 9 mm were labeled as doubtful, and < 5 mm was considered a negative response (American Thoracic Society, 1974). Newer recommendations for the interpretation of PPD skin tests take into account the clinical setting in which the observation is being made (Comstock et al., 1981). The old criteria remain useful guidelines for interpreting epidemiological studies, and were in effect when the currently available data on cutaneous responsiveness to PPD were obtained. We have therefore retained these values for this discussion. The appropriateness of their use with an individual patient should be determined based on the clinical setting.

Nash and Douglas (1980) reported that almost 25% of their patients with active tuberculosis had less than 10 mm of induration when tested with an intermediate-strength (5 TU) PPD. Twenty percent of their patients exhibited responses of less than 5 mm of induration. The average age of patients with negative responses to PPD was 61.5 years, compared with a 48.6-year average for the PPD-positive group. In vitro stimulation of the cultured peripheral blood lymphocytes of tuberculin-positive and negative patients revealed a small but statistically significant decrease in the proliferative response of cells from negative patients treated with low phytohemagglutinin concentrations. No difference was noted at high phytohemagglutinin concentrations. Zeitz et al. (1974) also reported decreased lymphocyte responsiveness to phytohemagglutinin in predominantly older patients with anergy and tuberculosis. Lymphocytes from five of their patients were retested after successful treatment of the infection. There was a significant increase in the response to both phytohemagglutinin and PPD. McMurray and Echeverri

(1978) observed mixed results in studies of 12 elderly tuberculosis patients who initially failed to respond to skin tests with a 250 TU PPD. After treatment, six patients developed positive skin tests and six did not.

These observations suggest that a portion of older patients have delayed cutaneous unresponsiveness to tuberculosis caused by the active infection, while a second group has decreased responsiveness attributable to aging. In vitro testing has demonstrated a decline in mitogen response by the lymphocytes of normal elderly patients (Phair et al., 1978b). Others, but not all investigators, have noted a decrease in the number of peripheral blood T lymphocytes in the elderly (Diaz-Jousnen et al., 1975). Thus, decreased immune cell responsiveness and numbers may both be factors in this age-related functional decline. The clinical importance of this last component stems from the way impaired cellular immunity could permissively contribute to the severity and extent of infection.

Buckley and White (1978) and Roberts-Thompson et al. (1974) have observed a correlation between decreased delayed cutaneous hypersensitivity and increased mortality in the elderly. In the latter study, mortality was significantly higher in those elderly subjects who responded to none or very few of the delayed hypersensitivity skin test antigens, compared with those subjects with multiple positive responses.

A clinical illustration of the protective function of delayed-type hypersensitivity is presented in a report by Stead (1981). Residents of a nursing home who had previously had positive skin tests to tuberculin protein did not develop active disease during an outbreak of tuberculosis, but there was a high incidence of active infection in PPD converters. Likewise, when bacille Calmette Guérin (BCG) vaccination is used as prophylaxis against tuberculosis, protection from infection is related to the presence of cutaneous delayed hypersensitivity (Collins, 1972).

Accessory Immune Function

Certain accessory systems are important in the implementation of the immune response. These systems include neutrophils and other formed blood elements, the complement system, and vasoactive compounds present in body fluids. Palmblad and Haak (1978) reported normal neutrophil bactericidal activity as well as a slight but statistically insignificant increase in serum concentrations of the third and fourth components of the complement system in 15 elderly volunteers. Small but significant elevations in C3 were also found by Thompson and Buckley (1973). Nagaki and his co-workers (Nagaki et al., 1980) examined the complement system in more detail and found increases in total hemolytic complement, C1q, C4, C3, C5, and C9 as well as a decrease in factor B in serums from apparently healthy older subjects. Phair and his associates (Phair et al., 1978b) detected elevations in C3 and properdin, but normal concentrations of factor B in 70 healthy, elderly volunteers. Phair et al. (1978c) also found impaired neutrophil function in a small subset of elderly patients.

INFECTION

The immunological dysfunction of the aged is associated with an increased prevalence of infectious diseases (Center for Disease Control, 1980). Preventable infections are a significant source of morbidity in the elderly and very frequently predispose to or cause death. Tuberculosis, influenza, tetanus, and pneumococcal pneumonia are among the common preventable infections which continue to afflict older patients, often in a far more devastating fashion than found in younger persons. A renewed effort to control these infectious diseases is a worthy goal of geriatric medicine. Effective use of available forms of preventative medicine will require a vigorous educational effort to overcome patient and physician resistance.

Before turning to these specific forms of intervention, it may be useful to review several general principles that apply to the clinical evaluation of the infected older patient. First, since the signs and symptoms of infection are largely dependent upon the vigorous response of an intact immune system, the usual clinical evidence of infection may be reduced, obscured, or even absent. The elderly patient with meningitis may not have meningismus. The patient with peritonitis may lack a rigid abdomen. Fever and leukocytosis may be inappropriately absent (Gladstone and Recco, 1976). A heightened index of suspicion and awareness that the immune response is often altered or attenuated in the aged are needed to identify these instances of active infection. Second, physicial violation of primary barriers against the spread of infectious agents may modify the clinical findings. Examples of this problem include aspiration pneumonia, decubitus ulcers, colonic diverticulitis, and perirectal or vaginal infections. Third, the ambient flora of geriatric patients may differ from that of younger persons, making infection with unusual organisms more common. For example, Phair and his associates (Phair et al., 1978c) observed in older patients an increased incidence of oropharyngeal colonization with gram-negative bacilli and *Staphylococcus aureus*. Since the ambient oral flora correlates with the organisms isolated from patients with pneumonia, this has important clinical implications (Johanson et al., 1979; Johanson et al., 1972).

Once the presence of an infection is identified, treatment must be prompt and effective. The increased clinical fragility of the aged often dictates empiric therapy, precluding continued observation and selection of antimicrobials on the basis of a final microbiological diagnosis. Indeed, the eventual outcome of the illness may be determined early in the course of the infection by the physician's knowledge of the spectrum of organisms that could account for the preliminary clinical and laboratory findings, including gram stains of appropriate specimens. A vigorous effort should be made to isolate the responsible pathogen, particularly in patients with severe or unusual infections. These attempts should include cultures of the blood in instances of sepsis and of the relevant body fluids and external secretions in localized infections. A precise microbiological diagnosis and antibiotic sensitivities are useful in evaluating those elderly patients who respond suboptimally, and in all patients where the shortest course of the least toxic antibiotic is desired.

The information base available for making clinical judgments about initial antibiotic therapy has increased in complexity in recent years. This complexity stems from the increased spectrum of organisms known to infect older persons, the availability of many different antibiotics, our awareness of how antibiotics act and interact, and limitations imposed by the differing side effects of antimicrobial agents. For example, recognition of the increased susceptibility of the aged to *Legionella pheumophilia* and *Mycoplasma pneumoniae* has predicated the increased use of erythromycin, often in conjunction with other antimicrobial agents. The potential gain in the spectrum of pathogens covered by multiple drug regimens must be balanced against an awareness of how one antibiotic can occasionally interfere with the bactericidal action of other antibiotics against specific organisms (Cohn et al., 1980). Similar judgments are necessary with respect to the choice of potentially toxic antibiotics in the presence of possible kidney or hepatic impairment in the aged. These problems are particularly vexing when aminoglycoside antibiotics are used (Gladstone and Recco, 1976; Lutwick, 1980).

Finally, antibiotic therapy and other supportive measure are of minimal value in the face of severe immune dysfunction in the aged. Effective means for identifying those older patients who are at increased risk of infection are needed in order to better guide preventive forms of immunological intervention. It is hoped that the judicious use of blood products and other replacement or immunopotentiating therapy could then guide appropriate prophylactic intervention in the infection-prone aged.

Tuberculosis

Tuberculosis is of special interest because of the high incidence and severity of infection by *M. tuberculosis* in the elderly (Center for Disease Control, 1980). In a recent year, the case rates for tuberculosis were 17.1 per 100,000 for white persons and 99.0 per 100,000 for nonwhite persons over age 65. By contrast, the case rates were 8.9 and 65.7 per 100,000 for whites and nonwhites respectively, aged 25-44 (Sbarbaro, 1975). Gelb and his associates (Gelb et al., 1973) reported the clinical outcomes of 109 patients with treated miliary tuberculosis. The mortality rate was 40% in patients 41 years of age or older, compared with 18% in patients under 41 years of age. Stead (1981) reported that following exposure to a single index case, 45% of 104 elderly nursing home patients developed evidence of infection with tuberculosis. Eight patients developed clinical disease. The extent of clinical illness may have been reduced in Stead's study by vigorous efforts to provide prompt isoniazid (INH) prophylaxis to all known coverters and PPD-positive individuals whose prior skin test status was unknown.

Even limited tuberculosis in the aged is a cause for concern because of the increased toxicity in the elderly of the drugs used to treat that infection, in particular isoniazid (INH) (American Thoracic Society, 1974). The most common serious adverse effect of INH treatment is hepatitis (Kopanoff et al., 1978). The mechanism of isoniazid-induced liver dysfunction is not known, but it does not appear to represent an allergic response (Black et al., 1975).

Rare fatalities have occurred from INH-induced hepatitis, so that some authors initially suggested periodically measuring serum transaminase values in patients receiving INH alone or in combination with other antituberculous agents (Byrd et al., 1974). However, transient liver function abnormalities occur far more often than clinically significant changes in patients treated with isoniazid. Scharer and Smith (1969) demonstrated elevations of serum transaminase levels of up to 10 times the normal value in 10% of a group of patients receiving isoniazid prophylaxis. The two patients with the highest elevations were discontinued from the drug with a return to normal levels. INH was restarted and eventually they completed a course of therapy without difficulty. Seven patients with transaminase values up to five times the upper limit of normal were continued on isoniazid without ill effect. Over time, despite continued treatment, there was spontaneous reversion of their abnormal laboratory studies to normal.

Recently, the American Thoracic Society and the Center for Disease Control recommended that routine periodic serum transaminase measurements *should not be performed* on patients receiving INH (American Thoracic Society, 1974). Instead, they advised monthly contact with the patient to detect clinical symptoms of toxicity. Specifically, they suggested the following information be sought:

1. Symptoms consistent with those of liver damage or other toxic effects; that is, unexplained anorexia, nausea, or vomiting of greater than 3-day duration, fatigue or weakness of greater than 3-day duration, persistent paresthesia of the hands and feet.
2. Signs consistent with those of liver damage or other toxic effects; that is persistent dark urine, icterus, rash, elevated temperature greater than 3-day duration without explanation.
3. Other signs or symptoms the patient may report.

Currently, 1 year of INH, 300 mg per day, is recommended for several categories of patients, including "recent PPD converters" (American Thoracic Society, 1974). Clinical evidence suggests this is particularly important in the elderly. Stead (1981) reported that 2 of 5 elderly PPD converters who were not treated with isoniazid developed active tuberculosis, whereas none of the 36 converters who received a year's course of isoniazid, 300 mg per day, developed evidence of active infection.

In determining whether or not an elderly patient is a PPD converter, the so-called booster effect must be taken into account (Thompson et al., 1979). This term relates to the decrease over time in the response to intradermal PPD. On initial testing, the diameter of the area of induration may measure less than 10 mm and thus be read as negative. However, the patient is sensitized or "boosted" by the test itself. When rechallenged, there is an increase in the size of the reaction. This is falsely interpreted as "conversion" from a negative to a positive PPD. The incidence of this phenomenon increases with increasing age. Therefore, older patients whose baseline PPD status is being determined for the first time should have the test placed twice. The second test should be placed at least 1 week after the first and should serve as the recorded value.

Drug selection in the treatment of active tuberculosis in the elderly requires careful evaluation of the patient's social and environmental influences, as well as the extent of disease. With a view towards increased patient compliance, the American Thoracic Society and the Center for Disease Control recently issued a statement that patients being treated for active tuberculosis may be treated for only 9 months if both isoniazid and rifampin are used (Iseman et al., 1980). Since both rifampin and isoniazid may be hepatotoxic (Addington, 1979; Lees et al., 1970), the clinician must decide whether the advantage of a shorter course of therapy outweighs the increased risk of liver damage in an individual older patient.

Immunization

Prophylactic immunization can reduce the severity of and even prevent many of the common infectious problems of the aged. There are two general types of immunization, passive and active. Passive immunization refers to the administration of serum containing preformed specific antibodies to an exposed subject. Treatment with homologous serum is preferred since the use of sera from heterologous species (e.g., horse serum) is associated with a high incidence of serum sickness. An example of passive immunization with homologous serum is the use of human tetanus immune globulin in a previously unimmunized patient who has a high-risk exposure to tetanus, such as a traumatic wound (Fraser, 1976). Active immunization refers to use of a vaccine to provoke the generation of protective antibodies by the patient's own immune system. Active immunization has two main beneficial effects. Once formed, circulating antibodies offer protection against the antigenic pathogen or toxin; and on reexposure, the patient will develop a much more rapid, vigorous, anamnestic immune response.

For reasons cited previously, elderly patients may have intact secondary antigen responses but exhibit impaired ability to respond to antigens de novo. This makes "elective" exposure in the form of immunization particularly desirable. The impaired ability of older persons to develop a primary response to an infecting organism does not mean that vaccination will also be ineffective. As we will discuss, there is both serological and clinical evidence for the efficacy of vaccinating the elderly.

We have selected for examination in this chapter influenza, pneumococcal, and diptheria vaccination. A number of other vaccines are available, but their use is generally limited to persons with increased risk of exposure to a particular organism or to younger age groups. The newest vaccine in this category is for the prevention of hepatitis B. Over one-third of the geriatric patients in a recent study were found to have serum antibodies against this virus (Finkelstein et al., 1981).

This suggests that screening for the specific antibody is probably cost effective in the elderly population, before administering this expensive vaccine. This same study found that 94% of the subjects had antibodies to hepatitis A. This population was drawn from a New York City clinic, an area known to have a higher incidence of hepatitis A infection. Nevertheless, these data suggest that, at least for urban populations, passive immunization with immune serum globulin may be less important for the elderly subject exposed to hepatitis A.

Influenza

It has been estimated that 150,000 influenza-A-related deaths occurred in the United States between 1968 and 1979 (Center for Disease Control, 1979). The vast majority of those fatalities were elderly. The Immunization Committee of the Infectious Diseases Association of America has projected that during that time period 100,000 deaths would have been prevented by universal immunization of the aged. These sobering statistics require that all persons involved with older persons be familiar with the history and use of influenza vaccine.

One of the earliest studies pertaining to the serological response of the elderly to influenza vaccination was by Saslaw and his associates (Saslaw et al., 1966). They studied 440 institutionalized veterans, some of whom received annual influenza vaccination and some of whom did not. Vaccinated subjects had higher antibody titers to multiple strains than subjects not vaccinated. In 1967, Lamb et al. demonstrated the serological effectiveness of influenza vaccine in 554 elderly subjects using a standard aqueous and a depot-type vaccine. As in other studies (Phair et al., 1978a), the antibody response was usually greatest in the subjects with the lowest initial antibody titers.

When the specific antibody titers measured in vaccinated elderly subjects have been compared with those found in other age groups, the results have been inconsistent among different virus strains. Larger, smaller, and similar titer responses to those found with the young have been reported (Fulk et al., 1970; Ferry et al., 1976; Cate et al., 1976; Sabin, 1974). This is thought to reflect both age-related changes in the immune system as well as prior experience with the same or related virus strains by the elderly subjects.

Antibody titers do not necessarily correlate with protection, and so a number of authors have examined the clinical efficacy of various influenza vaccines. Ruben et al. (1974) studied an epidemic of A/England influenza in a home for the aged where approximately 50% of the residents had been vaccinated against the A/Hong Kong strain. The attack and death rates were comparable for both the vaccinated and unvaccinated residents. However, the illness was shorter and milder in the vaccinated population. The partial protection provided by immunization was interpreted as a result of antigenic similarities between the two virus strains. Another group (Miller et al., 1975) vaccinated 150 long-term residents of a chronic-care facility against influenza A (H3N2). They used either live attenuated vaccine or killed parenteral vaccine. The killed vaccine had fewer side effects and demonstrable efficacy in preventing infection. Howells et al. (1975) reported less bronchopneumonia and lower mortality in a group of elderly influenza vaccinees when compared with a control population of fellow residents in several domiciliary facilities. The difference did not become significant until the third year of annual vaccination. Whether this was due to better coverage in that year of the annual differences in influenza virus strains, or whether repetitive annual vaccination produced more effective immunization is uncertain. The results of immunizing over 5000 persons with the 1976 A/New Jersey/76 vaccine provided further evidence of the overall effectiveness and general lack of side effects of influenza vaccination in the elderly (Parkman et al., 1976).

Additional work has been directed at enhancing the serological response to influenza vaccination using adjuvants, depot preparations (Lamb et al., 1967), or nasal immunization (Fulk et al., 1969; Kasel et al., 1969). None of these approaches is clinically applicable at the present time.

In summary, it has been demonstrated that influenza vaccination will produce a positive antibody response in elderly patients. The titer of the response may be greater or less than that found in a younger population, depending on the vaccinee's previous experience with related virus strains. Vaccination reduces the severity and possibly decreases the incidence of influenza infection. Since the incidence and mortality of influenza infection are increased in the elderly, all persons 65 years of age and older should be vaccinated against influenza (Burnery, 1960). Because it is well known that changes occur in the antigenic composition of prevalent influenza virus strains from year to year, annual vaccination is indicated to heighten protection against exposure to the most likely current viral strains (Morris, 1965).

During the 1976 swine flu vaccination campaign, there was a small increase in the incidence of the Guillain-Barré syndrome in vaccinated persons. This was a more serious problem among the elderly. Because of the implications of this finding, the association between the Guillain-Barré syndrome and influenza vaccination was investigated further. Practicing neurologists in the United States were surveyed during the winters of 1978-1979 and 1979-1980. No increase in the incidence of the Guillain-Barré syndrome was found among vaccinees (Center for Disease Control, 1980). Vaccination can therefore be considered to be of essentially negligible risk and should not be withheld from older patients because of fear of this complication. The Center for Disease Control (1979) cites the following potential side effects from the influenza virus vaccine:

1. Local redness and induration at the site of injection for 1 or 2 days in less than one-third of vaccinees.
2. Fever, malaise, or myalgia lasting for 1-2 days. These side effects are most commonly found in children.

3. Immediate hypersensitivity reactions. This is thought to represent a reaction to a component of the vaccine, the most likely offender being egg protein from the culture medium that the virus was initially grown in. Patients with a history of anaphylaxis after ingesting eggs should not be given influenza vaccine.

4. In recognition of the increased incidence of the Guillain-Barré syndrome in vaccinees during the 1976 immunization campaign, this disorder is listed as a potential side effect of vaccination. In order to keep this problem in perspective, it is important to remember that the incidence in 1976 was 10 cases for every 1 million persons vaccinated. Only 5% of those cases resulted in fatality. By contrast, it has been estimated that over 150,000 excess deaths occured in the United States between 1968 and 1979 due to influenza A epidemics (Center for Disease Control, 1979).

A successful vaccination program must, of course, be based on more than clinical efficacy. Aho (1979) studied 122 elderly persons to determine their reasons for participating or not participating in the national swine flu immunization campaign. Physician influence played a major role in encouraging vaccination.

During the winter of 1981-1982, the potency of the vaccine was doubled to 15 μg/0.5 ml for each antigen in the trivalent vaccine. As always, one dose was required for persons over age 29 (Center for Disease Control, 1981a). The value of this increase in dose remains to be determined.

If an influenza epidemic occurs among an elderly, unvaccinated, closed population, consideration should be given to the use of amantadine hydrochloride. This antiviral compound provides protection against infection, but will not interfere with a patient's ability to respond to concurrent vaccination (Delker et al., 1980). Amantadine is not a substitute for prophylactic vaccination.

Tetanus and Diphtheria

With the advent of tetanus immunization, there has been a progressive decline in the incidence of tetanus in the general population. However, the case rate for the elderly continues to be high. In the most recent year for which figures are available, the case rate of tetanus was three times as high in persons over 60 than in any other segment of the population (Center for Disease Control, 1980). Ruben et al. (1978) reported that only 51% of a nursing home population had protective tetanus antitoxin titers and only 59% had effective diphtheria antitoxin titers. In the second part of their study, all patients who had no previous history of immunization were vaccinated with two doses of the commercial adult diphtheria-tetanus (dT) toxoid. While some patients did not respond adequately to the first immunization dose, all patients developed protective antitoxin levels after the second immunization. Side effects were minimal. Inadequate antitoxin levels were also found by Crossley and his co-workers in their study of 183 elderly persons living in Minnesota (Crossley et al., 1979). Only 41% of the men over age 59 and 29% of the women over age 40 had protective serum levels of tetanus antitoxin. By contrast, over 85% of a group of younger subjects had adequate titers. Patient recall of previous dT toxoid injections correlated well with serum antibody levels. Eighty-three percent of the patients who said that they had been immunized at least twice had protective tetanus antitoxin levels. Adequate diphtheria antitoxin activity was less frequently found, even in the multiply immunized population. This may reflect the prior use of tetanus toxoid rather than the combined vaccine. Finally, Kishimoto and his co-workers showed a decreased but still present response to tetanus toxoid injection in elderly volunteers (Kishimoto et al., 1980).

In short, elderly patients commonly have decreased tetanus and diphtheria antitoxin levels, but they will respond to vaccination. They should be considered candidates for routine tetanus and diphtheria immunization. Those patients with no history of immunization should receive two immunizing injections. Patients who have been immunized but whose last booster was given 10 or more years previously should receive a single dose of tetanus and diphtheria toxoid (Fraser, 1976). There is no evidence that giving routine injections more often than every 10 years is beneficial. Indeed, frequent dT immunization has been associated with immune-complex-type illness (Edsall et al., 1967). If important questions remain about a patient's antitoxin status, serum levels can easily be measured.

The United States Public Health Service Advisory Committee on Immunization Practices has published recommendations concerning appropriate tetanus prophylaxis for patients with new wounds that place them at additional risk of disease (Fraser, 1976). They are the same for the elderly as for younger persons. However, the geriatrician must keep in mind that tetanus can come not only from the obvious forms of trauma that affect all age groups, but also from such unexpected places as the common pressure sore or decubitus ulcer (Rueller and Cooney, 1981).

Pneumococcal Vaccination

Despite the essentially universal in vitro effectiveness of penicillin against *Streptococcus pneumoniae*, evidence suggests that pneumococcal infection continues to be a frequently fatal problem for the elderly. Austrian and Gold (1964) reviewed the experience with pneumococcal bacteremia over a 10-year period at the Kings County Hospital. There were 529 instances of pneumococcal bacteremia, with a mortality rate that increased from 0% for the 12 to 19-year age group to 18% for bacteremic patients aged 50-59, 43% for those aged 60-69, and a maximum of 83% in patients greater than 90 years of age. In bacteremic patients with no other evidence of extrapulmonary infection, the mortality rate was 28% for those over age 50, compared with 6-8% in a comparable younger group.

Finland (1979), in a study at Boston City Hospital, reported similar results. During the time period from 1951-1972, patients over the age of 60 accounted for 45% of the episodes of pneumococcal bacteremia at that institution. At the same time, the mortality rate for bacteremic patients over age 60 was 48%. This compared with a mortality rate of 22% in bacteremic patients aged 30-59, and 2% in bacteremic patients aged 0-25 years.

The precise reason for the failure of a substantial number of patients, particularly elderly patients, to respond to appropriate antimicrobial therapy is unknown. The studied patients were drawn from an inner-city population, and many had chronic illnesses. This may have accounted for the high mortality observed. Others have proposed that there is a point in an episode of pneumococcal pneumonia when irreversible physiological damage occurs. Beyond that time, even the introduction of an appropriate antimicrobial will fail to prevent the patient's death. Austrian and Finland propose that this point is passed much earlier and more frequently in the elderly (Austrian, 1975; Finland, 1979).

At present, the only way to potentially further reduce the incidence of fatal pneumococcal pneumonia in the elderly is to prevent the initial infection. Recently, a vaccine has been introduced that contains polysaccharide capsular material from the 12 most common strains of *S. pneumoniae*. These strains represent at least 80% of all of the cases of bacteremic pneumococcal disease reported in the United States (Center for Disease Control, 1978). The package insert has recommended routine vaccination for persons 50 years of age or older (Merck, Sharp, and Dohme, 1977).

The actual efficacy of the current pneumococcal vaccine has not been carefully evaluated in older age groups, and it has been observed that the vaccine is less than optimally effective in other high-risk populations (Broome et al., 1980). A study by Kauffman (1947) would appear to at least partly negate concern for the vaccine's efficacy in the elderly.

Kauffman (1947) vaccinated over 5000 persons against pneumococcal polysaccharide types 1, 2, and 3, and a comparable population was maintained as controls. Essentially all of the immunized patients and controls were over 50 years of age. There were 99 episodes of pneumonia in the vaccinated group and 227 in the control group. The mortality rate in the vaccinees was 6.2 per 1000 compared with 19.0 per 1000 among the controls. This study was performed before penicillin became available, but it suggests that elderly patients are capable of developing a significant protective antibody response after pneumococcal vaccination.

More recently, two large, controlled studies were conducted to assess the efficacy of a dodecavalent pneumococcal vaccine in institutionalized and in ambulatory populations (Austrian, 1980). Several thousand persons were in each trial. While there was serological evidence of effectiveness in each study, consistent benefit could not be demonstrated in terms of the type and frequency of respiratory infections. The author attributed this to the relatively low incidence of pneumococcal infection in the study groups. However, a low incidence of disease may indicate a limited need for vaccination.

The American College of Physicians (1982) and the Center for Disease Control (1982) have each issued statements suggesting that universal vaccination of all elderly persons is not justified based on current data. Others have suggested that vaccination of the entire population over age 65 would indeed be cost effective (Willems et al., 1980). Perhaps the most prudent approach at present is selective vaccination of patients with other recognized risk factors (e.g., chronic lung disease) or whose socioeconomic status or health care history suggests that they are not likely to receive proper medical attention for a respiratory infection. Unfortunately, the latter group may be least likely to be offered the vaccine. The topic of pneumococcal vaccination, particularly as it relates to efficacy, was recently reviewed by Schwartz (1982).

As the current pneumococcal vaccine is relatively new, the absolute duration of immunity is unknown. Revaccination is not recommended at the present time (Center for Disease Control, 1981b).

HYPERSENSITIVITY DISEASE

Hypersensitivity diseases include asthma, seasonal rhinitis, atopic dermatitis, contact dermatitis, and drug allergy. Disagreement exists about the actual prevalence and precise character of these conditions in the elderly, since the immunological dysfunction responsible for allergic or hypersensitivity disease in older persons causes illness that differs somewhat from that found in the young. Difficulties in definition also stem from the way the various allergic diseases are defined. For example, asthma, asthmatic bronchitis, and chronic bronchitis represent a spectrum of disorders that reflect the degree to which several common mechanisms contribute to the pathophysiology of the illnesses observed. The resulting clinical similarities often prevent precise differentiation between these related conditions (Gross, 1980).

Classically, allergic diseases are mediated by the homocytotropic antibody IgE. Other mechanisms have been suggested and implicated (Pepys and Hutchcroft, 1975), but are not known to be a prevalent cause of allergy. Contact dermatitis is caused by a cell-mediated immune reaction (Morgan and Keeran, 1970; Hanifin, 1979; DeWeck, 1977), although IgE may play a role in initiating the disease (Gershon et al., 1975).

Human homocytotropic antibodies are bound to mast cells. Reaction with specific antigen, or with anti-IgE, provokes release of various chemical mediators from the cell. Examples of these mediators include histamine and slow-reacting substance of anaphylaxis (SRS-A). The chemical mediators are responsible for the changes in tissues which cause clinical disease.

Delespesse et al. (1977b) measured the serum IgE concentrations in a group of apparently healthy residents of an old-age home. The values were compared with those of a control population of blood donors and laboratory staff, all of whom were less than 60 years of age. The older patients tended to have significantly lower total serum IgE concentrations as a group, although there was considerable overlap between the older and younger subjects. Both groups were then immunized with diphtheria toxoid, and their specific serum IgE response was followed with a radioallergosorbent (RAST) test. IgE antibodies to diphtheria toxin were much more commonly induced in the younger patients. Finally, a reverse Prausnitz-Kustner reaction was done in the two subject groups. This test employs rabbit anti-IgE to provoke the release of mediators from cutaneous mast cells. Although the amount of anti-IgE required to produce a reaction was comparable in the two groups, the size of the reaction was greater in younger subjects. A decrease in the elderly volunteers' responsiveness to histamine was excluded, since both groups developed comparably sized wheals when tested with intradermal histamine. These data suggest that older patients produce less homocytotropic IgE in response to an extrinsic allergen exposure, and comparably sensitized mast cells from older persons respond to allergens with less mediator release.

Johansson (1968), Wittig et al. (1980), and Orren and Dowdle (1975) all reported declining serum IgE levels with increasing age. The cross-sectional study by Wittig et al. (1980) provided additional insight. Normal controls had a relatively small decline in serum IgE levels with increasing age. Older patients with asthma exhibited a severalfold decrease from an average peak of 548 IU/ml in the 6 to 15-year age group to 172 IU/ml in the over-40 age group. At that age, the average serum IgE concentration in patients with asthma was still elevated in comparison with normal subjects at any age. The number of asthmatic patients with IgE levels less than 100 reached a minimum at age 16-20 years with a gradual increase from that age. Likewise, as the age increased from the teenage years to the over-40 age group, the percentage of asthmatic patients with few or no positive immediate hypersensitivity skin tests and low serum IgE levels increased from approximately 10 to over 40%. Since all of the patients over 40 were grouped together, it is not possible to know whether the trend toward less evidence of atopy became more pronounced with further increases in age. Patients with allergic rhinitis had serum IgE concentrations that fell between those detected in patients with asthma and healthy subjects. IgE levels were highest in patients with asthma and eczema. A large amount of variation in serum IgE concentrations existed in all groups.

Barbee et al. (1976) measured the reactivity of 3101 randomly selected subjects to cutaneous tests for immediate hypersensitivity. There was an age-related decrease in the cutaneous response to allergens.

An additional factor important in the pathogenesis of allergic disease is the innate predisposition of the atopic patient to develop signs and symptoms of illness following exposure to allergens. Equally atopic individuals, as determined by immediate hypersensitivity allergen skin tests, may have asthma, seasonal allergic rhinitis, atopic dermatitis, or be without symptoms entirely (Hagy and Settipane, 1971; Block et al., 1978). The capacity to develop an immediate hypersensitivity disease has been referred to as "hyperreactivity" in asthmatic patients. It is not completely understood, but considerable descriptive information, particularly in asthma, has been accumulated about it (Fish et al., 1980).

Deal and his associates (Deal et al., 1980) studied the effect of cold-air hyperpnea on asymptomatic asthmatics, subjects with season rhinitis, and normal controls. Whereas the cold-air challenge had no effect on the controls, there was a small drop in expiratory flow rates in patients with seasonal rhinitis, and a large decrease in patients with asthma. Similar differences in reactivity have been demonstrated in patients with asthma and those with hay fever using mecholyl (a parasympathetic agonist) and histamine (Townley et al., 1965). By contrast, inhalation of small quantities of known allergens does not always produce airway obstruction in asthmatics, and conversely may cause a significant fall in expiratory flow in some patients with hay fever (Townley et al., 1965; Ahmed et al., 1981).

Smith et al. (1980) measured the effect of topical carbamylcholine chloride (a parasympathetic agonist) on pupillary constriction in several groups of patients and in normal controls. They demonstrated a comparable increase in cholinergic responsiveness in those subjects with allergic asthma, allergic rhinitis, and in asymptomatic atopy. Of particular relevance to the finding common in older asthmatic patients, immediate hypersensitivity allergen skin test negative asthmatics showed a significantly greater increase in cholinergic responsiveness than either normals or atopic asthmatics.

Using similar techniques, this same group has demonstrated a marked increase in pupillary alpha-adrenergic responsiveness in allergic asthmatics and a smaller increase in patients with allergic rhinitis (Henderson et al., 1979). They and numerous other groups have demonstrated a decrease in the responsiveness of beta-adrenergic receptors in diverse tissues in subjects with atopy, including those with dermatitis, as well as those who are asymptomatic (Shelhamer et al., 1980; Szentivanyi, 1980). Szentivanyi (1980) reviewed the potential reasons for these observations and suggested a shift in the balance between beta- and alpha-adrenergic receptors in the atopic person. Under some circumstances, infectious agents augment this imbalance towards increased alpha-adrenergic and cholinergic activity.

Available evidence suggests decreased beta-adrenergic responsiveness occurs in the elderly (Roth, 1979; Schocken and Roth, 1977), and animal studies indicate increased alpha-adrenergic responsiveness with increasing age (Fleisch et al., 1970). The possibility exists that exaggerated age-dependent changes in the responsiveness of elements of the autonomic nervous system are responsible for the development of much of the "allergic" disease of the elderly.

Allergic respiratory diseases and hypersensitivity dermatitis are the best understood of the allergic disorders of older persons. For that reason, they will be discussed in more detail in the following sections. In-depth reviews of the allergic or immediate hypersensitivity process and its management can be found in standard allergy textbooks, such as those edited by Patterson (1980) or Middleton et al. (1978).

Allergic Respiratory Diseases

Incidence and Characteristics

The exact incidence and nature of allergic respiratory illness in the geriatric population remains controversial. With advanced age, nonallergic factors such as tobacco abuse and occupational exposure confound the interpretation of obstructive respiratory symptoms. Many clinicians contend that the older patient with asthma presents in a different fashion than the child or young adult (Ghory and Patterson, 1980; Taub, 1975; Lovell, 1970; Criep, 1970; Guerrant, 1978; Hanneuse et al., 1978). Older patients are said to have less evidence of an IgE-mediated allergic component, are less likely to respond to disodium chromoglycolate (Campbell and Tandon, 1969; Guerrant, 1978), and frequently require corticosteroids to control disabling symptoms. Several studies have been conducted to examine this problem more closely.

Schachter and Higgins (1976) demonstrated a trimodal distribution in the age of onset of asthma in male patients. The highest incidence of illness occurred in the group 0-4 years of age. The incidence declined until the fourth and fifth decades when a second peak was noted. The incidence again declined during the sixth decade, but increased beginning at 60 years of age. The incidence of illness in the oldest groups approached that found in young children. Elderly females had a similar pattern but with a less significant rise in disease incidence in the seventh decade and beyond. By contrast, allergic rhinitis showed a gradual decline in the rate of onset up to the oldest age group. There was a small but statistically insignificant increase in incidence at that point. Wittig et al. (1978) reviewed the records of over 2000 patients to determine the age of onset of asthma or allergic rhinitis. Approximately 10% of their patients developed disease after the age of 40 years. Burr et al. (1979) interviewed persons over the age of 70 in a small town in Wales, exclusive of residents of domiciliary facilities. Only 6.5% of the persons interviewed gave a history of current (2.9%) or past (3.6%) asthma. Current asthma was much more common among men (5.1%) than in women (1.8%). In a review of 11,551 patients with asthma, Ford (1969) reported that environmental causes could be identified in only 12% of individuals aged 60 years and older. By contrast, in patients with asthma ranging in age from 15 to 29 years and 30 to 44 years, Ford found identifiable environmental causes in 83% and 72% respectively.

Early evidence, as well as clinical observation, suggested that patients who developed asthma at a later age had more severe disease (Ogilvie, 1962). Hall and Henderson studied 180 patients over 15 years of age who were hospitalized because of asthma (1966). Patients were divided into three groups based on their current age as well as the age of onset of their disease (over 40/disease after 40; under 40/disease before 40; over 40/disease before 40). Late-onset asthmatics had more severe disease, a higher incidence of ear, nose, and throat problems, and more of them were on corticosteroids at the time of their admission. A family history of atopy or an allergic etiology was more commonly found in the patients with disease onset before age 40. There was only a small difference between the three groups in the number of patients responding to intradermal allergen skin tests for immediate hypersensitivity, amount of peripheral eosinophilia, number of patients with a history of adverse drug reactions, and admission white blood cell counts. Lee and Stretton (1972) found similar evidence of increased disease severity in their elderly asthmatics. All 15 of the patients they reported developed asthma at age 60 or later. Fourteen required corticosteroid therapy for control of their symptoms. Corticosteroids reduced the sputum volume and eosinophil count, and resulted in improvement in the patients' expiratory flow rates. All of their patients who produced sputum had significant sputum eosinophilia. Most of their patients had smoked in the past and lived in an industrial environment. It was Lee and Stretton's opinion that many of the subjects had had chronic bronchitis which abruptly deteriorated with the onset of superimposed asthma. Guerrant (1978) studied a group of asthmatic patients being treated at the University of Virginia Medical Center. Out of 117 patients, 57 developed asthma before age 40 and 19 after age 60. He found that atopic disease was much less common in the older asthmatics. Silbert and Dudani (1979) reported on 160 patients over age 60 seen in their practice for allergic respiratory diseases. A majority of the patients gave a history of allergic-type respiratory symptoms as children or young adults. In most cases, the symptoms were less severe than at the present time. Emotional factors appeared to be important in the precipitation of illness. Positive skin tests to pollens and other common allergens were common as were persistent mild upper respiratory tract symptoms. Hanneuse et al. (1978) examined a variety of laboratory and clinical characteristics in a population of 326 allergic patients. They reported a peak in total serum IgE at about age 15 with a gradual decline from that point. This trend was paralleled by an age-associated decline in radioallergosorbent (RAST) scores to selected allergens. Blood eosinophilia declined with age as well. Older asthmatics less often responded to disodium cromoglycolate and were more frequently corticosteroid dependent.

Mucus clearance, perhaps related to automonic dysfunction, may also be abnormal in the elderly with lung disease. Santa Cruz et al. (1974) demonstrated that tracheal mucus velocity was depressed from a value of 21.5 mm/min in young normal volunteers to 1.7 mm/min in patients aged 57-71 with chronic obstructive lung disease. Subcutaneous terbutaline, a beta-adrenergic agonist, had no effect on the mucus clearance rate in the normal controls but caused an increase of 114% in the patients with obstructive lung disease.

Treatment

The treatment of asthma in the elderly is similar to that for younger patients. Management can be directed at avoidance of the allergen, blocking the binding of the allergen to homocytotropic antibody, inhibition of the release of mediators, blocking the binding of the mediator to the target organ, or blocking or reversing the target organ effect (Webb-Johnson and Andrews, 1977; Van Arsdel and Paul, 1977).

Drugs that block H1 histamine receptors, such as chlorpheneramine and diphenhydramine, have played a major role in the alleviation of allergic symptoms of the skin and upper respiratory tract. Their use in asthma remains controversial and is generally not recommended (Goth, 1978). Antihistamines are associated with an increased incidence of dizziness, sedation, and hypotension in the elderly, and a specific warning to that effect may be found on the package of inserts of these drugs (Medical Economics Company, 1981). It is often helpful to give a small first dose of the selected antihistamine and to give the first and largest dose at bedtime. Patients should be warned of the potential side effects, and advised to limit activities accordingly.

Sympathomimetic drugs are of several types, related to the general category of activity (alpha-adrenergic, beta-adrenergic, or mixed). Beta-adrenergic drugs can be further divided into beta-1- and beta-2-stimulating subtypes. Beta-2 receptor stimulation mediates bronchodilatation as well as augments mucocilliary clearance (Santa Cruz et al., 1974). Beta-1 receptors are found on the myocardium and elsewhere. Since cardiac stimulation may be particularly undesirable in the elderly, nonspecific beta agonists such as ephedrine and isoproterenol have been replaced by relatively more specific beta-2 agents such as terbutaline, metaproteranol, and isoetharine. More recently, a third generation of beta-2 agonists, such as salbutamol, have come on the market. It is suggested that they have even less cardiac-stimulating effect with equal bronchodilating efficacy (Jack and Harris, 1978; Webb-Johnson and Andrews, 1977; Milner and Ingram, 1971; Riding et al., 1970). Clinical differences between the beta-2-selective drugs have not been quantitated. Therefore, the most cost-effective regimen remains to be established. The use of an alpha-adrenergic stimulant such as phenylephrine with a beta-adrenergic stimulant offers no advantage over the pure beta-adrenergic agonist, but can produce additional side effects (Spector et al., 1977).

Methylxanthines are an important group of drugs in the treatment of obstructive airways disease. They are metabolized by the liver and excreted by the kidney. The serum half-life is prolonged in the elderly. For this reason, the Food and Drug Administration has recommended that the maintenance dose in elderly patients be reduced, particularly in the presence of congestive heart failure or renal disease. Table 1 summarizes the current dosage guidelines for aminophylline and theophylline in elderly patients (Food and Drug Administration, 1980). These are only guidelines. Serum theophylline levels should be measured periodically in all patients.

Theophylline inhibits the action of phosphodiesterase, the enzyme that breaks down intracellular cyclic adrenesine monophosphate (AMP). Cyclic AMP is the intracellular messenger for beta-adrenergic stimulation (Ellis, 1978). An additive effect occurs when theophylline is used with a beta-adrenergic agonist (Wolfe et al., 1978). This effect is especially important in older persons with bronchospastic disease because lower doses of both drugs can be used with a consequent decrease in side effects. Theophylline has also been demonstrated to be of value in steroid-dependent asthmatics (Nassif et al., 1981). Because of the prolonged half-life of theophylline in the elderly, long-acting preparations may often allow for steady serum levels with a twice-daily dose. If necessary to facilitate administration, theophylline-granule-containing capsules can be opened, and the contents sprinkled on food.

Table 1 Aminophylline Dosage in the Elderly

Group[a]	Maintenance dose first 12 hr (mg/kg/hr)	Maintenance dose after 12 hr (mg/kg/hr)
Older patients	0.6	0.3
Patients with congestive heart failure, liver disease	0.5	0.1-0.2

[a] All patients not on theoyphylline receive a 6 mg/kg loading dose.
Source: Adapted from *FDA Drug Bulletin, 10*(1):5, 1980.

Cromolyn sodium inhibits the release of mediators by mast cells. This drug is not effective in the majority of elderly patients, for reasons that are not clearly known. Presumable mast cell products have a reduced role in this decrease in older persons.

Corticosteroids are supplemental drugs used to treat acute and chronic airway obstruction that is refractory to maximally tolerated bronchodilator therapy. Inhaled corticosteroids in effective doses do not cause systemic side effects. At higher doses significant absorption with adrenal suppression and other adverse reactions can occur. Inhaled corticosteroids are preferred to oral preparations for the treatment of asthma whenever possible. They may also be used by nasal inhalation for rhinitis. When oral steroids are required, an alternate-day regimen and the lowest lowest dose possible should constantly be pursued. If benefit cannot be demonstrated, they should be discontinued. The mechanism of action of corticosteroids in asthma is unknown. They are thought to potentiate the action of adrenergic agonists.

In young subjects, immunotherapy is of demonstrated efficacy for allergic rhinitis, and is probably useful in selected asthmatics (Patterson, 1979; Norman, 1980). In elderly patients with asthma, immunotherapy was thought effective in uncontrolled studies by Dudani et al. (1980) and by Guerrant (1978). Guerrant found that 6 of 15 (40%) patients over age 40 with a history of allergen-exposure-related symptoms improved on immunotherapy. By contrast, only 3 of 17 (18%) patients of similar age and allergic history, but without current exposure-related symptoms were improved. None of 23 patients with wheezing and without any evidence of allergic disease improved on immunotherapy. The mechanism of action of immunotherapy is unknown, although numerous biological changes have been documented (Norman, 1980).

Hypersensitivity Dermatitis

The prevalence of atopic dermatitis in the elderly is not clearly defined. It has been suggested that atopic dermatitis does not occur at all in people over age 65

(Morgan and Keeran, 1970). However, persistent symptoms with follow-up as long as 20 years have been noted in persons who had had severe atopic dermatitis as children (Roth and Kierland, 1964). As we have previously discussed, there is an age-related decline in the development of allergen-related symptoms and elevated IgE levels in patients with asthma (Wittig et al., 1980). Too few patients were tested in that study to determine whether or not the same phenomenon occurs in patients with eczema. However, the paucity of patients found by that group with atopic dermatitis after age 40 (2), compared with the number with asthma (52) or allergic rhinitis (21) suggests that atopic dermatitis is rare in the geriatric population. Since atopic dermatitis has been associated with abnormalities of both humoral and cell-mediated immunity (Hanifin and Lobitz, 1977), problems commonly found in the elderly, other factors must account for the development of disease.

Contact dermatitis is a cell-mediated phenomenon (deWeck, 1977). It appears to be present in the elderly in equal frequency to that found in younger patients but is less severe (Hanifin, 1979). This is consistent with the decline in other delayed hypersensitivity phenomena in the aged.

Immunotherapy and food avoidance have not been shown to be effective in elderly patients with hypersensitivity dermatitis. This suggests that IgE-mediated mechanisms do not play a significant role. Physical factors, such as drying of the skin, seem to be more important in the pathophysiology of dermatitis in the aged. Older patients often benefit from therapy designed to maintain skin moisture. When cellular immune mechanisms are involved, judicious use of topical corticosteroids may be of value. Avoidance of irritants and sensitizing agents is also advisable (Lantis and Lantis, 1975; Morgan and Keeran, 1970). Management is otherwise similar to that used in younger patients.

DISORDERS OF HOMEOSTASIS

Autoimmunity and Neoplasia

The latter decades of life are associated both with increased autoimmune phenomena and a high incidence of neoplasia. Both of these groups of disorders represent malfunction of the older person's immunological regulation of homeostasis. Some autoimmune processes, such as the destruction of erythrocytes that have reached the end of their natural life span, occur at all ages and represent useful physiological mechanisms. Other phenomena are without known pathological significance, such as the increased frequency of serum rheumatoid factor or cryoglobulins in otherwise asymptomatic elderly persons. By contrast, autoimmune illnesses, such as rheumatoid arthritis, may produce substantial moribidity and on occasion mortality in older age groups. Similar observations can be made about the various neoplastic processes that occur. Benign monoclonal gammopathies are felt to be without clinical significance, but multiple myeloma, amyloidosis, and soft tissue neoplasms can have serious consequences for older persons. Contemporary gerontology considers these superficially unrelated phenomena as reflecting a common failure of immunoregulation (Yunis and Greenberg, 1974; Walford, 1974; Makinodan et al., 1975; Kay, 1980).

This review will address certain generic alterations required in the approach to the aged patient, as well as some of the more important drugs used to treat these conditions. Detailed discussion of the management of these disorders is beyond the scope of this chapter, and the reader is again asked to consult the appropriate textbooks for more information.

Therapy

Management of the elderly patient with homeostatic immune dysfunction requires a recognition that the aged differ in important ways from younger patients. These differences include life expectancy, general medical condition, and quality of life. A high-risk, potentially disabling procedure can optimally offer only a limited additional amount of useful life to an octogenarian, whereas a much younger patient may have several decades added by a similarly successful intervention. Thus, a pneumonectomy may be indicated for a 45-year-old man with bronchogenic carcinoma, but be inappropriate for his 85-year-old counterpart. At that point, the risk of surgery is greater, and the patient's projected life span, even with complete removal of the tumor, is less. The same principles can be applied to the management of other types of neoplasia, such as carcinoma of the breast.

Advanced age does not always deprive the older patient of radical intervention that might be offered to someone much younger. Cracchiolo (1980) points out that the insertion of a prosthetic joint is generally reserved for persons over age 65. This relates to the uncertain durability of joint prostheses as well as the increased likelihood that the older patient will not be as inclined to damage the joint with inappropriate levels of activity.

The second factor of importance in treating the elderly with disorders of immunoregulation is their response to pharmacological therapy (Bluestone, 1980; Hollingsworth, 1980). Older persons may absorb, metabolize, or excrete drugs poorly; and drugs may have greater primary or side effects in the elderly patient. If symptoms are masked by other medical problems or the patient is a poor historian, it may be more difficult to determine the true need for or efficacy of a particular compound. Last, older patients may have difficulty in keeping track of a number of medications or, particularly with some of the rheumatic diseases, have difficulty with safety caps that are on most prescription and nonprescription drugs.

Comprehensive information on the pharmacology of the treatment of disorders of immunoregulation may be found in the work of Hollingsworth (1980) and Bluestone (1980), as well as in the symposium edited by Crooks and Stevenson (1977), and the text by Villaverde and MacMillan (1980). More general information appears in the text by Gilman et al. (1980) and in the American Medical Association's book on drug evaluations (1977). Because of the high incidence of polypharmacy in the elderly, drug interactions may be a particular problem in this age group. The book by Cohen and Armstrong (1974), as well as the periodic summary of adverse drug reactions that appears in *The Medical Letter* (1981) may also be valuable references.

Salicylates

Aspirin is one of the oldest and most commonly used drugs in the world. Because of its analgesic and anti-inflammatory effects, acetylsalicylic acid has had wide use in the treatment of inflammatory diseases, particularly rheumatoid arthritis. Whereas the relationship of plasma salicylate levels to the administered dose of aspirin is generally linear, the metabolism and clearance of this drug from the serum can vary from individual to individual. A greater percentage of drugs such as aspirin, which is partly bound to albumin, may be found unbound in the elderly. This is due to lower serum albumin levels, as well as competition for albumin-binding sites when multiple drugs are given (Wallace et al., 1976).

It has been recommended in rheumatoid disease that the salicylate dose should be increased until side effects are noted, with reduction from that point to the highest tolerated level (American Medical Association, 1977). This approach may not be appropriate in the elderly. Bluestone (1980) points out that the high-frequency hearing loss which frequently accompanies old age may mask the development of tinnitus, a common manifestation of salicylate intoxication. Hollingsworth (1980) observes that the elderly patient with salicylism may complain of dizziness, hearing loss, drowsiness, or a feeling of excitement. The patient may also have hyperpnea. It seems most reasonable to begin with a relatively low dose of aspirin, with gradual increments guided by careful clinical observation and perhaps serum salicylate levels.

A number of nonaspirin salicylate drugs have been marketed for the treatment of arthritis. These drugs are quite expensive, and there is little evidence that they offer any advantage over aspirin (*The Medical Letter*, 1978).

Nonsteroidal Anti-Inflammatory Drugs

Drugs are available for the treatment of inflammatory diseases in the elderly that have anti-inflammatory action and are neither salicylates nor corticosteroids. These drugs have been grouped as nonsteroidal anti-inflammatory drugs. This category originally included only phenylbutazone (Butazolidin) and indomethacin (Indocin). In recent years a number of newer agents have been introduced including naproxen (Naprosyn), ibutrofen (Motrin), tolmetin sodium (Tolectin), fenoprofen calcium (Nalfon), sulindac (Clinoril), meclofenamate sodium (Meclomen), and zomepirac sodium (Zomax). The last, zomepirac, is recommended primarily for analgesia rather than for its anti-inflammatory effect.

Because of the massive amounts of aspirin consumed on an annual basis in the United States, a substantial investment has been made to develop and market these newer drugs. They are all much more expensive than aspirin. The proponents of the most recent preparations argue that they are often as effective as aspirin, with fewer side effects.

Like aspirin, the nonsteroidal anti-inflammatory drugs block the synthesis of prostaglandins by cyclooxygenase. They share many side effects with aspirin, although the incidence may be less. These include gastrointestinal bleeding, prolongation of the bleeding time due to inhibition of platelet function, and renal damage (*The Medical Letter*, 1980b; Flower et al., 1980; Wilkins and O'Brien, 1974; Pinals et al., 1977). Flower et al. (1980) also suggest that these drugs may have an effect on male fertility and should not be used in men with "marginal fertility." This may be important for some geriatric patients.

Phenylbutazone preceded by many years the introduction of the other drugs which have been discussed. Pemberton (1954) demonstrated an age-related increase in side effects with this drug, ranging from 23% in the third decade of life to 60% in patients 61-70 years of age. Whether this is related to the demonstrated prolongation of the plasma half-life of phenylbutazone in the elderly is unknown (O'Malley et al., 1971). The most serious of all side effects are aplastic anemia and agranulocytosis. The manufacturer recommends that phenylbutazone be used for no more than a week in patients over 60 years of age. Whereas it may be useful for limited periods in the treatment of gout (Hollingsworth, 1980), some suggest that any use of phenylbutazone in the elderly is "inadvisable" (Flower et al., 1980).

Indomethacin has also been used in the past for a variety of inflammatory diseases. It may be of value in the treatment of acute gout, but it offers little benefit in the long-term management of other forms of inflammatory arthritis.

In summary, the new nonsteroidal anti-inflammatory drugs may be effective and well tolerated in inflammatory conditions in the elderly when aspirin has not been effective or cannot be used. These drugs are not, however, without side effects, and trials of the various agents may be necessary to arrive at an appropriate medication and dose.

Corticosteroids

Systemic corticosteroid therapy has been used in the management of a broad spectrum of inflammatory conditions, including rheumatoid arthritis, systemic lupus erythematosis, temporal arthritis, polymyalgia rheumatica, and inflammatory bowel disease. In addition, corticosteroids are useful in the treatment of some neoplastic diseases such as the lymphomas.

As with other drugs, there is very little specific data about the effects of corticosteroids on the elderly. Associated side effects include adrenal suppression, fluid retention, hyperglycemia, increased susceptibility to infection, possibly peptic ulceration, myopathy, mental confusion, cataracts, osteoporosis, and vertebral compression fractures (Haynes and Murad, 1980). Many of these problems are commonly found in the aged. Systemic corticosteroids may therefore create difficulties both in the diagnosis and management of elderly patients. Local corticosteroids, such as beclomethasone for bronchospasm, various steroid creams and ointments for dermatological problems, and the intra-articular corticosteroids for localized inflammatory joint and other musculoskeletal problems, are preferred whenever possible. Relative contraindications to treatment with systemic corticosteroids exist in those patients who already have manifestations of osteoporosis, hypertension, congestive heart failure, or diabetes.

Significant systemic absorption of topical corticosteroids can occur. Even when this route of administration is employed, patients should be treated with the lowest effective concentration and potency.

Some of the synthetic corticosteroids have substantially less mineralocorticoid or fluid-retaining effect than the older drugs. Prednisone has a relative sodium-retaining potency that is 80% that of cortisol, but has four times the anti-inflammatory activity. Dexamethasone has 25 times the anti-inflammatory activity of cortisol, but no sodium-retaining action (Haynes and Murad, 1980).

Miscellaneous Anti-Inflammatory Drugs

Other anti-inflammatory drugs are used in the treatment of the elderly. These include gold, penicillamine, and the antimalarials. Space does not permit discussion of all of these agents, as well as the many antineoplastic drugs used in this population. Almost all of these compounds are associated with significant side effects that may be exaggerated when they are used in the aged.

IMMUNOLOGICAL RECONSTITUTION

A number of experimental approaches have been taken with laboratory animals towards reversing the decline in immune function which occurs with advanced age (Makinodan and Kay, 1980). In human studies, phamacological interventions that reverse age-associated immune dysfunction show promise, but are not yet of demonstrable efficacy. The work done with zinc and levamisole represents different examples of the type of studies that have been performed and the nature of the results that have been reported.

Zinc

Duchateau et al. (1981) recently reported a controlled study of the effects of daily zinc sulfate on selected parameters of immune function in elderly persons. The treated group developed a small but significant increase in the percentage of peripheral blood T lymphocytes, an increase in the number and size of positive delayed hypersensitivity skin test reactions, and an enhanced specific immunoglobulin response to tetanus immunization. These changes were not associated with increases in the in vitro lymphocyte response to phytohemagglutinin, con-conavalin A, or pokeweed mitogen. This is the only study of its type of zine im-munopotentiation in the elderly, although supportive data are available from other observations.

Pekarek and his associates (Pekarek et al., 1979) reported a case of a young male with a diet deficient in both calories and zinc, and a markedly reduced serum zinc level. His cutaneous response to dinitrochlorobenzene and in vitro lymphocyte response to phytohemagglutinin were grossly abnormal. After only 3 weeks of zinc therapy, both of these parameters of cell-mediated immunity were normal. This was associated with healing of a decubitus ulcer and clearing of lo-calized seborrhea. Of note, he did not change his other dietary intake or gain weight until 3 months after commencing zinc supplementation.

Golden and his group (Golden et al., 1978) studied the effect of topical zinc sulphate on the cutaneous delayed hypersensitivity response of 10 malnourished children. Patients were tested simultaneously with two intradermal injections of a *Candida* antigen. One injection site was covered with zinc sulfate ointment, and the second with a placebo. Zinc-tested sites had a significantly greater response to intradermal *Candida albicans*. There was a significant correlation between the pa-tients' serum zinc levels and the ratio of the response between the treated and the untreated sides.

A recent abstract reported an improved in vitro response to mitogens after repletion therapy of zinc-deficient patients. In the two patients tested, this was associated with a substantial increase in serum thymopoietin levels (Cunningham-Rundles et al., 1979). The role of thymic hormones in zinc-associated immuno-deficiency is uncertain, but they too have been linked with the immune dysfunc-tion of the elderly.

An inherited disorder of zinc malabsorption, acrodermatitis enteropathica, has been described (Moynahan, 1974). Patients with this disorder have frequent infections and a variety of abnormalities of immune function (Weston et al., 1977).

Lindeman et al. (1971) reported an age-related decline in serum zinc concen-trations in both males and females, along with a statistically insignificant increase in red blood cell zinc levels. There was considerable variability in the individual data. These results suggest the possibility of clinically unrecognized zinc deficiency resulting in minimal immunological dysfunction in the elderly.

It is unlikely that zinc deficiency accounts for all of the changes that occur in the immune responses of older persons. However, zinc is relatively nontoxic, easy to administer, and inexpensive (Aggett and Harris, 1979). Longitudinal studies are indicated to determine its ultimate role.

Levamisole

Levamisole is an anthelmintic which has been studied for several years because of suggestions that the drug had immunostimulating potential. Verhaegen and associates examined the effect of levamisole on the delayed cutaneous hypersensitivity responses of elderly subjects (Verhaegen et al., 1973). They reported that 5 of the 12 anergic patients who received levamisole converted their intradermal PPDs to positive compared with none of the control anergic patients. There was no difference between the groups in in vitro tests of lymphocyte function. Another group examined the effect of levamisole on elderly subjects' delayed hypersensitivity responses to tuberculin; specific immunoglobulin responses to influenza A, influenza B, and the Sendai virus; and serum IgA levels (Renoux et al., 1973). Statistically significant changes were noted in all three areas tested. Others have confirmed improvement in delayed hypersensitivity skin test responses in levamisole-treated elderly subjects unassociated with significant alterations in in vitro immune function (Pasquier et al., 1975).

Recently, Delespesse and colleagues failed to show a significant augmentation by levamisole of elderly subjects' IgG response to diphtheria toxin and confirmed the lack of significant in vitro effect on the lymphocyte response to phytohemagglutinin (Delespesse et al., 1977). This group did show a slight increase in the treated subjects' isohemagglutinin titers.

In summary, levamisole appears to have some mild immunopotentiating effect in the aged. Whether this effect can be translated into clinical activity remains to be demonstrated.

ACKNOWLEDGMENTS

The authors want to thank Julie Farr, Lori Tripp, and Elsie Morris for their excellent secretarial assistance in the preparation of this chapter.

REFERENCES

Addington, W. W. (1979). The treatment of pulmonary tuberculosis. *Arch. Intern. Med. 139*: 1391-1395.

Aggett, P. J., and Harris, J. T. (1979). Current status of zinc in health and disease states. *Arch. Dis. Child. 54*: 909-917.

Ahmed, T., Fernandez, R. J., and Wanner, A. (1981). Airway responses to antigen challenge in allergic rhinitis and allergic asthma. *J. Allergy Clin. Immunol. 67*: 135-145.

Aho, W. R. (1979). Participation of senior citizens in the swine flu innoculation program: an analysis of health belief model variables in preventive health behavior. *J. Gerontol. 34*: 201-208.

American College of Physicians (1982). Pneumococcal vaccine recommendation. *Ann. Intern. Med. 96*: 206-207.

American Medical Association (1977). *AMA Drug Evaluations*, 3d ed. Publishing Sciences Group, Inc., Littleton, Mass.

American Thoracic Society (1974). Preventive therapy of tuberculosis infection. *Am. Rev. Resp. Dis. 110*: 371-374.

Austrian, R. (1975). Random gleanings from a life with the pneumococcus (Maxwell Finland Lecture). *J. Infect. Dis. 131*: 474-484.

Austrian, R. (1980). *Surveillance of Pneumoccocal Infection for Field Trials of Polyvalent Pneumococcal Vaccines.* National Institutes of Health, Bethesda, Maryland, Report DAB-VDP-12-84, pp. 1-84.

Austrian, R., and Gold, J. (1964). Pneumococcal bacteremia with especial reference to bacteremic pneumococcal pneumonia. *Ann. Intern. Med. 60*: 759-776.

Baer, H., and Bowser, R. T. (1963). Antibody production and development of contact skin sensitivity in guinea pigs of various ages. *Science 140*: 1211-1212.

Barbee, R. A., Lebowitz, M. D., Thompson, H. C., and Burrows, B. (1976). Immediate skin test reactivity in a general population sample. *Ann. Intern. Med. 84*: 129-133.

Battershill, J. H. (1980). Cutaneous testing in the elderly patient with tuberculosis. *Chest 77*: 188-189.

Black, M., Mitchell, J. R., Zimmerman, H. J., Ishak, K. G., and Epler, G. R. (1975). Isoniazid-associated hepatitis in 114 patients. *Gastroenterology 69*: 289-302.

Block, S. A., Lee, W. Y., Remigio, L. K., and May, C. D. (1978). Studies of hypersensitivity reactions to foods in infants and children. *J. Allergy Clin. Immunol. 62*: 327-334.

Bluestone, R. (1980). The diagnosis and management of rheumatic disease in the elderly—a special challenge. In *Aging, Immunity and Arthritic Disease (Aging, Vol. II)*, M. M. B. Kay, J. Galpin, and T. Makinodan (Eds.). Raven Press, New York, pp. 183-194.

Broome, C. V., Facklem, R. R., and Fraser, D. W. (1980). Pneumococcal disease after pneumococcal vaccination. *N. Engl. J. Med. 303*: 549-552.

Buckley, C. E., III, and Dorsey, F. C. (1970). The effect of aging on human serum immunoglobulin concentrations. *J. Immunol. 105*: 964-972.

Buckley, C. E., III, and Dorsey, F. C. (1971). Serum immunoglobulin levels throughout the life-span of healthy man. *Ann. Intern. Med. 75*: 673-682.

Buckley, C. E., III, and Roseman, J. M. (1976). Immunity and survival. *J. Am. Geriatr. Soc. 24*: 241-248.

Buckley, C. E., III, and Trayer, H. R. (1972). Serum IgD concentrations in sarcoidosis and tuberculosis. *Clin. Exp. Immunol. 10*: 257-265.

Buckley, C. E., III, and White, D. H. (1978). Aging and immunocompetence skin testing. In *Recent Advances in Gerontology, International Congress Series No. 469*, H. Orimo, K. Shimada, M. Iriki, and D. Maeda (Eds.). Excerpta Medica, Princeton, N.J., pp. 444-449.

Buckley, C. E., III, Buckley, E. G., and Dorsey, F. C. (1974). Longitudinal changes in serum immunoglobulin levels in older humans. *Fed. Proc. 33*: 2036-2039.

Burnet, F. M. (1970). An immunological approach to aging. *Lancet 2*: 358-360.

Burney, L. E. (1960). Influenza immunization. *Pub. Health Rep. 75*: 944.

Burr, M. L., Charles, T. J., Roy, K., and Seaton, A. (1979). Asthma in the elderly: an epidemiological survey. *Br. Med. J. 1*: 1041-1044.

Byrd, R. B., Kaplan, P. D., and Gracey, D. R. (1974). Treatment of pulmonary tuberculosis. *Chest 66*: 560-567.

Campbell, A. H., and Tandon, M. K. (1969). A trial of disodium chromoglycolate in older asthmatics. *Med. J. Aust. 2*: 535-537.

Cate, T. R., Kasel, J. A., Couch, R. B., Six, H. R., and Knight, V. (1977). Clinical trials of bivalent influenza A/New Jersey/76—A/Victoria/75 vaccines in the elderly. *J. Infect. Dis. 1977*: 5518-5525.

Center for Disease Control (1978). Pneumococcal polysacharide vaccine. *Morbid. Mortal. Week. Rep. 27*: 29-31.

Center for Disease Control (1979). Influenza vaccine. *Morbid. Mortal. Week. Rep. 28*(20): 213-239.

Center for Disease Control (1980). Annual Summary 1979: reported morbidity and mortality in the United States. *Morbid. Mortal. Week. Rep. 28*(54): 1-119.

Center for Disease Control (1981a). Influenza vaccine 1981-82. *Morbid. Mortal. Week. Rep. 30*(23): 279-287.

Center for Disease Control (1981b). Pneumococcal polysacharride vaccine. *Morbid. Mortal. Week. Rep. 30*(33): 410-419.

Center for Disease Control (1982). Pneumococcal polysaccharide vaccine. *Ann. Intern. Med. 96*: 203-205.

Cohen, S. N., and Armstrong, M. F. (1974). *Drug Interactions: A Handbook for Clinical Use*. Williams and Wilkins, Baltimore.

Cohn, J. R., Buckley, C. E., III, Hohl, C., Tyson, G., and Niesh, D. (1982). Response to intradermal human PPD, avian PPD and six recall antigens in a nursing home population. *Am. Rev. Resp. Dis. 125*: 178s.

Cohn, J. R., Jungkind, D. L., and Baker, J. (1980). In vitro antagonism by erythromycin of the bactericidal action of antimicrobials against common respiratory pathogens. *Antimicrob. Agents Chemother. 18*: 872-876.

Collins, F. M. (1972). Acquired resistance to mycobacterial infections. *Adv. Tuberc. Res. 18*: 1-30.

Comstock, G. W., Daniel, T. M., Snider, D. E., Jr., Edwards, P. Q., Hopewell, P. C., and Vandiere, H. M. (1981). The tuberculin skin test: official statement of the American Thoracic Society. *Am. Rev. Resp. Dis. 124*: 356-363.

Cracchiolo, III, A. (1980). Reconstructive surgery in the elderly arthritic. In *Aging, Immunity and Arthritic Diseases* (*Aging*, Vol. II), M. M. B. Kay, J. Galpin, and T. Makinodan (Eds.). Raven Press, New York, pp. 231-249.

Crawford, J., and Cohen, H. (1981). Disorders of amyloid disposition. In *Protein Abnormalities: Diagnostic and Clinical Aspects*, S. Ritzman (Ed.). Little, Brown, Boston.

Criep, L. H. (1970). The management of bronchial asthma in the aged. *Geriatrics 25*(9): 135-145.

Crooks, J., and Stevenson, I. H. (1977). *Drugs and the Elderly*. University Park Press, Baltimore.

Crossley, K., Irvine, P., Warren, J. B., Lee, B. K., and Mead, K. (1979). Tetanus and diphtheria immunity in urban Minnesota adults. *JAMA 242*: 2298-2300.

Cunningham-Rundles, C., Cunningham-Rundles, S., Garafalo, J., Iwata, T., Incefy, G., Twomey, J., and Good, R. A. (1979). Increased T lymphocyte function and thymopoietin following zinc repletion in man. *Fed. Proc. 38*: 1222.

Deal, E. C., Jr., McFadden, E. R., Jr., Ingram, R. H., Jr., Breslin, F. J., and Jaeger, J. J. (1980). Airway responsiveness to cold air and hyperpnea in normal subjects and in those with hay fever and asthma. *Am. Rev. Resp. Dis. 121*: 621-628.

Delespesse, G., de Maubeuge, J., Kennes, B., Nicaise, R., and Govaerts, A. (1977b). IgE mediated hypersensitivity in aging. *Clin. Allergy 7*: 155-160.

Delespesse, G., Vrijens, R., de Maubeuge, J., Hudson, D., Kennes, B., and Govaerts, A. (1977a). Influence of levamisole on the immune response of old people. *Int. Arch. Allergy Appl. Immunol. 54*: 151-157.

Delker, L. L., Moser, R. H., Nelson, J. D., Rodstein, M., Rolls, K., Sanford, J. P., and Swartz, M. N. (1980). Amantadine: Does it have a role in the prevention and treatment of influenza? A National Institutes of Health concensus development conference. *Ann. Intern. Med. 92*: 256-258.

de Weck, A. L. (1977). Immune responses to environmental antigens that act on the skin: the role of lymphokines in contact dermatitis. *Fed. Proc. 36*: 1742-1747.

Dhar, S., Shastri, S. R., and Lenora, R. A. K. (1976). Aging and the respiratory system. *Med. Clin. North Am. 60*(6): 1121-1139.

Diaz-Jousnen, E., Williams, R. C., and Strickland, R. G. (1975). Age related changes in T and B cells. *Lancet 1*: 688-689.

Duchateau, J., Delespesse, G., Vrijens, R., and Collet, H. (1981). Beneficial effects of oral zinc supplementation on the immune response of old people. *Am. J. Med. 70*: 1001-1004.

Dudani, N., Silbert, N. E., Belcher, S. M., Wang, C. S., and Andosca, J. B. (1980). Respiratory tract allergy of acute onset in an ambulatory geriatric group. *Ann. Allergy 45*: 23-25.

Edsall, G., Elliott, M. W., Peebles, T. C., Levine, L., and Eldred, M. C. (1967). Excessive use of tetanus toxoid boosters. *JAMA 202*: 111-113.

Eickhoff, T. C. (1971). Immunization against influenza: rationale and recommendations. *J. Infect. Dis. 123*: 446-454.

Ellis, E. F. (1978). Theophylline and its derivatives. In *Allergy Principles and Practice*, Vol. 1, E. Middleton, Jr., C. E. Reed, and E. F. Ellis (Eds.). C. V. Mosby, St. Louis, pp. 434-453.

Ferry, B. J., Evered, M. G., and Morrison, E. I. (1976). Antibody responses to influenza virus subunit vaccine in the aged. *Med. J. Aust. 1*: 540-542.

Finkelstein, M. S., Freedman, M. L., Shenkman, L., and Krugman, S. (1981). Evidence of prior hepatitis B and hepatitis A virus infection in an ambulatory geriatric population. *J. Gerontol. 36*: 302-305.

Finland, M. (1979). Pneumonia and pneumococcal infections, with special reference to pneumococcal pneumonia (Amberson Lecture). *Am. Rev. Resp. Dis. 120*: 481-502.

Fish, J. E., Ankin, M. G., Kelly, J. F., and Peterman, V. I. (1980). Comparison of responses to pollen extract in subjects with allergic asthma and nonasthmatic subjects with allergic rhinitis. *J. Allergy Clin. Immunol. 65*: 154-161.

Fleisch, J. H., Maling, H. M., and Brodie, B. B. (1970). Evidence for existance of alpha-adrenergic receptors in mammalian trachea. *Am. J. Physiol. 218*: 596-599.

Flower, R. J., Moncada, S., and Vane, J. R. (1980). Analgesic-antipyretics and anti-inflammatory agents: drugs employed in the treatment of gout. In *Goodman and Gilman's The Pharmacological Basis of Therapeutics*, A. G. Gilman, L. S. Goodman, and A. Gilman (Eds.). Macmillan, New York, pp. 682-728.

Food and Drug Administration (1980). I.V. dosage guidelines for theophylline products. *FDA Drug Bull. 10*(1): 4-6.

Ford, R. M. (1969). Aetiology of asthma: a review of 11,551 cases (1958-1968). *Med. J. Aust. 1*: 628-631.

Fraser, D. W. (1976). Preventing tetanus in patients with wounds. *Ann. Intern. Med. 84*: 95-97.

Fulk, R. V., Fedson, D. S., Huber, M. A., Fitzpatrick, J. R., Howar, B. F., and Kasel, J. A. (1969). Antibody responses in children and elderly persons following local or parenteral administration of an inactivated influenza virus vaccine, A2/Hong Kong/68 variant. *J. Immunol. 102*: 1102-1105.

Fulk, R. V., Fedson, D. S., Huber, M. A. Fitzpatrick, J. R., and Kasel, J. A. (1970). Antibody responses in serum and nasal secretions according to age of recepient and method of administration of A2/Hong Kong/68 inactivated influenza virus vaccine. *J. Immunol. 104*: 8-13.

Gelb, A. F., Leffler, C., Brewin, A., Mascatello, V., and Lyons, H. A. (1973). Milliary tuberculosis. *Am. Rev. Resp. Dis. 108*: 1327-1333.

Gershon, R. K., Askenase, P. W., and Gershon, M. D. (1975). Requirement for vasoactive amines for production of delayed type hypersensitivity skin reactions. *J. Exp. Med. 142*: 732-747.

Ghory, A. C., and Patterson, R. (1980). Treating asthma in the elderly. *Geriatrics 35*(8): 32-38.

Gilman, A. G., Goodman, L. S., and Gilman, A. (1980). *Goodman and Gilman's The Pharmacological Basis of Therapeutics.* Macmillan, New York.

Girard, J. P., Paychere, M., Cuevas, M., and Fernandes, B. (1977). Cell mediated immunity in an aging population. *Clin. Exp. Immunol. 27*: 85-91.

Gladstone, J. L., and Recco, R. (1976). Host factors and infectious diseases in the elderly. *Med. Clin. North Am. 60*(6): 1225-1240.

Golden, M. N. H., Golden, B. E., Harland, P. S. E. G., and Jackson, A. A. (1978). Zinc and immunocompetence in protein energy malnutrition. *Lancet 1*:1226-1228.

Goth, A. (1978). Antihistamines. In *Allergy Principles and Practice*, Vol. 1, E. Middleton, Jr., C. E. Reed, and E. F. Ellis (Eds.). C. V. Mosby, St. Louis, pp. 454-463.

Gross, L. (1965). Immunological defect in aged population and its relationship to cancer. *Cancer 18*: 201-204.

Gross, N. J. (1980). What is this thing called love?—Or, defining asthma. *Am. Rev. Resp. Dis. 121*: 203-204.

Grossman, J., Baum, J., Gluckman, J., Fusner, J., and Condemi, J. J. (1975). The effect of aging and acute illness on delayed hypersensitivity. *J. Allergy Clin. Immunol. 55*: 268-275.

Guerrant, J. L. (1978). Asthma in older patients. *Va. Med. 105*: 775-778.

Hagy, G. W., and Settipane, G. A. (1971). Prognosis of positive allergy skin tests in an asymptomatic population. *J. Allergy Clin. Immunol. 48*: 200-211.

Hall, J. W., and Henderson, L. L. (1966). Asthma in the aged. *J. Am. Geriatr. Soc. 14*: 779-794.

Hanafin, J. M., and Lobitz, W. C., Jr. (1977). Newer concepts of atopic dermatitis. *Arch. Dermatol. 113*: 663-670.

Hanifin, J. M. (1979). Eczematous conditions in the elderly: common and curable. *Geriatrics 34*(1): 29-38.

Hanneuse, Y., Delespesse, G., Hudson, D., de Halleux, F., and Jacques, J. M. (1978). Influence of aging on IgE mediated reactions in allergic patients. *Clin. Allergy 8*: 165-174.

Haynes, R. C., Jr., and Murad, F. (1980). Adrenocorticotropic hormone; adrenocortical steroids and their synthetic analogues: inhibitors of adrenocortical steroid biosynthesis. In *Goodman and Gilman's The Pharmacological Basis of Therapeutics*, A. G. Gilman, L. S. Goodman, and A. Gilman (Eds.). Macmillan, New York, pp. 1466-1496.

Henderson, W. R., Shelhamer, J. H., Reingold, D. B., Smith, L. J., Evans, R., III, and Kaliner, M. (1979). Alpha-adrenergic hyperresponsiveness in asthma. *N. Eng. J. Med. 300*: 642-647.

Hollingsworth, J. W. (1980). Rehabilitation and conservative management of joint disease in the elderly. In *Aging, Immunity and Arthritic Disease* (*Aging*, Vol. II), M. M. B. Kay, J. Galpin, and T. Makinodan (Eds.). Raven Press, New York, pp. 211-229.

Howells, C. H. L., Vesselinova-Jenkins, C. K., Evans, A. D., and James, J. (1975). Influenza vaccination and mortality from bronchopneumonia in the elderly. *Lancet 1*: 381-383.

Iseman, M. D., Albert, R., Locks, M., Raleigh, J., Sutton, F., and Farer, L. S. (1980). Guidelines for short course tuberculosis chemotherapy. *Am. Rev. Resp. Dis. 121*: 611-614.

Jack, D., and Harris, D. M. (1978). Beta-adrenergic agents. In *Allergy Principles and Practice*, Vol. I, E. Middleton, Jr., C. E. Reed, and E. F. Ellis (Eds.). C.V. Mosby, St. Louis, pp. 407-427.

Johanson, W. G., Pierce, A. K., Sanford, J. P., and Thomas, G. D. (1972). Nosocomial infection with gram negative bacilli. *Ann. Intern. Med. 77*: 701-706.

Johanson, W. G., Jr., Woods, D. E., and Chaudhuri, T. (1979). Association of respiratory tract colonization with adherence of gram-negative bacilli to epithelial cells. *J. Infect. Dis. 139*: 667-673.

Johansson, S. G. O. (1968). Serum IgND levels in healthy children and adults. *Int. Arch. Allergy 34*: 1-8.

Kasel, J. A., Hume, E. B., Fulk, R. V., Togo, Y., Huber, M., and Hornick, R. B. (1969). Antibody responses in nasal secretions and serum of elderly persons following local or parenteral administration of inactivated influenza virus vaccine. *J. Immunol. 102*: 555-562.

Kaufman, P. (1947). Pneumonia in old age. *Arch. Intern. Med. 77*: 518-531.

Kay, M. M. B. (1980). Immunological aspects of aging. In *Aging, Immunity and Arthritic Disease*, (*Aging*, Vol. II), M. M. B. Kay, J. Galpin, and T. Makinodan (Eds.). Raven Press, New York, pp. 33-78.

Kishimoto, S., Tomino, S. Mitsuya, H., Fujiwara. H., and Tsuda (1980). Age related decline in the *in vitro* and *in vivo* synthesis of antitetanus toxoid antibody in humans. *J. Immunol. 125*: 2347-2352.

Kopanoff, D. E., Snider, D. E., and Caras, G. J. (1978). Isoniazid-related hepatitis: a U.S. Public Health Service cooperative study. *Am. Rev. Resp. Dis. 117*: 991-1001.

Lamb, G. A., Feldman, H. A., and Flescher, R. (1967). Antibody-inducing effects of aqueous and depot influenza vaccines in the elderly. *Am. J. Med. Sci. 254*: 513-527.

Lantis, L. R., and Lantis, S. D. H. (1975). Allergic dermatoses in the older patient. *Geriatrics 30*(2): 75-84.

Lee, H. Y., and Stretton, T. B. (1972). Asthma in the elderly. *Br. Med. J. 4*: 93-95.

Lees, A. W., Allan, G. W., Smith, A. J., Tyrrell, W. F., and Fallon, R. J. (1970). Toxicity from rifampicin plus isoniazid and rifampicin plus ethambutol therapy. *Tubercl 52*: 182-189.

Lindeman, R. D., Clark, M. L., and Colmore, J. P. (1971). Influence of age and sex on plasma and red-cell zinc concentrations. *J. Gerontol. 26*: 358-363.

Lovell, R. G. (1970). Problems of allergy with advancing age. *Geriatrics 25*(9): 101-103.

Lutwick, L. I. (1980). Principles of antibiotic use in the elderly. *Geriatrics 35*(2): 54-60.

Makinodan, T., Heidrick, M. L., and Nordin, A. A. (1975). Immunodeficiency and autoimmunity in aging. *Birth Defects 11*(1): 193-198.

Makinodan, T., and Kay, M. M. B. (1980). Age influences on the immune system. *Adv. Immunol. 29*: 287-330.

McMurray, D. N., and Echeverri, A. (1978). Cell mediated immunity in anergic patients with pulmonary tuberculosis. *Am. Rev. Resp. Dis. 118*: 827-834.

McMurray, D. N. (1980). Mechanisms of anergy in tuberculosis. *Chest 77*: 4-5.

Medical Letter (1978). Non-aspirin salicylate products for arthritis. *20*(22): 100.

Medical Letter (1980a). Non-steroidal anti-inflammatory drugs for rheumatoid arthritis. *22*(7): 29-31.

Medical Letter (1980b). Meclofenamate sodium (Meclomen): a new antiarthritic agent. *22*(26): 111-112.

Medical Letter (1981). Adverse interactions of drugs. *23*(5): 17-28.

Merck, Sharp, and Dohme (1977). Package insert for pneumovax, circular number DC 7014801.

Middleton, E., Jr., Reed, C. E., and Ellis, E. F. (1978). *Allergy Principles and Practice*. C.V. Mosby, St. Louis.

Miller, L. W., Hume, E. B., O'Brien, F. R., Togo, Y., and Hornick, R. B. (1975). Alice strain live influenza (H3N2) vaccine in an elderly population. *Am. J. Epidemiol. 101*: 340-346.

Milner, A. D., and Ingram, D. (1971). Bronchodilator and cardiac effects of isoprenaline, orciprenaline and salbutamol aerosols in asthma. *Arch. Dis. Child. 46*: 502-507.

Morgan, R. J., and Keeran, M. (1970). Allergic skin problems in older individuals. *Geriatrics 25*(9): 146.

Morris, J. A. (1965). Correlation of influenza antibody with immunity. In *New Research on Influenza: Studies with Normal Volunteers*, V. Knight, moderator. *Ann Intern. Med. 62*: 1307-1325.

Moynahan, E. J. (1974). Achrodermatitis enteropathica: a lethal inherited human zinc-deficiency disorder. *Lancet 2*: 399-400.

Nagaki, K., Hiramatsu, S., Inai, S., and Sasaki, A. (1980). The effect of aging on complement activity (CH50) and complement protein levels. *J. Clin. Lab. Immunol. 3*: 45-50.

Nash, D. R., and Douglas, J. E. (1980). Anergy in active pulmonary tuberculosis. *Chest 77*: 32-37.

Nassif, E. G., Weinberger, M., Thompson, R., and Huntley, W. (1981). The value of maintenance theophylline in steroid-dependent asthma. *N. Engl. J. Med. 304*: 71-75.

Norman, P. S. (1980). An overview of immunotherapy: implications for the future. *J. Allergy Clin. Immunol. 65*: 87-96.

Ogilvie, A. G. (1962). Asthma: a study in prognosis of 1,000 patients. *Thorax 17*: 183-189.

O'Malley, K., Crooks, J., Duke, E., and Stevenson, I. H. (1971). Effect of age and sex on human drug metabolism. *Br. Med. J. 3*: 607-609.

Orren, A., and Dowdle, E. B. (1975). The effects of sex and age on serum IgE concentrations in three ethnic groups. *Int. Arch. Allergy Appl. Immunol. 48*: 824-835.

Pakarek, R. S., Sanstead, H. H., Jacob, R. A., and Barcome, D. F. (1979). Abnormal cellular immune responses during acquired zinc deficiency. *Am. J. Clin. Nutr. 32*: 1466-1471.

Palmblad, J., and Haak, A. (1978). Aging does not change blood granulocyte bactericidal capacity and levels of complement factors 3 and 4. *Gerontology 24*: 381-385.

Parkman, P. D., Galasso, G. J., Top, F. H., Jr., and Nobel, G. R. (1976). Summary of clinical trials of influenza vaccines. *J. Infect. Dis. 134*: 100-107.

Pasquier, P., Vidal, M., Couture, J., Niel, G., Floc'h, F., and Werner, G. H. (1975). Action du levamisole sui la restauration de l'immunitie cellulaire chez l'homme. *Nouv. Presse Med. 3*: 2736.

Patterson, R. (1979). Clinical efficacy of allergen immunotherapy. *J. Allergy Clin. Immunol. 64*: 155-158.

Patterson, R. (1980). *Allergic Diseases: Diagnosis and Management*. Lippincott, Philadelphia.

Pemberton, M. (1954). Use of phenylbutazone in rheumatoid arthritis. *Br. Med. J. 1*: 490-493.

Pepys, J., and Hutchcroft, B. J. (1975). Bronchial provocation tests in etiologic diagnosis and analysis of asthma. *Am. Rev. Resp. Dis. 112*: 829-859.

Phair, J., Kauffman, C. A., Bjornson, A., Adams, L., and Linnemann, C., Jr. (1978a). Failure to respond to influenza vaccine in the aged. *J. Lab. Clin. Med. 92*: 822-828.

Phair, J. P., Kauffman, C. A., Bjornson, A., Gallagher, J., Adams, L., and Hess, E. V. (1978b). Host defenses in the aged: evaluation of components of inflammatory and immune responses. *J. Infect. Dis. 138*: 67-73.

Phair, J. P., Kauffman, C. A., and Bjornson, A. (1978c). Investigation of host defense mechanisms in the aged as determinants of nosocomial colonization and pneumonia. *J. Reticuloendothel. Soc. 23*: 397-405.

Pinals, R. S., Runge, L. A., Jabbs, J. M., and Maddi, V. I. (1977). New nonsteroidal anti-inflammatory drugs. *NY State J. Med. 77*: 1268-1270.

Public Health Services Advisory Committee on Immunization Practices (1972).

Diphtheria and tetanus toxoids and pertussis vaccine. *Morbid. Mortal. Week. Rep. 21 (Suppl. 25)*: 5-7.

Radl, J., Sepers, J. M., Skvaril, F., Morell, A., and Hijmans. W. (1975). Immunoglobulin patterns in humans over 95 years of age. *Clin. Exp. Immunol. 22*: 84-90.

Renoux, G., Renoux, M., Morand, P., and Dartigues, P. (1973). Action immunostimulante du levamisole sur les personne agees. *Rev. Med. Tours 7*: 797-801.

Riding, W. D., Dinda, P., and Chatterjee, S. S. (1970). The bronchodilator and cardiac effects of five pressure packed aerosoles in asthma. *Br. J. Dis. Chest 64*: 37-46.

Roberts-Thompson, I. C., Whittingham, S., Youngchaiyad, U., and Mackay, I. R. (1974). Aging, immune response and mortality. *Lancet 2*: 368-370.

Roth, G. S. (1979). Hormone receptor changes during adulthood and senescence: significance for aging research. *Fed. Proc. 38*: 1910-1914.

Roth, H. L., and Kierland, R. R. (1964). The natural history of atopic dermatitis. *Arch. Dermatol. 89*: 209-214.

Rowky, M. J., Buchanan, H., and Mackay, I. R. (1968). Reciprocal change with age in antibody to extrinsic and intrinsic antigens. *Lancet 2*: 24-26.

Ruben, F. L., Johnston, F., and Streiff, E. J. (1974). Influenza in a partially immunized aged population. *JAMA 230*: 863-866.

Ruben, F. L., Nagel, J., and Fireman, P. (1978). Antitoxin responses in the elderly to tetanus-diphtheria (Td) immunization. *Am. J. Epidemiol. 108*: 145-149.

Rueller, J. B., and Cooney, T. G. (1981). The pressure sore: pathophysiology and principles of management. *Ann. Intern. Med. 94*: 661-666.

Sabin, A. B. (1947). Antibody response of people of different ages to two doses of uncentrifuged, Japanese B encephalitis vaccine. *Proc. Soc. Exp. Biol. Med. 65*: 127-130.

Santa Cruz, R., Landa, J., Hirsch, J., and Sackner, M. A. (1974). Tracheal mucous velocity in normal man and in patients with obstructive lung disease: effects of terbutaline. *Am. Rev. Resp. Dis. 109*: 458-463.

Saslaw, S., Carlisle, H. N., and Perkins, R. L. (1966). Effect of dosage and influenza vaccine content on antibody response in an aged population. *Am. J. Med. Sci. 251*: 195-206.

Sbarbaro, J. A. (1975). Tuberculosis: the new challenge to the practicing clinician. *Chest (Suppl.) 68*: 436-443.

Schachter, J., and Higgins, M. W. (1976). Median onset of asthma and allergic rhinitis in Tecumseh, Michigan. *J. Allergy Clin. Immunol. 57*: 342-351.

Schaller, J. G. (1975). Immunodeficiency and autoimmunity. *Birth Defects 11(1)*: 173-184.

Scharer, L., and Smith, J. P. (1969). Serum transaminase elevations and other hepatic abnormalities in patients receiving isoniazid. *Ann. Intern. Med. 71*: 1113-1120.

Schocken, D. D., and Roth, G. S. (1977). Reduced β-adrenergic receptor concentrations in aging man. *Nature 267*: 856-858.

Schwartz, J. S. (1982). Pneumococcal vaccine: clinical efficacy and effectiveness. *Ann. Intern. Med. 96*: 208-220.

Shelhamer, J. H., Metcalfe, D. D., Smith, L. J., and Kaliner, M. (1980). Abnormal adrenergic responsiveness in allergic subjects: analysis of isoproterenol-induced cardiovascular and plasma cyclic adenosine monophosphate responses. *J. Allergy Clin. Immunol. 66*: 52-60.

Silbert, N. E., and Dudani, N. (1979). Epidemiology of respiratory disorders in a geriatric age group. *Ann. Allergy 43*: 26-31.

Smith, L. J., Shelhamer, J. H., and Kaliner, M. (1980). Cholinergic nervous system and immediate hypersensitivity. *J. Allergy Clin. Immunol. 66*: 374-378.

Spector, S. L., Hudson, L., and Petty, T. L. (1977). Effect of Bronkosol and its components on cardiopulmonary parameters in asthmatic patients. *J. Allergy Clin. Immunol. 59*: 371-376.

Stead, W. W. (1981). Tuberculosis among elderly persons: an outbreak in a nursing home. *Ann. Intern. Med. 94*: 606-610.

Szentivanyi, A. (1980). The radioligand binding approach in the study of lymphocyte adrenoceptors and the constitutional basis of atopy. *J. Allergy Clin. Immunol. 65*: 5-11.

Taub, S. J., (1975). The diagnosis and treatment of asthma in the elderly. *Eye Ear Nose Throat Mon. 54*: 248-251.

Thompson, J., and Buckley, C. E., III (!973). Serum β1A levels in older humans. *J. Gerontol. 28*: 434-440.

Thompson, N. J., Glassroth, J. L., Snider, D. E., Jr., and Farer, L. S. (1979). The booster phenomenon in serial tuberculin testing. *Am. Rev. Resp. Dis. 119*: 587-597.

Townley, R. G., Dennis, M., and Itkin, I. H. (1965). Comparative action of acetyl-beta-methylcholine, histamine and pollen antigens in subjects with hay fever and patients with bronchial asthma. *J. Allergy 36*: 121-137.

Van Arsdel, P. P., Jr., and Paul, G. H. (1977). Drug therapy in the management of asthma. *Ann. Intern. Med. 87*: 68-74.

Verhaegen, H;. DeCree, J., Verbruggen, F., Hoebeke, J., DeBrabander, M., and Brugmans, J. (1973). Immune responses in elderly anti-negative subjects and the effect of levamisole. *Verb. Dtsch. Ges. Inn. Med. 79*: 623-628.

Villaverde, M. M., and MacMillan, C. W. (1980). *Ailments of Aging*. Van Nostrand Reinhold, New York.

Vitetta, E. S., and Uhr, J. W. (1977). IgD and B cell differentiation. *Immunol. Rev. 37*: 50-88.

Walford, R. L. (1974). Immunologic theories of aging: current status. *Fed. Proc. 33*: 2020-2027.

Wallace, S., Whiting, B., and Runcie, J. (1976). Factors affecting drug binding in plasma of elderly patients. *Br. J. Clin. Pharmacol. 3*: 327-330.

Webb-Johnson, D. C., and Andrews, J. L. (1977). Bronchodilator therapy. *N. Engl. J. Med. 297*: 476-482, 758-764.

Weston, W. L., Huff, J. C., Humbert, J. R., Hambidge, K. M., Neldner, K. H., and Walravens, P. A. (1977). Zinc correction of defective chemotaxis in achrodermatitis enteropathica. *Arch. Dermatol. 113*: 422-425.

Willkins, R. F., and O'Brien, W. M. (1974). Non-steroidal anti-inflammatory drugs (NSAID). *Bull. Rheuma. Dis. 24*: 770-777.

Willems, J. S., Sanders, C. R. Riddiough, M. A., and Bell, J. C. (1980). Cost effectiveness of vaccination against pneumococcal pneumonia. *N. Engl. J. Med. 303*: 553-559.

Wittig, H. J., Belloit, J., de Fillippi, I., and Royal, G. (1980). Age-related serum immunoglobulin E levels in healthy subjects and in patients with allergic disease. *J. Allergy Clin. Immunol. 66*: 305-313.

Wittig, H. J., McLaughlin, E. T., Leifer, K. L., and Belloit, J. D. (1978). Risk factors for the development of allergic disease: analysis of 2,190 patient records. *Ann. Allergy 41*: 84-88.

Wolfe, J. D., Tashkin, D. P., Calvarese, B., and Simmons, M. (1978). Bronchodilator effects of terbutaline and aminophylline alone and in combination in asthmatic patients. *N. Engl. J. Med. 298*: 363-367.

Yunis, E. J., and Greenberg, L. J. (1974). Immunopathology of aging. *Fed. Proc. 33*: 2017-2019.

Yunis, E. J., Fernandes, G., and Greenberg, L. J. (1975). Immune deficiency, autoimmunity and aging. *Birth Defects 11*(1): 185-192.

Zeitz, S. J., Ostrow, J. H., and Van Arsdel, P. P., Jr. (1974). Humoral and cellular immunity in the anergic tuberculosis patient. *J. Allergy Clin. Immunol. 53*: 20-26.

Part III
Aging: Neurochemistry and Behavior

Part III
Aging: Neurochemistry and Behavior

10

Structure and Function of the Aged Hypothalamoneurohypophysial System

Vernon J. Choy* / *University of California, Berkeley, California*

INTRODUCTION

Despite the demonstrated diverse actions of the neurohypophysial peptides, classically represented by vasopressin, oxytocin, and their associated neurophysins, and now including somatostatin and the enkephalins, little is known of how the mammalian hypothalamoneurohypophysial system (HNS) is affected by age. Most of the data concern vasopressin; virtually nothing has been reported for somatostatin and enkephalin. The gap in our knowledge is unfortunate because of the many biological consequences of possible deficits in neurohypophysial function and control. The purpose of this chapter is to examine the alterations in both the structure and function of the HNS in the old individual. The normal HNS and its products will be described in moderate detail so that these can be related to the age-altered system. However, a full review of the HNS can be found elsewhere (Soloff and Pearlmutter, 1979).

NEUROSECRETION

Concepts of Neurosecretion

Neurosecretory systems can be broadly defined to include neurons whose axon terminals represent the sites of storage and release of specific materials synthesized

---

*Present affiliation: Postgraduate School of Obstetrics and Gynaecology, The University of Auckland, Auckland, New Zealand

elsewhere in the cell. The products of these cells are true hormones, although some of them do not circulate throughout the organism. Together with associated glial cells and blood vessels, neurosecretory systems form neurohemal organs. Examples of these organs are the median eminence and neurohypophysis of mammals, and the urophysis of fish. Extensive monographs may be consulted for more detailed descriptions on the subject (Maddrell and Nordmann, 1979; Lederis and Veale, 1978; Bargmann and Scharrer, 1970; Knowles and Vollrath, 1974; Bargmann et al., 1978).

Neurosecretory neurons are characterized by their production and release of chemical mediators which reach target organs via vascular channels. These channels are, for example, the general circulation in the case of the posterior pituitary hormones, or the hypophysial portal systems in the case of the hypothalamic hormones. In the HNS neurons, defined by the pioneering studies of Bargmann and Scharrer (1952), the hormones are the peptides, vasopressin and oxytocin. These neurons can be recognized at the light microscope level by a number of relatively specific histochemical techniques (chrome-hematoxylin-phloxine, chrome-alum-hematoxylin, paraldehyde-fuchsin) and at the ultrastructural level by the presence within the cells of neurosecretory granules (nsg). These nsg are membrane-bound vesicles usually about 100-300 nm in diameter with contents which are characteristically electron dense. A consequence of the large space between neurosecretory cell endings and their targets is that these cells must produce much larger amounts of transmitter substance than do conventional neurons. The products of mediation are not confined to the region of the axon endings since large amounts of neurosecretory material (nsm) are manufactured and stored in cell bodies. The structural appearance of the cells reflects this bias in that the cells contain extensive Golgi systems that spawn numerous nsg, which are consequently readily detectable by so-called Gomori procedures.

Neurosecretory granules must be transported from the cell body to the site of release at the axon endings. This involves a system of axonal transport which delivers the granules at an appropriate rate to the release site. Perturbation of axonal transport rate may cause aggregations of nsg within the axon; the axons then become coarse and varicose in appearance, and are punctuated by variously sized Herring bodies (Dellman and Rodriguez, 1970). Axoplasmic transport has been recently reviewed by Ochs (1977). Historically, nsm was considered to be elaborated in cell bodies prior to transportation to the posterior pituitary for storage and release into the bloodstream. The term "neurosecretion" was coined for this concept (Bargmann and Scharrer, 1952). It is now believed that certain processing steps occur within the granules. The dense core of the nsg increases in size during the trip from the cell body to the nerve ending in the neurohypophysis. The increase appears to be due to an internal transformation of the dense core contents. The work of Sachs and colleagues (1969) has led to the view that a large precursor undergoes enzymatic cleavage to free endogenous hormone within the nsg during transport. This concept has been proposed as a model of biosynthesis, translocation, processing, and release of peptides in peptidergic neurons (Gainer et al., 1977).

The Morphology of the HNS

The cytoarchitecture of the rat HNS under normal and experimental conditions has been extensively investigated and is similar to that of other species (Dierickx, 1980). As the name implies, this complex structure has components in the hypothalamus and in the neural lobe of the pituitary with a tract of nerve fibers joining the two parts.

The neural lobe of the pituitary contains an accumulation of axon terminals ending on blood capillaries and diffusely distributed pituicytes. The axon terminals are the storage site for vasopressin and oxytocin, together with the neurophysin proteins. However, the neurohypophysis is not exclusively oxytocinergic or vasopressinergic since some of the axons are known to contain other peptides, such as somatostatin or enkephalin. Most of the nerve fibers in the neurohypophysis are the terminals of axons from the magnocellular neurosecretory nuclei of the hypothalamus: the supraoptic nucleus (SON) and the paraventricular nucleus (PVN). These nuclei are composed of large neurosecretory neurons whose axons stream caudomedially to the floor of the third ventricle where they form the HNS fiber tract. This nerve tract traverses the internal region of the median eminence, a neurohemal organ rich in nerve terminals and blood vessels, to the pituitary stalk and the neurohypophysis. The SON and PVN also possess a parvocellular component, a rich capillary network, nerve fibers, and neuroglial cells. It has been suggested that enkephalin innervation of the neurohypophysis originates from the magnocellular nuclei (Rossier et al., 1979, 1980). Somatostatin innervation also appears to originate from the hypothalamus (Brownstein et al., 1975).

As already mentioned, light microscopic studies of tissue with Gomori methods have revealed the presence of nsm in the HNS, and have allowed extensive mapping of Gomori-positive elements throughout the hypothalamus and pituitary. Such histochemical procedures are of limited value for several reasons: first, Gomori stains depend on the presence of high concentrations of protein-bound disulfide groups and, therefore, stain any other structure that fulfills this criterion; second, it is not possible to distinguish oxytocin-containing neurons from vasopressin-containing neurons, since the procedure uses one of the associated disulfide-rich neurophysins as the chromophil rather than the hormones themselves. Recent improvements in immunologically based measuring techniques have provided major advances in this field of study. Radioimmunoassays can be used to quantify the amount of each hormone in specific brain structures and body fluids.

Immunohistochemical staining methods have applications both at the light microscope level as well as at the ultrastructural level (Buijs, 1980). With such immunostaining techniques it is possible, for example, to distinguish between oxytocin-containing and vasopressin-containing neurons. Further improvement has involved the use of antibodies specific for oxytocin-neurophysin and vasopressin-neurophysin to recognize the respective neurons. On this chemical basis, and on the basis of electrophysiological measurements, the neurons of the SON and PVN have been segregated into two types: those that contain oxytocin and those that contain vasopressin (Dierickx, 1980; Swaab et al., 1975). Similarly, an extensive enkephalinergic system parallels morphologically the neuroendocrine oxytocinergic and vasopressinergic systems (Micevych and Elde, 1980). The differential distribution of each type of neuron within the respective nuclei, the median eminence, and the neurohypophysis has now been described fully (Dierickx, 1980). A further result of these new procedures has been the novel localization of neurohypophysial hormones in numerous extra-HNS areas of the brain (Buijs et al., 1978; Buijs et al., 1980; Sterba et al., 1980).

Modulation of Neurohypophysial Function

Vasopressin is the antidiuretic hormone of all mammals. The main function of the hormone is to control water reabsorption in the kidney. Its secretion is controlled by several factors, including plasma osmolality and blood volume. It has been proposed that osmoreceptors are present in the hypothalamus to account for osmolar sensitivity (Verney, 1947); these are sensitive to the osmolality of the body fluids and, in some manner, control the release of vasopressin. It has been established that the SON does contain osmoreceptors (Sundsten and Sawyer, 1961; Woods et al., 1966), but it is not clear whether the magnocellular neurons are osmosensitive (Hayward and Vincent, 1970; Mason, 1980). Vasopressin secretion is controlled primarily by osmolar factors, as well as several secondary control mechanisms. These are blood pressure, circulating blood volume, pain, stress, emesis, and several humoral factors (Robertson, 1977; Robertson and Rowe, 1980; Valiquette, 1980).

Oxytocin neurons can be distinguished from vasopressin neurons by their specific position in the SON and PVN (Choy and Watkins, 1977). They can also be distinguished by their distinctive electrophysiological firing patterns (Hayward and Reaves, 1980). Oxytocin secretion may occur in response to secretory stimuli that are more specific for vasopressin (e.g., oxytocin secretion is affected by osmotic stress as well as by hemodynamic factors). In the vasopressin-deficient homozygous Brattleboro rat, pituitary oxytocin is depleted, presumably due to a compensatory hypersecretion of this remaining hormone. More specific secretory stimuli for oxytocin are suckling and coitus (Valiquette, 1980).

The diverse stimuli of oxytocin and vasopressin release suggest a rich innervation of the HNS from other parts of the brain. This is indeed true; the SON and PVN contain significant concentrations of monoamine neurotransmitters, substances that probably represent monoaminergic innervation. Histofluorescence and immunohistochemical investigations indicate these neurotransmitters are not in neurosecretory cells, but in nerve terminals that are closely apposed to the neurosecretory cell bodies (Palkovits and Brownstein, 1978; Khachaturian and

Sladek, 1980). The concentrations of these neurotransmitters are usually much higher in the PVN than in the SON. The presence of neurotransmitters in the neurosecretory nuclei represents the biochemical correlate of central nervous system modulation of the HNS at the level of the hypothalamus.

Apart from the modulation of HNS function at the level of the hypothalamus, hormone release may also be controlled at the axon terminal in the pituitary by endogenous opioids (Bisset et al., 1978; Brownell et al., 1980; Miller, 1980). Innervation of the posterior pituitary by enkephalinergic neurons in the SON and PVN may regulate the secretion of oxytocin and vasopressin (Rossier et al., 1979). For example, a stable analogue of enkephalin inhibits release of vasopressin in humans (Brownell et al., 1980); inhibition of stimulus-evoked vasopressin release is caused by morphine and beta-endorphin, and the inhibitory effects of enkephalin can be reversed by naloxone, the opioid agonist. These findings suggest the possible existence of inhibitory opiate receptors on the terminals of vasopressin fibers in the neurohypophysis. Comparison of the distribution of oxytocin and vasopressin with that of the enkephalins in the neurohypophysis of the rat has indicated that met-enkephalin is invariably associated with oxytocin terminals, and leu-enkephalin is often associated with vasopressin terminals. Perhaps the enkephalins are the copeptides of the oxytocin and vasopressin neurosecretory system, and they have a modulatory influence on neurohypophysial hormone release (Miller, 1980).

NEUROHYPOPHYSIAL HORMONES

Extrahypothalamic Localization and Action

Until recently, hypothalamic neurosecretory neurons were thought to have an exclusively regulatory function at the level of the pituitary. However, they are now known to have extensive projections to numerous areas of the brain (Buijs et al., 1978; Buijs et al., 1980; Glick and Brownstein, 1980; Kozlowski et al., 1978; Sterba et al., 1980) where their hormonal products may influence various central nervous system activities (Boer et al., 1980; Emson, 1979; Snyder, 1980). The evidence concerning the function of these projects is quite incomplete and often inferential; it is probable that they fill a neurotransmitter role. Certainly, behavioral effects involving memory and learning have been demonstrated for vasopressin, and analogues of these peptides (see Chaps. 15 and 16). It remains to be seen whether or not these neuropeptides can be liberated at central synapses to act on specific receptors on postsynaptic membranes and, therefore, qualify as true neurotransmitters.

Novel HNS hormones

Much of the previous discussion has concerned oxytocin and vasopressin, the active principles of the mammalian neurohypophysis. Their action on peripheral organs has been extensively characterized, although some of these functions are not well understood. Several other products are released by the posterior pituitary. The work of Sachs and co-workers (1969) suggests that each of the neurohypophysial hormones is synthesized as a precursor that contains one hormone, its associated neurophysin, and an undefined glycosylated remnant peptide (Nicholas et al., 1980). This "peptide fragment" may yet prove to be of greater importance than its present role as "disposable packaging."

Several other hormones may also be included in the present context. The endogenous opioids have already been mentioned. The hypophysiotropic hormone, somatostatin, has been detected in substantial concentrations in the neural lobe of the pituitary (Brownstein et al., 1975). Somatostatin has a well-known inhibitory action on the release of growth hormone from the anterior pituitary. In this capacity it reaches the pituitary from the hypothalamus by way of the portal vascular system of the median eminence. The functional significance of this substance to the neurohypophysis is not known, although it may represent a hypothalamo-neurohypophysio-adenohypophysial pathway.

EFFECT OF AGE ON THE MORPHOLOGY OF THE HNS

Introduction

Although age-related structural changes in various organs and some areas of the brain have been well documented, the data concerning changes in the HNS are sparse and not entirely consistent. It is, therefore, instructive to survey these data to identify where and by what means further studies might be undertaken. The question of whether deficiencies in the vasopressin control system are responsible for age-related changes in fluid balance, or whether such shifts provoke neurosecretory activity and changes in morphology, must be considered. As in all such investigations, it is most desirable to be able to relate functional alterations to structural changes. Despite the scattered nature of the data to be described below, some generalization can be formulated; there appears to be a decrease in the amount of nsm in the HNS, and the components of the HNS show conspicuous alterations that can be interpreted in several ways.

A survey of the current literature indicates that the aging rodent and, to a lesser extent, human, exhibits changes in salt and water metabolism, and that there is a redistribution of water among the various compartments of the body. This change in water balance cannot be attributed to nephron loss alone. What of HNS degeneration and cell loss? In the case of neuronal degeneration, a further concern that is not generally taken into account is the high regenerative capacity of neurosecretory neurons, which can survive the loss of large portions of axons without major impairment of function (Dellman, 1973). Conclusive evidence regarding HNS decline cannot, therefore, be provided from morphological measurements alone. Anatomical data must be supplemented by physiological and biochemical measurements.

Neurohypophysis

The concentration of nsm in the pituitary, determined from semiquantitative histochemical procedures, was first reported by Rodeck et al. (1960). These investigators found no difference between glands of young (3-6 months old) and old rats (12-24 months old), but Gomori-positive material was markedly diminished in the glands of rats more than 24 months old. Bioassay for the hormones in the pituitaries revealed no decrement in vasopressin concentration, but a slight decrease in oxytocin, thereby inducing a significant difference between vasopressin:oxytocin ratios for the old and young rats. A later report describing a similar experiment (Morrison and Staroscik, 1964) suggested that the amount of nsm in the rat pituitary increased markedly with age, perhaps due to degenerative changes (Green and Van Breeman, 1955). The different conclusions may be explained by the lack of agreement as to what age should be considered "old"; Rodeck and co-workers (1960) used rats more than 24 months old, whereas Morrison and Staroscik (1964), 19-month-old animals. This difference was further emphasized by Dunihue (1965), who discovered that nsm in the posterior lobe of young rats (10 months old) was abundant, but moderately to severely reduced in old rats (30 months old). The reduction in nsm concentration was accompanied by an increase in the number of pituicytes. Studies on human and cattle pituitaries either failed to find a relationship between the amount of nsm and age in humans (Currie et al., 1960), or a small decline in cattle (Nikitin, 1961).

The recent availability of highly specific immunohistochemical techniques has allowed further advances beyond the early studies. The vasopressin concentration of the pituitary declined progressively from young-adult rats (3-9 months) to old rats (12-24 months) (Watkins and Choy, 1980). Oxytocin and neurophysin concentrations also declined with age, but not so severely. However, even in rats more than 24 months old residual amounts of hormone persisted.

The bulk of the evidence favors the suggestion that with increasing age decreased quantities of neurohypophysial hormones are stored in the pituitary, which remains viable although in a depressed state. Quantitative ultrastructural analysis of the old mouse pituitary illustrates this conclusion (Wilkinson and Davies, 1981). Ultrastructural alterations include increased autophagic activity, increased perivascular space, decline in pituicyte volume, and decreased nsg size. However, the overall morphology of the neurohypophysis of the old mouse under physiologically defined resting conditions indicates maintenance of function (Wilkinson and Davies, 1981).

The data outlined are not meaningful alone, since decreased gland content may be a result of either a decrease in biosynthesis or an increase in secretory activity (Morris et al., 1979; Choy and Watkins, 1977). A detailed study of the HNS tract may yield some additional clues; changes in fiber tracts or decrease in hypothalamic nuclei content may indicate an impairment in synthesis and transport. On the other hand, measurements of plasma or urine concentrations are good indices of secretory activity. Unfortunately, experiments with radiolabeled amino acid precursors, to monitor protein biosynthesis and transport in the old specimens, have not been undertaken to pinpoint areas of functional decline.

Hypothalamus

An early survey of structural alterations in the brain (Warren, 1956) indicated that the nuclei of the rat hypothalamus show some of the most impressive and striking incidences of specificity of age changes seen anywhere in the nervous system. No clear evidence was seen of real degenerative changes in cells of the SON and PVN, nor was there an indication of cell destruction and an accumulation of age pigment in any of the cells. However, in some single nerve cells a decrease of Nissl substance accompanied by vacuolization, a decrease in cell size, and an apparent regression of the cell nucleus were found. This description was a confirmation of an earlier investigation which found no cell destruction in the SON and PVN of the senile human hypothalamus (Buttlar-von Brentano, 1954). Both of these studies were essentially anatomical in approach with no reference to the neurosecretory activity or to the nsm content of the cells. Improved histological techniques have led to the understanding that the HNS is affected by age, although agreement concerning the severity of these alterations is lacking. It is probable that a certain degree of age-dependent deterioration occurs in neurosecretory neurons (Polenov and Pavlovic, 1978), but the lack of uniformity in experimental protocol, age of animals, and area of the HNS studied has not allowed a resolution to the question of to what extent the HNS alters with advanced age.

Lin and co-workers (1976) reported minor alterations in the nuclear volume of neurons in the SON and PVN of old female and male rats, more than 22 months old, compared with young controls (3-5 months old). The nuclear volume of the hypothalamic neurons of old females was significantly smaller than that of young rats. However, the extent of decrease in the various areas was not the same, with the largest decrease in the SON (30% decrease) and a minor 10% decrease in the PVN. Frolkis and colleagues (1972) reported a similar reduction (6%) in the nuclear size of secretory neurons from 24-month-old rats compared with young controls. Morphometric data from young (3-6 months old), old (12-24 months old), and senile rats (> 24 months old) are compared in Table 1 (Watkins and Choy, personal communication). In the young and old group, nuclei from PVN neurons were significantly larger that nuclei from the SON. More importantly, in both the SON and PVN, neurons from the oldest rats had nuclei that were 20-25% smaller in diameter. The reduction in the nucleus size of neurosecretory neurons is considered by some investigators to be a sign of a decrease in functional activity (Polenov and Pavlovic, 1978). These data suggest that age changes of the HNS neurons are area-specific to a high degree. As will be seen below, a great deal more evidence supports this suggestion. A comparison of hypothalamic area volumes, neuron density, and neuron number in old and young female rats has shown no

Table 1 Stereological Measurements of Cell Nuclei from the Supraoptic Nucleus and Paraventricular Nucleus of the Rat Hypothalamus

Age (months)	Nucleus diameter $(\mu m)^a$			
	SON	p^b	PVN	p^b
3-6	$8.72 \pm 0.81(520)^c$		$9.08 \pm 0.78(520)$	$p_0 < 0.005$
12-24	$8.90 \pm 1.06(398)$	p_1 ns	$9.25 \pm 0.97(400)$	$p_0 < 0.005$ $p_1 < 0.005$
>24	$7.24 \pm 1.26(450)$	$p_1 < 0.005$ $p_2 < 0.005$	$7.22 \pm 1.24(460)$	p_0 ns $p_1 < 0.005$ $p_2 < 0.005$

[a]Serial transverse sections of the hypothalamus were stained for neurophysin. Selection of SON and PVN cells for measurement was by a systematic sampling procedure which required that a line in the microscope eyepiece micrometer passed over the cell nucleus.

[b]Statistical analysis by Student's t-test. p_0: SON vs. PVN; p_1: 12-24 months vs. 3-6 months: p_2: > 24 months vs. 12-24 months. ns, not significant.

[c]Mean ± standard deviation. Number in parentheses represents number of cells measured.

Source: W. B. Watkins and V. J. Choy, unpublished data.

significant neuron loss in the HNS. Area volume was greater in the old specimens, but neuron density was decreased; these changes were probably the consequences of continued brain growth (Hsu and Peng, 1978). The conclusion (Hsu and Peng, 1978) that the decreased antidiuretic response to osmotic stimuli in old rodents was not due to a decreased number of cells, but to decreased function of individual neurons or to changes in neuronal organization, will be explored in further detail below.

Neurosecretory material concentration may be unchanged in rats up to 24 months of age, but severely depleted in older animals (Rodeck et al., 1960). The depletion in nsm can be correlated with loss in vasopressin, oxytocin, and neurophysin storage. Moreover, the decrease in stainable material is probably more severe in the PVN than the SON, and is greater in oxytocinergic neurons than in vasopressinergic neurons (Watkins and Choy, 1980). Such age-related decreases in neurohypophysial hormone concentrations are not reported by all workers (Sladek et al., 1980), and are probably influenced by differences in experimental technique. For example, prolonged extraction in alcohol, and long-term treatment in hot paraffin, both essential histological procedures, may either leech out the peptides from the tissue or destroy the remaining immunoreactive principles. The problem of whether or not these losses occur more readily in the old than young specimens awaits a detailed biochemical solution. Are there altered forms of the hormones in the old HNS, and are these forms more susceptible to damage or dissolution? There is evidence that variant forms of hormones occur more commonly in old rats than in the young (Klug and Adelman, 1978; Nicolas et al., 1980).

Quantitative changes notwithstanding, it is generally agreed that the old HNS tract exhibits evidence of altered axoplasmic transport; axonal fibers appear varicose and dilated, and Herring bodies are larger (Watkins and Choy, 1980; Frolkis et al., 1972; Morrison and Staroscik, 1964; Pilgrim, 1970; Sladek et al., 1978; Sladek et al., 1980). Davies and co-workers (Davies and Fotheringham, 1980; Wilkinson and Davies, 1981), in a quantitative ultrastructural study of the 26-month-old mouse HNS, concluded that transport of nsg from the SON to the pituitary occurred at a reduced rate without evidence of activated protein synthesis. It, therefore, appears that decreased neuronal activity (depletion of hormones, decrease in nucleus size), along with reduced axonal transport (varicose axonal fibers), may be consistent with the reported decreased pituitary stores of hormones and the occurrence of at least one physiological correlate of depressed neurohypophysial function in old rats, diabetes insipidus. This may be an oversimplified generalization since alternative explanations can be formulated. For example, an altered relationship between synthesis and transport or transport and secretion may promote morphological changes in the rat HNS (Choy and Watkins, 1977; Krisch, 1980). It is also necessary to consider in greater detail the reported deterioration in selected regions of the HNS.

Comparison of old (26-34 months old) and young mouse hypothalami stained with a silver impregnation technique indicates that pathological changes in the SON and PVN are not frequent, although neuronal alterations suggestive of metabolic change may occur (Machados-Salas et al., 1977). Ultrastructural analysis led to the same conclusion (Davies and Fotheringham, 1980). Age pigment, however, may accumulate in these areas of the hypothalamus (Davies and Fotheringham, 1980; Machados-Salas et al., 1977; Pilgrim, 1970; Samorajski et al., 1968). Morrison and Staroscik (1964) described an increase in the number of vacuoles within the area of the magnocellular nuclei. Likewise, Frolkis and co-workers (1972) described some definite degenerative changes; neuron elongation, reduction in nuclear size, and some nuclear pyknosis. These signs of reduced functional activity were particularly clear in the peripheral cells of the HNS. Interestingly, oxytocinergic neurons are differentially positioned in the dorsal region of the SON and around the periphery of the PVN, and it is these that are most affected by age (Watkins and Choy, 1980). Structures suggestive of neuronal activation and degeneration in the HNS of 12 to 24-month-old rats are illustrated in Fig. 1. Structures similar to the vacuolated neurons in Fig. 1 have also been described by other investigators as being present in the primarily oxytocin-containing anterior commissural nucleus of 30-month-old rats (Sladek et al., 1980). Therefore, it is possible that at least some cells of the HNS are activated by the aging process and that some of these activated cells, perhaps through overactivation, may eventually degenerate. These cells can be seen in selected areas of the hypothalamus, and because of the progressive nature of the process, cells in different stages of activation and destruction will be observed. The various structures that might be found in the aged hypothalamus are illustrated in Fig. 2. Structures A-D are in different stages of the secretory cycle, whereas those structures of type E-F are in different stages of degeneration (Watkins and Choy, 1980). Age changes are highly area-specific in regard to hypothalamic regions as well as within each hypothalamic nucleus. Perhaps this area specificity partly accounts for the differences in the studies described above.

EFFECT OF AGE ON HNS FUNCTION

Introduction

Morphological observations are sometimes only meaningful when they can be correlated with function. This is particularly true in the present context. In general, deteriorative alterations in the structural components of the HNS may be consistent with observed age-related changes in water and electrolyte balance, and may even be linked with some of the changes in learning and memory processes, discussed elsewhere in this volume. However, this generalization, appropriate to lab-

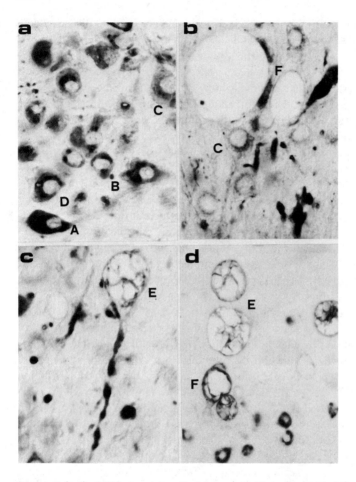

Figure 1 (a-d) HNS structures that are suggestive of neuronal degeneration. Samples illustrated were from 12 to 24-month-old rats. Cells were stained by immunohistochemical procedures for neurophysin: (a) Cells of type A-D from the PVN. These cells are in various stages of the neurosecretory cycle and are normal. (b) Structures of types C and F in the SON. F appears to be a vacuole with associated immunostaining and could result from cell destruction. (c) and (d) Degenerative structures of types E and F in the PVN. These appear to be the result of complete or partial vacuolization of neurosecretory cells. The interrelationship of these structures is illustrated in Fig. 2. (From Watkins and Choy, 1980, with permission of ANKHO International, Inc.)

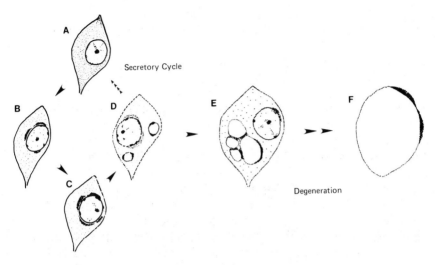

Figure 2 Different stages of neurosecretory cycle (A-D) and the life course (A-F) of magnocellular neurosecretory cells in the rat HNS. Small arrow head indicates recovery of a cell during a secretory cycle. (From Watkins and Choy, 1980, with permission of ANKHO International, Inc.)

oratory rodents, cannot be directly extrapolated to humans inasmuch as old people do not show clinical evidence of the diabetes insipidus of the old rat, and the sparse morphological data are not indicative of major HNS alterations. Nonetheless, in both species, definite changes do occur in the response of the HNS to secretory stimuli. These changes are not necessarily associated with vasopressin control of water balance, but may concern other functions of the hypothalamus. For example, posterior pituitary extract alone or in combination with cortisol appears to improve overall condition of old rats, and even produces a modest prolongation of the life span of these animals (Friedman and Friedman, 1963, 1964). The evidence that oxytocin may be a life-prolonging factor in the extract (Bodanszky and Engel, 1966) is consistent with the observed area-specific deterioration of oxytocinergic neurons (Watkins and Choy, 1980).

Salt and Water Balance

It has long been thought that a decline in neurohypophysial function might be an important event in the aging process (Findley, 1949). It was suggested by Findley (1949) that disease conditions such as obesity, hypertension, arteriosclerosis, diabetes mellitus, sexual impotence, osteoporosis, and muscular weakness are due to hypofunction of the neurohypophysis. These widespread consequences of HNS decline are not proven, although several alterations in senescent rat and human physiology could be explained in this manner.

Data concerning salt and water handling in aged rats are available (Friedman and Friedman, 1957a,b; Friedman et al., 1956; Friedman et al., 1960). In essence, the process of aging in the rat involves certain fundamental readjustments in water balance. This is also probably the case in humans, in whom body water steadily shifts from the intracellular to the extracellular phase. Older rats consistently excrete more water and tend to absorb more sodium under load. These changes are accentuated by previous dehydration and appear to be due to a change in renal function. However, the kidney in old rats is responsive to vasopressin stimulus (Turkington and Everitt, 1976), and the diminished reabsorption of water is readily reversed by pitressin. Therefore, the locus of decline could involve the HNS. Convincing evidence for possible HNS involvement has been provided from young rats with diabetes insipidus induced by neurohypophysial denervation. These animals have both an increased extracellular fluid volume and increased total extracellular sodium. Moreover, this preparation closely resembles the intact old rat with age-induced diabetes insipidus. In both experimental models, some of the observed symptoms can be alleviated and a normal fluid balance restored by administration of small doses of vasopressin (Friedman et al., 1960).

Tissue Hormone Levels

Radioimmunoassayed levels of hypothalamic vasopressin remain unchanged in the aged Fischer rat [cited as unpublished data by Sladek, in Sladek et al., (1980)]. This measurement of hypothalamic tissue, without attached median eminence, is notably different from another study that indicated an age-related decline in hypothalamic (including median eminence) vasopressin in the same strain of rats (Landfield et al., 1980). Such differences may be explained by changes in the distribution of vasopressin in the various components of the HNS, especially the median eminence; this would occur during, for example, a disturbance of axonal transport processes. Interestingly, no consistent difference in oxytocin content of the posterior pituitary could be demonstrated in Fischer 344 rats of various ages (3, 14, and 24 months old) (Landfield et al., 1980). Somatostatin values are not yet available for the glands from old animals. Met-enkephalin tends to increase with age in hypothalamus and posterior pituitary (Landfield et al., 1980). The relationship between decreases in these peptides levels and neurohypophysial responsiveness has yet to be explored. It is obvious from the above short outline that further measurements by both radioimmunoassay and bioassay of neurohypophysial hormone levels in the separate components of the HNS are necessary.

Modulation of Hormone Secretion

Most of the data available on the secretion of neurohypophysial hormones concern vasopressin release under normal and stressed conditions. Secretion data for oxytocin, somatostatin, and the enkephalins from old animals and humans are not available, mostly because of inadequate assay procedures.

The daily excretion of vasopressin and the basal plasma vasopressin concentration fall significantly in 30-month-old rats (Turkington and Everitt, 1976). It is reasonable to infer that these reductions reflect the amount of hormone released by the neurohypophysis. Restoration to normal values of salt and water balance in 24-month-old rats by administration of small doses of vasopressin certainly provides an excellent argument for such a decline (Friedman et al., 1960). The recent report (Frolkis et al., 1981) of a rise in the vasopressin contents in rat blood from 7.4 μU/ml plasma in mature rats (8-10 months old) to 28.0 μU/ml in senile rats (26-28 months old) is in direct contrast to the above findings. This single instance notwithstanding, the current consensus is that the concentrations of vasopressin in the circulation of old rats are less than normal.

Responsiveness of vasopressin release to appropriate stimulus is markedly different in aged rats and humans compared with normal adults. It is well known that vasopressin control is exquisitely sensitive to changes in the external and internal environments (Robertson and Rowe, 1980), and considering the multidirectional and heterochronological alterations that occur in the aging hypothalamus (Frolkis et al., 1972), different responses to stimuli might be expected. Young rats (8 months old) show a prompt falloff in urine volume with a concomitant increase in urine vasopressin concentration during a period of dehydration. Both responses are much slower in 24-month-old rats (Turkington and Everitt, 1976). In an earlier study, 24-month-old rats failed to respond to the osmotic stimulation applied by the intracarotid injection of 1.5% sodium chloride (Friedman et al., 1956). Dicker and Nunn (1958) confirmed that osmotic stimulation of the neurohypophysis can cause an antidiuretic response, but these investigators observed no decline with age, perhaps because their animals were not old enough (12 months old). The differences in the pattern of dehydration responses in old animals may be due to an impaired sensitivity of osmoreceptors (Turkington and Everitt, 1976). Maximal levels of vasopressin released during prolonged dehydration stress were always significantly less in old rats, so it is probable that the old animal produces less hormone. This reduced hormone output correlates well with the description of depleted concentrations of nsm in the neurohypophysis of old rats.

Conclusions about the relationship between aging and the HNS have been largely based on data derived from experiments conducted on laboratory animals.

Marked species differences make correlations with human physiology difficult. In humans, aging enhances the vasopressin release response to osmotic stimuli (Helderman et al., 1978), perhaps due to an increase in the sensitivity of the osmoregulatory system. Figure 3 illustrates the fact that for any given increase in plasma osmolality (induced by a hypertonic saline infusion), plasma vasopressin rises more in the old compared with young adults. The cause of age-related increase in osmoreceptor sensitivity is not known. In the same subjects (54-92 years old), baseline plasma vasopressin concentrations were not significantly different from those of normal adults (21-49 years old) after overnight dehydration. These values are in total contrast with those from old rats, which show a definite decline in plasma vasopressin. Not all vasopressin regulatory mechanisms are influenced in this way. Many older subjects show diminished or absent release of vasopressin following hemodynamic stimulation (Robertson and Rowe, 1980). When allowed to stand after 16 hr of complete bed rest, many young as well as elderly subjects show a significant drop in mean arterial pressure. In the young, this hypotensive stimulus results in a rise in plasma vasopressin. In many elderly subjects, however, the stimulus produces little or no change in the hormone concentrations. These

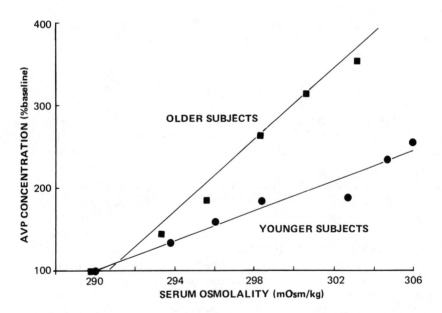

Figure 3 Correlation between serum osmolality and vasopressin concentration in young and old subjects during a 2-hr intravenous infusion of 3% saline at the rate of 0.1 ml/kg/min. The points represent mean values of osmolality and vasopressin at successive 20-min intervals in each age group. (Redrawn from Helderman et al., 1978.)

changes may be attributed to alterations in HNS modulation, rather than to abnormalities in the HNS itself.

Blood osmolality, blood volume, and blood pressure appear to be most important in the normal control of vasopressin release. The latter two influences are nonosmotic stimuli, as are emesis, glucopenia, and angiotensin. Some of these control mechanisms may be important only under certain conditions (Robertson, 1977), and although much is known about them in the adult individual (Bonjour and Malvin, 1970; Mouw et al., 1971; Schrier et al., 1979; Sladek and Joynt, 1978; Veale and Lederis, 1978), only scanty data have been obtained concerning how these processes are affected with age. However, the functional and morphological relationship between monoaminergic and peptidergic neurons (Khachaturian and Sladek, 1980) may have relevance in the mediation of HNS control by nonosmotic factors acting by way of interneurons. In that case, age-related alterations in peptidergic target neurons may occur in concert with alterations of afferent adrenergic fibers with a resulting decline and reorganization of these terminal fibers (Sladek et al., 1980). Further investigations are required, not only to clarify the relationship between aminergic and peptidergic neurons, but also to clarify how this relationship would be affected with age.

Opiates appear to inhibit the release of oxytocin and vasopressin by acting on nerve terminals in the neurohypophysis (Brownell et al., 1980; Iversen et al., 1980; Martin and Voigt, 1981; Michevych and Elde, 1980; Rossier et al., 1979). It is possible that these substances are capable of inhibiting hormone release in response to an osmotic stimulus, for example, by elevating the osmotic threshold for vasopressin release (Komai et al., 1979; Miller, 1975, 1980). Determinations of opiate content of brain and pituitary tissue from aged animals are rare. In summary, met-enkephalin content increases whereas hypothalamic endorphin content is reduced by about 50% in old rats (Barden et al., 1981; Dupont et al., 1980; Gambert et al., 1980). Pituitary endorphin content is slightly elevated in 20-month-old rats compared with 6-week-old rats. It is not known whether these alterations in opiate levels are universal, or whether they are implicated in altered HNS function. Nevertheless, the 50% reduction in PVN endorphin content (Barden et al., 1981) is consistent with reduced HNS activity, provided there exists a positive feedback between the two peptidergic systems. It is quite apparent from this discussion that some aspects of HNS modulation, and the effects of age on this kind of control, are not well characterized, and that the field remains a fertile area of research.

CONCLUSION

The HNS appears to be an excellent model for the study of development and aging of neuroendocrine systems. Its unique morphological features, particularly the ready accessibility of the various components in the hypothalamus and pituitary, recommend it as a candidate for intense scrutiny. Such study would perhaps yield clues as to the nature of the aging process in other neurosecretory systems and the central nervous system. The diverse actions of the hypothalamus are exemplified by the many functional roles of the HNS; these actions are both endocrine and neural, neuroendocrine. The HNS has well-characterized physiological actions on peripheral tissues through the mediation of its equally well-known hormones. However, in recent years new evidence has been collected to show that the subject of HNS physiology has not been exhaustively investigated, and that a whole new realm of neuroendocrinology awaits exploration. In this novel domain, peptides have neuroactive properties, and may well constitute a completely new class of neurotransmitter.

The discussion in this chapter, which has included an extensive description of the age-related changes of the HNS in the rat and also in a number of other mammals, may be completed with a small but broad conclusion. It seems that with advancing age, the HNS undergoes several alterations. These elusive alterations, variously reported as being nonexistent to severe, appear to include: (1) depletion of pituitary hormone stores; (2) disturbances of axonal transport; and (3) degeneration of specific populations of the nuclei that constitute the HNS. These morphological features of the aging HNS are accompanied by important shifts in the mechanisms that modulate the responses of the HNS to appropriate stimuli. These modulatory networks are not well understood, since they incorporate components and mediators that have only recently come to light. It is this aspect of HNS function that is expected to lead to further understanding of the aging process. This is possible since it is the multifunctional and complex actions of the hypothalamus that are implicated in age changes rather than a single central factor. Therefore, although the effects of age on the mammalian HNS are not fundamentally catastrophic in that survival is not drastically threatened, subtle alterations in this complex neuroendocrine region may be instrumental in the etiology of other age-associated conditions, such as postmenopausal hot flushes and hypertension.

ACKNOWLEDGMENTS

Some of the work in this review was financed by the Medical Research Council of New Zealand. Special thanks to Professor Paola S. Timiras for many helpful suggestions, Carol Farver for preparing the draft, and Mark Lewin for help in preparing the bibliography. This is dedicated to Janet Joe.

REFERENCES

Barden, N., Dupont, A., Labrie, F., Merand, Y., Rouleau., Vaudry, H., and Boissier, J. R. (1981). Age-dependent changes in the beta-endorphin content of discrete rat brain nuclei. *Brain Res. 208*: 209-212.
Bargmann, W., and Scharrer, E. (1952). The site of origin of the hormones of the posterior pituitary. *Am. Sci. 40*: 255-259.

Bargmann, W., and Scharrer, B. (1970). In *Aspects of Neuroendocrinology Vth International Symposium on Neurosecretion*, W. Bargman and B. Scharrer (Eds.). Springer-Verlag, New York.

Bargmann, W., Oksche, A., Polenov, A., and Scharrer, B. (1978). In *Neurosecretion and Neuroendocrine Activity: Evolution, Structure and Function. VIIth International Symposium on Neurosecretion*, W. Bargman, A. Oksche, A. Polenov, and B. Scharrer (Eds.). Springer-Verlag, New York.

Bisset, G. W., Chowdery, H. S., and Feldberg, W. (1978). Release of vasopressin by enkephalin. *Br. J. Pharm. 62*: 370-372.

Bodanszky, M., and Engel, S. L. (1966). Oxytocin and the life span of male rats. *Nature 210*: 751.

Boer, G. J., Swaab, D. F., Uylings, H. B. M., Boer, K., Buijs, R. M., and Velis, D. N. (1980). Neuropeptides in rat brain development. *Prog. Brain Res. 55*: 207-227.

Bonjour, J. P., and Malvin, R. L. (1970). Stimulation of ADH release by the renin-angiotensin system. *Am. J. Physiol. 218*: 1555-1559.

Brownell, J., del Pozo, E., and Donatsch, P. (1980). Inhibition of vasopressin secretion by a met-enkaphalin (FK 33-824) in humans. *Acta Endocrinol. 94*: 304-308.

Brownstein, M., Arimura, A., Sato, H., Schally, A. V., and Kizer, J. S. (1975). The regional distribution of somatostatin in the rat brain. *Endocrinology 96*: 1456-1461.

Buijs, R. M. (1980). Immunocytochemical demonstration of vasopressin and oxytocin in the rat brain by light and electron microscope. *J. Histol. Cytol. 28*: 357-360.

Buijs, R. M., Swaab, D. F., Dogterom, J., and van Leeuwen, F. W. (1978). Intra- and extrahypothalamic vasopressin and oxytocin pathways in the rat. *Cell Tiss. Res. 186*: 423-433.

Buijs, R. M., Velis, D. N., and Swaab, D. F. (1980). Extrahypothalamic vasopressin and oxytocin innervation of fetal and adult rat brain. *Prog. Brain Res. 53*: 159-167.

Buttlar-von Brentano, K. (1954). Zur Lebensgesichte des nucleus basalis, tuberomammilaris, supraopticus, und paraventricularis unter normalen and pathogenen bedingungen. *J. Hirnforsch. 1*: 337-419.

Choy, V. J., and Watkins, W. B. (1977). Immunocytochemical study of the hypothalamo-neurohypophysial system. II. Distribution of neurophysin, vasopressin and oxytocin in the normal and osmotically stimulated rat. *Cell Tiss. Res. 180*: 467-490.

Currie, A. R., Adamsons, H., and Van Dyke, H. B. (1960). Vasopressin and oxytocin in the posterior lobe of the pituitary of man. *J. Clin. Endocrinol. 20*: 947.

Davies, I., and Fotheringham, A. P. (1980). The influence of age on the hypothalamo-neurohypophyseal system of the mouse: A quantitative ultrastructural analysis of the supraoptic nucleus. *Mech. Ageing Develop. 12*: 93-105.

Dellman, H. D. (1973). Degeneration and regeneration of neurosecretory systems. *Int. Rev. Cytology 46*: 215-315.

Dellman, H. D., and Rodriguez, E. M. (1970). Herring bodies: an electron microscopic study of local degeneration and regeneration of neurosecretory axons. *Z. Zellforsch. III*: 293-315.

Dicker, S. E., and Nunn, J. (1958). Antidiuresis in adult and old rats. *J. Physiol. 141*: 332-336.

Dierickx, K. (1980). Immunocytochemical localization of the vertebrate cyclic nonapeptide neurohypophysial hormones and neurophysins. *Int. Rev. Cytology 62*: 119-185.

Dunihue, F. W. (1965). Reduced juxtaglomerular cell granularity, pituitary neurosecretory material, and width of the zone glomerular in aging rats. *Endocrinology 71*: 948-951.

Dupont, A., Lepine, J., Langelier, P., Merand, Y., Rouleau, D., Vaudry, H., Gros, C., and Barden, N. (1980). Differential distribution of beta-endorphin and enkephalins in rat and bovine brain. *Reg. Peptides 1*: 43-52.

Emson, P. C. (1979). Peptides as neurotransmitter candidates in the mammalian central nervous system. *Prog. Neurobiol. 13*: 61-116.

Findley, T. (1949). Role of the neurohypophysis in the pathogenesis of hypertension and some allied disorders associated with aging. *Am. J. Med. 7*: 70-84.

Friedman, S. M., and Friedman, C. L. (1957a). Salt and water balance in ageing rats. *Gerontologia 1*: 107-121.

Friedman, S. M., and Friedman, C. L. (1957b). Salt and water balance in relation to blood pressure in aging rats. *Gerontologia 1*: 127-141.

Friedman, S. M., and Friedman, C. L. (1963). Effect of posterior pituitary extracts on the lifespan of old rats. *Nature 200*: 237-238.

Friedman, S. M., and Friedman, C. L. (1964). Prolonged treatment with posterior pituitary powder in aged rats. *Exp. Gerontol. 1*: 37-48.

Friedman, S. M., Friedman, C. L., and Nakashima, M. (1960). Effect of pitressin on old-age changes of salt and water metabolism in the rat. *Am. J. Physiol. 199*: 35-38.

Friedman, S. M., Hinke, J. A. M., and Friedman, C. L. (1956). Neurohypophyseal responsiveness in the normal and senescent rat. *J. Gerontol. 11*: 286-291.

Frolkis, V. V., Bezrukov, V. V., Duplenko, Y. K., and Genis, E. D. (1972). The hypothalamus in aging. *Exp. Gerontol. 7*: 169-184.

Frolkis, V. V. Shevchuk, V. G., Golovchenko, S. F., Bogatskaya, L. N., Verzhikovskaya, N. V., and Medved, V. I. (1981). The effect of hormones on the heamodynamics in animals of different age groups. *Exp. Gerontol. 16*: 1-12.

Gainer, H., Peng Loh, Y., and Sarne, Y. (1977). Biosynthesis of neuronal peptides. In *Peptides in Neurobiology*, H. Gainer (Ed.). Plenum, New York, p. 183.

Gambert, S. R., Garthwaite, T. L., Pontzer, C. H., and Hagen, T. C. (1980). Age-related changes in central nervous system beta-endorphin and ACTH. *Neuroendocrinology 31*: 252-255.

Glick, S. M., and Brownstein, M. J. (1980). Vasopressin content of rat brain. *Life Sci. 27*: 1103-1110.

Green, J. D., and Van Breeman, V. L. (1955). Electron microscopy of the pituitary and observations on neurosecretion. *Am. J. Anat. 97*: 177-227.

Hayward, J. N., and Reaves, T. A. (1980). The endocrine brain: electrophysiological aspects. In *The Endocrine Functions of the Brain*, M. Motta (Ed.). Raven Press, New York.

Hayward, J. N., and Vincent, J. D. (1970). Osmosensitive single neurons in the hypothalamus of unanesthetized monkey. *J. Physiol.* (*Lond.*) *210*: 947-972.

Helderman, J. H., Vestal, R. E., Rowe, J. W., Tobin, J. D., Andres, R., and Robertson, G. L. (1978). The response of arginine vasopressin to intravenous ethanol and hypertonic saline in man: the impact of aging. *J. Gerontol. 33*: 39-47.

Hsu, H. K., and Peng, M. T. (1978). Hypothalamic neuron number of old female rats. *Gerontology 24*: 434-440.

Iversen, L. L., Iversen, S. D., and Bloom, F. F. (1980). Opiate receptors influence vasopressin release from nerve terminals in rat neurohypophysis. *Nature 284*: 350-353.

Khachaturian, H., and Sladek, J. R. (1980). Simultaneous monoamine histofluorescence and neuropeptide immunocytochemistry. III. Ontogeny of catecholamine varicosities and neurophysin neurons in the rat supraoptic and paraventricular nuclei. *Peptides 1*: 77-95.

Klug, T. L., and Adelman, R. C. (1978). Age-dependent accumulation of an immunoreactive species of thyrotropin (TSH) which inhibits production of thyroid hormones. *Adv. Exp. Med. Biol. 97*: 259-264.

Knowles, F., and Vollrath, L. (1974). *In Neurosecretion–The Final Neuroendocrine Pathway. VIth International Symposium on Neurosecretion*, F. Knowles and L. Vollrath (Eds.). Springer-Verlag, New York.

Komai, K., White, K., and Robertson, G. L. (1979). Opiates elevate the osmotic threshold for vasopressin release in rats. *Clin. Res. 27*: 254A.

Kozlowski, G. P., Brownfield, M. S., and Hostetter, G. (1978). Neurophysin and gonadotropin-releasing hormone (GnRH) containing hypothalamo-fugal neurosecretory systems. In *Current Studies of Hypothalamic Function*, K. Lederis and W. L. Veale (Eds.). Karger, Basel, pp. 15-26.

Krisch, B. (1980). Nongranular vasopressin synthesis and transport in early stages of rehydration. *Cell Tiss. Res. 207*: 89-107.

Landfield, P. W., Sundberg, D. K., Smith, M. S., Eldridge, J. C., and Morris, M. (1980). Mammalian aging. Theoretical implications of changes in brain and endocrine systems during mid- and late-life in rats. *Peptides 1* (*Suppl. 1*): 185-196.

Lederis, K., and Veale, W. L. (1978). In *Current Studies on Hypothalamic Function, 1978. Vol. 1, Hormones*, K. Lederis and W. L. Veale (Eds.). Karger, Basel.

Lin, K. H., Peng, Y. M., Peng, M. T., and Tseng, T. M. (1976). Changes in the nuclear volume of rat hypothalamic neurons in old age. *Neuroendocrinology 21*: 247-254.

Machado-Salas, J., Scheibel, M. E., and Scheibel, A. B. (1977). Morphological changes in the hypothalamus of the old mouse. *Exp. Neurol. 57*: 102-111.

Maddrell, S. H. P., and Nordmann, J. J. (1979). In *Neurosecretion*. Blackie, London.

Martin, R., and Voigt, K. H. (1981). Enkephalins co-exist with oxytocin and vasopressin in nerve terminals of rat neurohypophysis. *Nature 289*: 502-504.

Mason, W. T. (1980). Supraoptic neurons of rat hypothalamus are osmosensitive. *Nature 287*: 154-157.

Micevych, P., and Elde, R. (1980). Relationship between enkephalinergic neurons and the vasopressin-oxytocin neuroendocrinology system of the cat. An immunohistochemical study. *J. Comp. Neurol. 190*: 135-146.

Miller, M. (1975). Inhibition of antidiuretic hormone release in the rat by narcotic antagonists. *Neuroendocrinology 19*: 241-251.

Miller, M. (1980). Role of endogenous opioids in neurohypophysial function in man. *J. Clin. Endocrinol. Metab. 50*: 1016-1020.

Morris, J. F., Nordman, J. J., and Dyball, R. E. J. (1979). Structure function correlation in mammalian neurosecretion. *Int. Rev. Exp. Pathol. 18*: 1-75.

Morrison, A. B., and Staroscik, R. N. (1964). The neurosecretory substance in the neurohypophysis of the rat during maturation and aging. *Gerontologia 9*: 65-70.

Mouw, D., Bonjour, J. P., Malvin, R. L., and Vander, A. (1971). Central action of angiotensin in stimulating ADH release. *Am. J. Physiol. 220*: 239-242.

Nicolas, P., Camier, M., Laubner, M., Masse, M. J. O., Mohring, J., and Cohen, P. (1980). Immunological identification of high molecular weight forms common to bovine neurophysin and vasopressin. *Proc. Natl. Acad. Sci. USA 77*: 2587-2491.

Nikitin, V. N. (1961). Changes in the endocrine glands due to ageing. *Russ. Rev. Biol. 50*: 180.

Ochs, S. (1977). Axoplasmic transport in peripheral nerve and hypothalamo-neurohypophyseal systems. *Adv. Exp. Med. Biol. 87*: 13-40.

Palkovits, M., and Brownstein, M. J. (1978). Concentrations of neurotransmitters in the supraoptic and paraventricular nuclei of the rat. In *Neurosecretion and Neuroendocrine Activity*, W. Bargman, A. Oksche, A. Polenov, and B. Scharrer (Eds.). Springer-Verlag, Berlin, pp. 150-255.

Pilgrim, C. (1970). Altersbedingte anhaufung von lysosomalen residualkorpen in zellfortsatzen. *Z. Zellforsch. 109*: 573-582.

Polenov, A. L., and Pavlovic, M. (1978). The hypothalamo-hypophysial system in acipenseridae. VII. The functional morphology of the peptidergic neurosecretory cells in the preoptic nucleus of the sturgeon, Acipenser guldenstadt brandt. A quantitative study. *Cell Tiss. Res. 186*: 559-570.

Robertson, G. L. (1977). The regulation of vasopressin function in health and disease. *Rec. Prog. Horm. Res. 33*: 373-385.

Robertson, G. L., and Rowe, J. (1980). The effect of aging on neurohypophyseal function. *Peptides 1 (Suppl. 1)*: 159-162.

Rodeck, H., Lederis, K., and Heller, H. (1960). The hypothalamo-neurohypophyseal system in old rats. *J. Endocrinol. 21*: 225-230.

Rossier, J., Battenberg, Pittman, Q., Bayon, Koda, L., Miller, R., Guillemin, R., and Bloom, F. (1979). Hypothalamic enkephalin neurones may regulate the neurohypophysis. *Nature 277*: 653-655.

Rossier, J., Pittman, Q., Bloom, F., and Guillemin, R. (1980). Distribution of opiod peptides in the pituitary: a new hypothalamic-pars nervosa enkephalinergic pathway. *Fed. Proc. 39*: 2555-2560.

Sachs, H., Fawcett, P., Takahatake, Y., and Portanova, R. (1969). Biosynthesis and release of vasopressin and neurophysin. *Rec. Prog. Horm. Res. 25*: 447-491.

Samorajski, T., Ordy, J. M., and Rady-Reimer, P. (1968). Lipofuscin pigment accumulation in the nervous system of aging mice. *Anat. Rec. 160*: 555-574.

Schrier, R. W., Berl, T., and Anderson, R. J. (1979). Osmotic and nonosmotic control of vasopressin release. *Am. J. Physiol. 236*: F321-F332.

Sladek, C. D., and Joynt, R. J. (1978). Angiotensin stimulation of vasopressin release from the rat hypothalamo-neurohypophyseal system in organ culture. *Endocrinology 104*: 148-153.

Sladek, J. R., Khachaturian, H., Hoffman, G. E., and Scholer, J. (1980). Aging of central endocrine neurons and their aminergic afferents. *Peptides 1 (Suppl. 1)*: 141-157.

Sladek, J. R., McConnell, J., and McNeil, T. H. (1978). Integrated morphology of neuronal catecholamines and neurophysin in the aged macaque. *Adv. Exp. Biol. Med. 113*: 241-250.

Snyder, S. H. (1980). Brain peptides as neurotransmitters. *Science 209*: 976-983.

Soloff, M. S., and Pearlmutter, A. F. (1979). Biochemical actions of neurohypophysial hormones and neurophysin. In *Biochemical Actions of Hormones, Vol. VI*, G. Littwack (Eds.). Academic, New York, pp. 265-333.

Sterba, G., Naumann, W., and Hoheisel, G. (1980). Exohypothalamic axons of the classic neurosecretory systems and their synapses. *Prog. Brain Res. 53*: 141-158.

Sundsten, J. W., and Sawyer, C. H. (1961). Osmotic activation of neurohypophysial hormone release in rabbits with hypothalamic islands. *Exp. Neurol. 4*: 548-561.

Swaab, D. F., Pool, C. W., and Nijveldt, (1975). Immunofluorescence of vasopressin and oxytocin in the rat hypothalamo-neurohypophysial system. *J. Neural Trans. 36*: 195-215.

Turkington, M. R., and Everitt, A. V. (1976). The neurohypophysis and aging with special reference to the antidiuretic hormone. In *Hypothalamus, Pituitary and Aging*, A. V. Everitt and J. A. Burgess (Eds.). Charles C Thomas, Springfield, Ill., pp. 123-136.

Valiquette, G. (1980). Posterior pituitary hormones and neurophysins. In *The Endocrine Functions of the Brain*, M. Motta (Ed.). Raven Press, New York, pp. 385-417.

Veale, W. L., and Lederis, K. (1978). In *Current Studies on Hypothalamic Function, 1978. Vol. 2, Metabolism and Behavior*, K. Lederis and W. L. Veale (Eds.). Karger, Basel.

Verney, E. B. (1947). The antidiuretic hormone and the factors which determine its release. *Proc. Roy. Soc. Lond. (Biol.) 135*: 25-106.

Warren, A. (1956). Structural alterations in the nervous system. *J. Chron. Dis. 3*: 575-596.

Watkins, W. B., and Choy, V. J. (1980). The impact of aging on neuronal morphology in the rat hypothalamo-neurohypophysial system: an immunohistochemical study. *Peptides 1 (Suppl. 1)*: 239-245.

Wilkinson, A., and Davies, I. (1981). The influence of age on the hypothalamo-
    neurohypophyseal system of the mouse: a quantitative ultrastructural anal-
    ysis of the posterior pituitary. *Mech. Ageing Dev. 15*: 129-139.
Woods, J. W., Bard, P., and Bleir, R. (1966). Functional capacity of the deaffer-
    ented hypothalamus: water balance and responses to osmotic stimuli in de-
    cerebrate cat and rat. *J. Neurophysiol. 29*: 751-767.

11

Lesion-Induced Axon Sprouting in the Aged Central Nervous System: A Possible Endocrine Influence

Stephen W. Scheff / *University of Kentucky Medical Center, Lexington, Kentucky*

INTRODUCTION

Not many years ago it was believed that the central nervous system was a static system, being "hard-wired" early in development and essentially unchangeable in the mature animal. Over the past decade it has been shown that neuronal circuitry can be altered in the mature central nervous system and is not a phenomenon attributed only to the peripheral nervous system. In response to certain types of neuronal damage where a particular group of target neurons are partially denervated, residual afferents can form new functional connections and replace those which were lost. This process, commonly referred to as axon sprouting or reactive synaptogenesis, appears to be very widespread and not specific to one area (Cotman, 1978). Whereas the CNS is very well protected, injury does occur and often results in a loss of function. In many cases reactive synaptogenesis appears to be one of the factors underlying a restoration of the lost function following brain damage. Neuronal loss is a normal consequence of the aging process, as well as a prominent characteristic of common disorders of the aging nervous system such as stroke, tumors, and senile dementia. In view of this incidence of cell loss in the aged CNS, it is important to determine the capacity of the aged brain to support reactive synaptogenesis and to find ways to increase the probability that the most appropriate connections are made.

In order to gain new insights into the factor of aging on sprouting in the central nervous system, it was necessary to study a simple brain area. The hippocampus lends itself as a model system for such studies because its structure is relatively simple for a cortical area (Fig. 1). Anatomically, it is composed of only two major parts with the afferent fibers terminating in precise laminae. Additionally, both the afferent and efferent projections to the hippocampus have been well defined by a number of investigators (Ramon y Cajal, 1911; Lorente de No, 1934; Blackstad, 1956; Hjorth-Simonsen, 1972; Zimmer, 1971; Gottlieb and Cowan, 1972; Swanson et al., 1978). Finally, the hippocampus is easily accessible to experimental manipulation.

Within the hippocampal formation of the rat lies the dentate gyrus, an area composed primarily of granule cells. In this chapter I will report on experiments concerned with axon sprouting in the dentate gyrus of young mature and aged animals. First, it is necessary to briefly describe some of the organization of this brain structure. The dentate gyrus consists of one major cell type, granule cells, with dendrites arborizing in a zone called the molecular layer. The few afferent fibers to this area have a precise laminar arrangement when terminating upon the apical dendrites of the granule cells. The inner one-fourth of the molecular layer is termed the commissural-associational (C-A) zone. This area receives commissural fibers arising from the CA3-CA4 pyramidal cells of the contralateral hippocampus by way of the hippocampal commissure. This same inner terminal field also receives fibers arising from the ipsilateral CA3-CA4 pyramidal cells which make up an

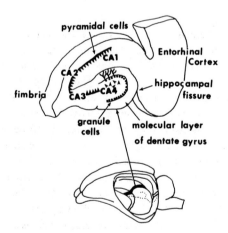

Figure 1 Schematic diagram showing the location of the hippocampal formation and a hippocampal chip. The hippocampal formation consists of the hippocampus proper, where the pyramidal cells are the major cell type, and the dentate gyrus, where the granule cells are the major cell population. Granule cell dendrites ramify in the molecular layer.

intrahippocampal associational system (Blackstad, 1956; Zimmer, 1971; Gottlieb and Cowan, 1972; Hjorth-Simonsen and Laurberg, 1977; Swanson and Cowan, 1977; Swanson et al., 1978). The outer three-quarters of the granule cell dendritic tree is innervated by a massive projection from the entorhinal cortex (Blackstad, 1958; Raisman et al., 1965; Hjorth-Simonsen and Jeune, 1972; Matthews et al., 1976) and a sparser input from the septum (Meibach and Siegel, 1977; Lewis and Shute, 1967; Mosko et al., 1973; Swanson and Cowan, 1977). In addition, this same terminal field receives a very minor input from brain-stem nuclei such as locus ceruleus and midbrain raphe nuclei (Segal and Landis, 1974). A prominent feature of this afferent lamination is the absence of overlap between the entorhinal input and the commissural-associational input (Fig. 2). This lamination pattern represents one of the most striking examples of synaptic specificity in the mature nervous system. The entorhinal, commissural, associational, and septal afferent inputs to the dentate gyrus account for the vast majority of the synapses in this area.

One common experimental procedure to study reactive synaptogenesis in the dentate gyrus is to unilaterally remove the entorhinal cortex and, over time, examine the denervated area of the dentate gyrus ipsilateral to the lesion. This preparation has one extraordinary advantage: because of the unique circuitry of the hippocampal formation, each animal can serve as its own control since the projection of the entorhinal cortex is almost entirely unilateral (Goldowitz et al., 1975; Hjorth-Simonsen and Zimmer, 1975).

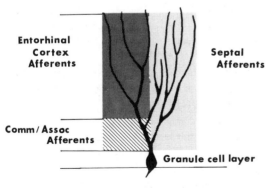

Figure 2   Diagram of four of the major afferents to the dentate granule cells. The inputs are strictly ordered on the dendrites with the entorhinal and septal afferents occupying the outer three-quarters of the molecular layer, and the commissural and associational afferents terminating on the inner one-quarter. There is very little overlap between the entorhinal afferents and the commissural and associational afferents.

REACTIVE SYNAPTOGENESIS FOLLOWING PARTIAL DENERVATION

Fiber Growth in Young-Adult Animals

In young-adult rats a unilateral lesion of the entorhinal cortex removes approximately 85% of the terminals from the distal three-fourths of the granule cell dendrites ipsilateral to the lesion (Matthews et al., 1976). This loss takes only a few days, but requires weeks before the neuropil begins to approach the same synaptic density as observed preoperatively. Reactive synaptogenesis is responsible for restoring the denervated zone to near-normal levels. With the light microscope it is possible to examine some of the afferent systems responsible for the reinnervation. The initial response one observes with this type of lesion is the appearance of hypertrophied astrocytes and the proliferation of microglia throughout the denervated area in the dentate gyrus. In addition, there appear numerous degenerating terminals in the area normally innervated by the entorhinal afferents. Electron microscopic examination of the outer three-fourths of the molecular layer ipsilateral to the lesion demonstrates a marked reduction in the density of intact synapses to a level which is only 12-14% of those normally present in this brain area. Accompanying this reduction in synapses is an increase in degenerative debris and dying terminals. This loss of synaptic input, to the dendrites of the granule cells following removal of the entorhinal cortex, is transient and is followed by the growth and formation of new connections. Over time, the number of normal-appearing synaptic contacts in this region of the molecular layer is restored to approximately 85% of preoperative levels. The new synapses originate primarily from (1) septal afferents, (2) afferents of the contralateral entorhinal cortex, and (3) commissural-associational pyramidal cells which normally project primarily to the inner one-fourth of the granule cell dendrites (Cotman and Lynch, 1976; Cotman and Nadler, 1978). The reaction of the commissural and associational afferents is perhaps the best documented case of reactive synaptogenesis in the central nervous system.

In response to the entorhinal lesion (Fig. 3), the commissural and associational fibers expand outward along the dendritic tree of the granule cell so as to increase their original territory by as much as 30-40% (Lynch et al., 1976, 1977; Scheff et al., 1977, 1978b). This expanded C-A fiber zone in the operated animals continues to form a very discrete lamina as in the normal preoperative animals. The cholinergic projection from the septal nuclei and the projection from the contralateral entorhinal cortex proliferate entirely in the denervated area and withdraw from the area of expansion now occupied by the commissural and associational fibers (Cotman and Nadler, 1978; Nadler et al., 1977; Storm-Mathisen, 1974). The C-A fibers establish a new boundary which is further up on the dendritic tree, actually invading part of the former zone of the ipsilateral entorhinal input. As a result of the postlesion reorganization, a new laminar distribution is created on the apical dendrite of the granule cell. It is important to note here that not all afferents to the granule cell dendritic tree respond after this type of lesion. The monoaminergic

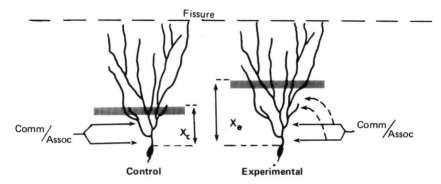

Figure 3 Schematic drawing of the method used to determine outward expansion of the commissural-associational (C-A) fiber plexus. Camera lucida drawings are made of the area of termination of the C-A afferents. The projection of these afferents contralateral to the entorhinal lesion respresents the normal or preoperative width of the afferent zone (X_c). Ipsilateral to the entorhinal ablation, the C-A zone expands outward (X_e) towards the hippocampal fissure. The growth of this fiber plexus is expressed as a percent increase in width of the denervated side over the contralateral or control side. Shrinkage of the outer portion of the molecular layer following the entorhinal ablation is not a factor since only the absolute width of the C-A projection is measured.

fibers from the locus ceruleus do not increase in abundance following an entorhinal lesion (Cotman and Nadler, 1978).

The commissural-associational system is ideally suited for studies designed to test factors, such as aging, which might affect the rate and magnitude of the sprouting response. The C-A fiber growth proceeds at a specific rate and the magnitude of growth is quantifiable. Many techniques have been utilized to study C-A outgrowth, and they provide substantial documentation for sprouting of the system following a lesion of the entorhinal cortex (Lynch et al., 1973, 1977; Goldowitz and Cotman, 1980; West et al., 1979; Scheff et al., 1977, 1978b; Lee et al., 1977). Moreover, this anatomical response is accompanied by an altered physiological response. Neurophysiological studies demonstrate that the commissural and associational systems have not only sprouted but have formed new synapses that are functional (West et al., 1975).

Reactive Fiber Growth in Aged Animals

A series of studies was undertaken to determine the affect of age on reactive fiber growth in the hippocampus (Scheff et al., 1980b). All of the aged animals reported in these studies were 24 to 27-month-old Sprague-Dawley rats acquired from the National Institute of Aging, and they were compared with 3 to 4-month-old animals of the same strain.

Prior to experimental removal of the entorhinal cortex, a group of animals was examined to determine whether or not any anatomical differences occurred as a result of the aging process. In both age groups all the major cytoarchitectonic fields of the hippocampus could be readily identified. Whereas no detailed cell count was made of the pyramidal and granule cell layers, it was determined that all areas appeared to have a full complement of cells. In addition, small cell bodies, which were lightly stained, were numerous and uniformily scattered throughout the molecular layer of the dentate gyrus. Some coronal brain sections were stained for the enzyme acetylcholinesterase (AChE). The distribution of AChE activity was identical between the two age groups, and suggests that the density of cholinergic septohippocampal afferents was equivalent.

Tissue prepared with the Holmes fiber method demonstrated a rich fiber plexus in the molecular layer. There appeared to be no discontinuities in this brain region of aged vs. young-adult animals. No evidence of neurofibrillary tangles or argyrophyllic senile plaques were detected. Thus, the commissural and associational and the entorhinal afferents to the dentate gyrus appeared equivalent for the two age groups. In contrast to the above similarities, the aged animals were found to have more astrocytes in the molecular layer of the dentate gyrus (Table 1). The older animals had astrocytes which were dramatically hypertrophied throughout the molecular layer in agreement with Landfield et al. (1977). Finally, catecholaminergic innervation to the dentate gyrus was examined using a modification of the glyoxalic acid histofluorescence method. Whereas there did not appear to be any reduction in the overall pattern of catecholaminergic fibers or the intensity of fluorescence, the aged animals did manifest an abundance of yellow-brown autofluorescent material throughout the hippocampus and septal area. This material was intracellular, appearing as fine granules, and may be related to pigments known to accumulate with age. Electron microscopic analysis of the dentate gyrus also failed to reveal any major differences between the two age groups. Qualitatively, the neuropil ultrastructure agreed with previous descriptions given by others in younger animals (Matthews et al., 1976; Laatsch and Cowan, 1966). Quantitatively the aged animals have slightly fewer synapses in the molecular layer of the dentate gyrus, but this difference was not significant between the two age groups. This finding disagrees with that of Geinisman and Bondareff (1976) who report a 27% decrease in synapses in the dentate gyrus. This difference between the two studies might possibly be explained by different species of animals used and sampling techniques. Whereas there does appear to be a minor age-dependent loss of synapses in aged rats, the distribution of the loss varies between rat strains. In summary, there appear to be no dramatic age-dependent alterations in the hippocampal dentate gyrus.

In order to study the capacity of the aged brain to support reactive synaptogenesis, the entorhinal cortex was unilaterally removed in a procedure identical to that employed for the younger animals. At various times following this removal,

Table 1 Number of Astrocytes in the Outer Molecular Layer of the Dentate Gyrus in Unoperated Animals at 3 Months of Age and 25-27 Months of Age[a]

Age	3 Months old	25-27 Months old
	68	78
	56	92
	52	90
	61	108
	63	87
	50	89
	53	
	50	
	62	
X	57.22	90.6
S.D.	6.49	9.79
n	9	6

[a]Each number represents the mean value for a single animal at that age. Counts were made from coronal sections using a standard grid. Values for each subject are means obtained from six sections per animal.
Source: Modified from Scheff et al., 1980b.

animals were examined using both light and electron microscopic techniques. First, brains were examined, using a modified Fink-Heimer stain, 2 days following the entorhinal lesion. The pattern of degeneration products in aged animals was identical to that found in younger animals (Fig. 4). Next, brains were stained for the enzyme AChE to assess reactive growth of the septohippocampal afferents. The AChE pattern in young-adult animals 12 days postlesion is characterized by a wide dark band of staining in the outer half of the molecular layer of the dentate gyrus as previously reported (Cotman et al., 1973; Lynch et al., 1972; Nadler et al., 1977). The reactive pattern found in the aged animals appeared qualitatively different from that of the younger animals. Whereas the aged animals still featured the darker band in the outer portion of the molecular layer, it was not as intense as that observed in the younger animals. These results cannot be explained on the basis of differences in shrinkage of the molecular layer between the two age groups. Measurements failed to reveal a significant difference in width of the molecular layer following the entorhinal lesion.

Brain sections were also stained with the Holmes method to reveal changes in the commissural and associational fibers. Camera lucida drawings were made of at least six sections from each brain of both experimental and control sides. The removal of the entorhinal cortex resulted in a 21.7% increase in the width of the

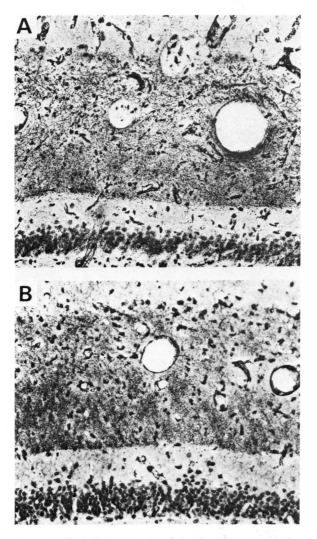

Figure 4 Fink-Heimer stain of the dentate gyrus molecular layer 2 days following ablation of the entorhinal cortex ipsilaterally. The top photograph (a) was taken from a 27-month-old rat, and the bottom picture (b) was taken from a 2-month-old animal. Note the similarity in the pattern of degenerative debris. (From Scheff et al., 1980b.)

commissural-associational fiber plexus in the younger animals. The outgrowth in the older animals was significantly reduced, showing only a 13.4% increase (Fig. 5). It is interesting to note that considerable variation occurred in the aged animal group. In some animals the response was nearly identical to that of the younger rats, whereas other aged animals demonstrated practically no outgrowth of the fiber plexus. This variability was not correlated with any obvious abnormal feature of the dentate gyrus anatomy or to the size and location of the entorhinal lesion.

Electron microscopic examination of the dentate gyrus at various intervals following the lesion revealed a major difference between the two age groups in the reinnervation process (Hoff et al., 1981a). In the younger animals a significant repopulation of lost synaptic contacts occurs within 10 days following the damage. As shown in Fig. 6, the aged animals do not show an equivalent reaction within the same time course. By 10 days after the damage, the aged brains show very little synapse replacement. By 60 days after the damage, the aged animals do demonstrate considerable reinnervation, but still are significantly behind the younger animals. The aged animals continue to lag behind the younger ones throughout the reinnervation process. Eventually, however, the older group does achieve preoperative levels of synaptic density. In light of the fact that the preoperative synaptic densities in the two age groups are not significantly different, the apparent decrease in rate of replacement cannot be explained by preoperative differences in density. Finally, the reinnervated neuropil of the aged rats did not appear qualitatively different from preoperative controls.

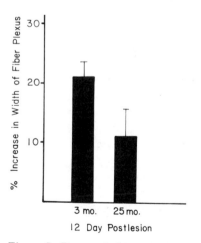

Figure 5 Bar graph demonstrating the percentage in outgrowth of the commissural-associational fiber plexus for aged and young-adult rats. Note the significant reduction in outgrowth for the older animals, indicating a reduction in reactive growth capacity. (From Cotman and Scheff, 1979.)

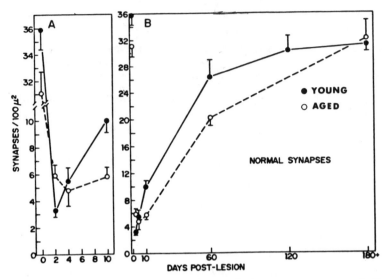

Figure 6   Graph showing the time course of synapse reappearance in the outer molecular layer of the dentate gyrus following an ipsilateral entorhinal lesion. Note that the aged animals (open dots) always lag behind the younger animals (closed dots) during the reinnervation process. (From Hoff et al., 1981a.)

MECHANISM FOR REDUCED REACTIVE GROWTH

The reduction in the capacity of the aged brain to support reactive growth might be due to a number of factors: (a) inability of target cells to accept new synaptic contacts, (b) the loss of growth capacity of afferents which form the new contacts, or (c) a significant change in the neuropil environment creating a situation which is not complimentary to the reactive growth process. This change may be due to the lack of some growth-promoting substance or the lack of inhibition of a growth retardant. Whatever the mechanism may be, it appears to affect a large variety of neuronal types within the hippocampal formation. Whereas there is no single answer to the question of what factor or factors are responsible for the reduction in the growth capacity, some clues have been gained with hormone studies. Endocrine studies have attempted to create in part a physiological condition somewhat equivalent to that of the aged animal.

It has been recently shown that circulating levels of glucocorticoids in aged animals are considerably elevated as compared with young-adult animals (Landfield et al., 1978; Riegle and Hess, 1972; Tang and Phillips, 1978). Since the hippocampal formation and, in particular, the dentate gyrus has specific receptor sites for corticosterone (Stumpf, 1971; McEwen et al., 1969; Pfaff et al., 1976), it was hypothesized that elevated corticosterone might affect the growth response. This may help to explain in part some of the age-related changes observed in the hippocampus.

In a recent series of experiments (Scheff et al., 1980a) the effect of glucocorticoids on axon sprouting in the hippocampus was investigated. Cortisol (hydrocortisone) 5 mg/kg was administered subcutaneously to a group of young-adult (3 month old) rats. The animals were pretreated 6 days before and for 6 or 15 days after removal of the entorhinal cortex. A second group of animals served as controls and received the vehicle and removal of the entorhinal cortex. A third group was treated with the hormone but was given no lesion. The brains were then examined for changes in morphology indicating a change in reactive synaptogenesis. Animals treated with cortisol and killed 6 days after the surgery demonstrated no significant change in the septohippocampal pathway as determined by AChE staining. By 15 days postlesion, the cortisol-treated animals did show a significant change in AChE staining and were determined to be equivalent to control animals with equivalent survival time. This change in the staining pattern indicated that, whereas sprouting of the septohippocampal afferents does occur in cortisol-treated animals, it does so at a slower rate than the sprouting response observed in control animals.

In addition to the septohippocampal afferents, the normally robust response of the commissural-associational system was also markedly influenced by the addition of cortisol treatment. In young-adult animals without hormone treatment, a lesion of the entorhinal cortex normally elicits a 17 and 22% outgrowth of the C-A fiber plexus at postoperative days 6 and 15, respectively. Animals treated with hormone consistently showed a significant decrease in the outgrowth of the C-A fiber plexus at both survival times. The cortisol treatment resulted in a maximum outgrowth of only 13.5% (Fig. 7). These results demonstrate that exogenous

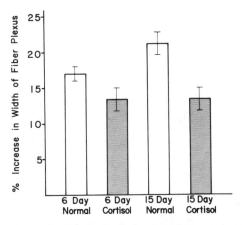

Figure 7   Bar graph showing the reduction in outgrowth of the commissural-associational fiber plexus as a result of treatment with hydrocortisone (Cortisol). Normal animals were treated with saline. Both normal and cortisol-treated animals were given unilateral lesions of the entorhinal cortex. (From Scheff et al., 1980a.)

glucocorticoids can influence lesion-induced axon sprouting in the hippocampus. If one compares the results of sprouting in young-adult (3 month old) rats given steroid treatment with the response observed in aged (24-27 month old) animals, there is a striking similarity in the reduction of the reactive growth response (Fig. 8).

Examination of coronal sections through the hippocampus from animals treated only with cortisol and given no lesion revealed a very unusual astrocytic response. The astrocytes appeared hypertrophied despite the fact that no lesion was performed in these animals. The astrocytic processes were thickened and cell bodies irregular in shape. The effect was observed not only in the dentate gyrus but throughout the hippocampal formation. Normally, astrocytes are known to exhibit such hypertrophy only in response to brain injury. Electron microscopic analysis has failed to show any massive degeneration process as a result of the hormone treatment which might elicit such an astrocyte response. It is important to note that these cortisol-treated animals showed the morphological change of astrocytes identical to those described in aged animals.

The previous experiments demonstrated that the sprouting reaction in the dentate gyrus could be altered with a steroid which is not physiological to the rat. Scheff et al. (1982) tested whether or not chronic changes in a physiological glucocorticoid, corticosterone, might also alter axon sprouting. Young-adult rats were adrenalectomized and administered steroid therapy in the form of pellets containing different concentrations of corticosterone (CORT). The CORT pellets, in conjunction with adrenalectomies, allowed a precise regulation of the circulating levels of corticosterone. The serum concentration of CORT was maintained at one of four different levels: 3.5 μg/100 ml, 14.0 μg/100 ml, 28.0 μg/100 ml, and

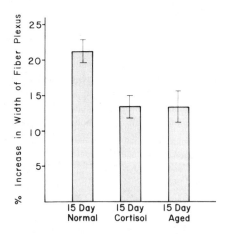

Figure 8 Bar graph comparing the outgrowth of the commissural-associational fiber plexus following a unilateral entorhinal lesion in 3-month-old rats with and without cortisol treatment and in 25-month-old untreated rats.

less than 0.1 μg/100 ml. This last group was given cholesterol pellets in place of CORT pellets. In addition, a control group which received a sham adrenalectomy and no steroid treatment was included. Five days following implantation of the pellets, the animals were subjected to a unilateral removal of the entorhinal cortex. Following a 15-day survival time, the animals were killed and the brains analyzed for changes in brain morphology. A detailed, quantitative analysis of the reactive outgrowth of the C-A fiber plexus was performed. Blood samples were collected for verification of serum CORT levels with a radioimmunoassay.

The different levels of CORT had a significant influence on the outgrowth of the C-A fiber plexus when compared with animals given a sham adrenalectomy and a unilateral lesion of the entorhinal cortex (Fig. 9). First, adrenalectomized animals given cholesterol in place of CORT (< 0.1-μg/100-ml group) did not differ from the control animals. The group which was maintained at 14-μg CORT/100-ml serum also did not differ from either of these two control groups. However, the 28-μg CORT animals did show a significant reduction in the C-A sprouting response when compared with the other experimental animals. This finding supports the results previously obtained with the administration of hydrocortisone. Finally, animals maintained at 3.5 μg CORT also showed a reduction in the outgrowth of the C-A fiber plexus. This reduction in the growth response observed in the 3.5-μg animals might possibly be due to a unique interaction with the levels of adrenocorticotropic hormone (ACTH) and this particular circulating level of CORT.

This study confirmed the previous results demonstrating that animals with increased levels of glucocorticoids consistently show a significant decrease in out-

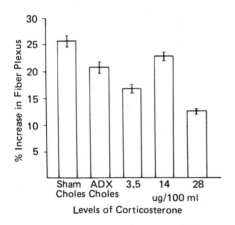

Figure 9 Bar graph showing changes in the commissural-associational fiber plexus 15 days after unilateral removal of the entorhinal cortex in young adrenalectomized (ADX) animals. Corticosterone level is expressed in μg corticosterone/ 100 ml serum. Animals maintained at extremely high levels of corticosterone show a significant reduction in fiber outgrowth. (From Scheff and Cotman, 1982.)

growth of C-A fibers. Coupled with the depressed sprouting response was a morphological change in the astrocytes. This included an increase in astrocyte cell number within the dentate gyrus molecular layer as well as an apparent hypertrophy of astrocytes. This change in morphology is particularly interesting since it can be obtained from animals which received only the steroid therapy and no lesion. This astrocyte condition is found normally in aged animals which have elevated corticosterone levels. In summary, the steroid hormones appear to exert some control over axon sprouting in the hippocampus. The reduction observed in young animals treated with steroids correlates very closely with that found in aged animals. The hippocampus, however, may be the only area of the CNS which is affected by this steroid treatment. It was necessary then to test the generality of these previous findings.

In order to test the generality of not only the steroid treatment but also the factor of aging on reactive growth, the reactions of central catecholaminergic fibers in the septum and the anomalous growth of sympathetic fibers were examined. The septum was used because the sprouting response in this area is quite robust and analysis is simple.

The septal nuclei receive two main inputs. One input arises from the hippocampus and projects to the septum via the fimbria fornix. The other afferent projection courses by way of the medial forebrain bundle and carries catecholaminergic fibers arising from the locus ceruleus and brain-stem nuclei (Moore and Bloom, 1979). If the fimbria fornix is cut unilaterally, the septum is partially deprived of its hippocampal afferents. Following this lesion there is a marked change in the distribution of the adrenergic innervation to the septum ipsilateral to the lesion (Moore et al., 1971; Scheff et al., 1978a; Reis et al., 1978). This growth response also has a specific time course. The first detectable change occurs at about 15 days postlesion, increasing by about 30 days postlesion, and persisting through at least 100 days (Moore et al., 1974). The response is of considerable magnitude and easily followed by histofluorescence methods.

In these same animals it is also possible to examine the reaction of peripheral catecholaminergic fibers in the brain. Recently, Loy and Moore (1977) and Stenevi and Bjorklund (1978) reported that catecholaminergic fibers originating from the superior cervical ganglion grow into certain denervated zones of the dentate gyrus when the fimbria fornix is damaged. This response has since been replicated (Loy et al., 1980; Scheff et al., 1978a; Crutcher et al., 1979). Very coarse and intensely fluorescent catecholaminergic fibers innervate the inner molecular layer and hilar region of the dentate gyrus. This very unusual growth of the sympathetic system follows a very defined time course. Within the first 2 weeks, sympathetic innervation can be observed in the medial portions of the hippocampal formation, and as time progresses, the anomalous catecholaminergic innervation can be found more laterally as far as the CA3 area of the hippocampal pyramidal cells.

Both young-adult and aged (24-27 month old) rats demonstrated equivalent fluorescence in the lateral portions of the septum along the border of the lateral ventricle (Scheff et al., 1978a). The only difference preoperatively between the two groups was the presence of a yellow-brown autofluorescent material found throughout the CNS of the aged animals. By 30 days after the frimbria transection in the younger animals, the catecholaminergic (CA) fibers had proliferated in the denervated septal area in agreement with previous reports. The same operation performed on the older animals elicited a qualitatively similar response in the lateral septal area, but a response which was quantitatively less pronounced. These results indicated that the CA fibers still have the capacity to grow in the aged brain but to a reduced degree. Next, the reaction of the sympathetic neurons was investigated. In the young-adult animals, coarse and intensely fluorescent CA fibers characteristic of sympathetic origin innervated the dentate gyrus molecular layer and the hilar region. In the aged brains only one animal was observed to have this anomalous growth response and that animal showed only a few fibers innervating the most medial tip of the dentate gyrus. In all of the other aged animals this anomalous sympathetic innervation was absent. The results of these experiments involving the sympathetic innervation of the dentate gyrus and reactive growth in the septum indicate that the reduction in plasticity found with age also affects the peripheral nervous system and can be found in more than one area of the central nervous system.

In order to test whether or not steroids could affect this CA sprouting, young-adult animals were adrenalectomized and maintained at either 14-μg CORT/100-ml serum or 28-μg CORT/100-ml serum as in the previous experiments. Additional animals were sham-adrenalectomized and given cholesterol pellets. All of the animals were then subjected to a transection of the fimbria. After a postoperative period of 30 days, the brains were analyzed for changes in CA innervation.

In all the animals maintained at the high (28 μg CORT) levels, there was a significant reduction in sprouting of the anomalous CA innervation. The 28-μg rats showed two very significant changes as compared with the control animals. First, the extent of growth was significantly reduced. In many cases, it mimicked the extent found in the aged animals (Fig. 10). Second, the fibers were much finer in appearance than those found in the two other groups. Animals maintained at 14 μg CORT showed the anomalous growth which was equivalent in extent to that of the control animals, but the fibers appeared thinner and not as coarse as previously observed. These results then demonstrate that the glucocorticoids can also affect sprouting in systems other than the central nervous system.

CONCLUSION

The above findings show a number of important features about the aged central nervous system and imply that hormonal factors may play an integral part in synaptic remodeling. Whereas the overall pattern of connections between the two age groups was determined not to be significantly different, there does appear to be a difference in their functional capacity. The two groups respond quite differently

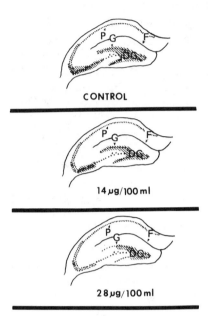

CONTROL

14 μg/100 ml

28 μg/100 ml

Figure 10 Schematic diagram of the hippocampal formation showing area of innervation (dashed lines) by sympathetic fibers following a fimbria-fornix lesion. Control animals received only a sham adrenalectomy. In the control animals the shaded area encompasses most of the dentate gyrus (DG) and part of the pyramidal cells (P) in area CA3. The 14 μg/100 ml and 28 μg/100 ml indicate animals maintained at that serum concentration of circulating corticosterone. Whereas these animals show some growth, it is not to the same extent as that observed in the control animals. (F) indicates the hippocampal fissure.

to damage. In the young-adult animals residual afferents in the denervated zone quickly replace lost synaptic contacts. Replacement in aged animals progresses at a much slower rate, and in the case of an anomalous growth pattern, it may not occur at all.

It is not surprising that aged animals do not show a significant loss of synapses preoperatively, since the present rate of replacement of lost contacts is adequate to replace those which would be lost during the aging process or as a consequence of natural synaptic turnover as proposed by Cotman et al. (1981) and Hoff et al. (1981b). It is interesting to note that, whereas the rate of replacement was slower for the aged animals, they were able to restore the neuropil following massive damage. Whereas the reasons for the diminished rate of plasticity are not known, the recent work with hormones appears to be providing some clues.

This ability to quickly replace lost synaptic contacts may be particularly important if such growth underlies some type of restitution of function following damage. Based upon the present findings, one would predict that a significantly longer convalescence would be required by the aged animals and perhaps those animals treated with hormones, if one was to actualize complete recovery. However, in some cases, the neural damage leads to truly anomalous growth such as that reported by Goldowitz and Cotman (1978) or that previously mentioned with the superior cervical ganglion. In such cases this elicited growth may interfere with normal function and, hence, reactive synaptogenesis would be detrimental. In such cases the aged animals and those animals treated with high levels of steroids would be at an advantage in retarding the formation of new contacts.

Glucocorticoids are of tremendous clinical value in the reduction and prevention of cerebral edema following brain damage. However, the exact mechanism for this is not known. One possible mechanism would be through a membrane stabilization or by a suppressive response on fibroblast, one aspect of the inflammatory response (Gray et al., 1971). Steroids could influence the sprouting response through a membrane stabilization by preventing the extension of filopodia and the formation of sprouts in search of new contacts. Unsicker et al. (1978) demonstrated that glucocorticoids impair the outgrowth of processes in tissue-cultured sympathetic neurons and adrenal chromaffin cells. Alternatively, steroids may alter reactive growth indirectly through their affect on astrocytes. Whereas the role of astrocytes in the sprouting response is not completely understood, it is believed that they can participate in the regulation of neuron growth and influence the synthesis of neurotransmitters. Steroids have been shown to have marked affects on astrocytes.

Whatever the mechanisms are which regulate synaptogenesis in the aged animal, they appear to allow at least some compensation following damage. The similarities in experimental results from both aged animals and young-adult animals treated with high levels of steroids suggest that (1) the endocrine system may play a very important role in the functional properties of the aged brain and (2) steroid hormones may be a means to regulate reactive synaptogenesis.

REFERENCES

Blackstad, T. W. (1956). Commissural connections of the hippocampal region in the rat with special reference to their mode of termination. *J. Comp. Neurol.* *105*: 417-537.

Blackstad, T. W. (1958). On the termination of some afferents to the hippocampus and fascia dentata: An experimental study in the rat. *Acta Anat. Basel 35*: 202-214.

Cotman, C. (1978). *Neuronal Plasticity*. Raven Press, New York.

Cotman, C. W., and Lynch, G. S. (1976). In *Neuronal Recognition*. S. Barondes (ed.). Plenum, New York.

Cotman, C. W., and Nadler, J. V. (1978). Reactive synaptogenesis in the hippocampus. In *Neuronal Plasticity*, C. W. Cotman (Ed.). Raven Press, New York, pp. 227-271.

Cotman, C. W., and Scheff, S. W. (1979). Compensatory synapse growth in aged animals after neuronal death. In *Mechanisms of Aging and Development*, B. L. Strehler (Ed.). Elsevier Seqoia S.A., Lausanne, pp. 103-117.

Cotman, C. W., Matthews, D. W., Taylor, D., and Lynch, G. (1973). Synpatic rearrangement in the dentate gyrus: histochemical evidence of adjustments after lesions in immature and adult rats. *Proc. Natl. Acad. Sci. USA 70*: 3473-3477.

Cotman, C. W., Nieto-Sampedro, M., and Harris, E. W. (1981). Synapse replacement in the adult nervous system of vertebrates. *Physiol. Rev. 6*: 684-784.

Crutcher, K. A., Brothers, L., and Davis, J. N. (1979). Sprouting of sympathetic nerves in the absence of afferent input. *Exp. Neurol. 66*: 778-783.

Geinisman, Y., and Bondareff, W. (1976). Decrease in the number of synapses in the senescent brain: A quantitative electron microscopic analysis of the dentate gyrus molecular layer in the rat. *Mech. Aging Dev. 5*: 11-23.

Goldowitz, D., and Cotman, C. W. (1978). Induction of extensive fimbrial branching in the adult rat brain. *Nature 275*: 64-67.

Goldowitz, D., and Cotman, C. W. (1980). Do neurotrophic interactions control synapse formation in the adult rat brain? *Brain Res. 181*: 325-344.

Goldowitz, D., White, W., Steward, O., Cotman, C. W., and Lynch, G. (1975). Anatomical evidence for a projection from the entorhinal cortex to the contralateral dentate gyrus of the rat. *Exp. Neurol. 47*: 433-441.

Gottlieb, D., and Cowan, W. (1972). Evidence for a temporal factor in the occupation of available synaptic sites during development of the dentate gyrus. *Brain Res. 41*: 452-456.

Gray, J. B., Pratt, W. B., and Aronow, L. (1971). Effects of glucocorticoids on hexose uptake by mouse fibroblasts in vitro. *Biochemistry 10*: 277-284.

Hjorth-Simonsen, A. (1972). Projection of the lateral part of the entorhinal area to the hippocampus and fascia dentate. *J. Comp. Neurol. 146*: 219-231.

Hjorth-Simonsen, A., and Jeune, B. (1972). Origin and termination of the hippocampal perforant path in the rat studied by silver impregnation. *J. Comp. Neurol. 144*: 215-232.

Hjorth-Simonsen, A., and Laurberg, S. (1977). Commissural connections of the dentate area in the rat. *J. Comp. Neurol. 174*: 591-606.

Hjorth-Simonsen, A., and Zimmer, J. (1975). Crossed pathways from the entorhinal area to the fascia dentate. I. Normal in rabbits. *J. Comp. Neurol. 161*: 57-70.

Hoff, S. F., Scheff, S. W., Benardo, L. S., and Cotman, C. W. (1981). Lesion-induced synaptogenesis in the dentate gyrus of aged rats: I. Loss and reacquisition of normal synaptic density. *J. Comp. Neurol. 205*: 246-252.

Hoff, S. F., Scheff, S. W., Kwan, A., and Cotman, C. W. (1981). A new type of lesion-induced synaptogenesis: I. synaptic turnover in non-denervates zones of the dentate gyrus in young adult rats. *Brain Res. 222*: 1-13.

Laatsch, R. H., and Cowan, W. M. (1966). Electron microscopic studies of the dentate gyrus of the rat. I. Normal structure with special reference to synaptic organization. *J. Comp. Neurol. 128*: 359-396.

Landfield, P. W., Rose, G., Sandles, L., Wohlstadter, T., and Lynch, G. (1977). Patterns of astroglial hypertrophy and neuronal degeneration in the hippocampus of aged memory-deficient rats. *J. Gerontol. 32*: 3-12.

Landfield, P. W., Waymire, J. C., and Lynch, G. (1978). Hippocampal aging and adrenocorticoids: Quantitative correlations. *Science 202*: 1098-1102.

Lee, K., Stanford, E., Cotman, C. W., and Lynch, G. S. (1977). Ultrastructural evidence for bouton sprouting in the adult mammalian brain. *Exp. Brain Res. 29*: 475-485.

Lewis, P. R., and Shute, C. S. D. (1967). The cholinergic limb system: Projection to hippocampal formation, medial cortex, nuclei of the ascending reticular system, and the subfornical organ and supraoptic crest. *Brain 90*: 521-540.

Lorente de No, R. (1934). Studies on the structure of the cerebral cortex. II. Continuation of the study of the ammonic system. *J. Psych. Neurol. 46*: 113-177.

Loy, R., and Moore, R. Y. (1977). Anomalous innervation of the hippocampal formation by peripheral sympathetic axons following mechanical injury. *Exp. Neurol. 57*: 645-651.

Loy, R., Milner, T. A., and Moore, R. Y. (1980). Sprouting of sympathetic axons in the hippocampal formation: Conditions necessary to elicit ingrowth. *Exp. Neurol. 67*: 399-411.

Lynch, G., Gall, C., and Cotman, C. W. (1977). Temporal parameters of axon "sprouting" in the brain of the adult rat. *Exp. Neurol. 54*: 179-183.

Lynch, G., Gall, C., Rose, G., and Cotman, C. W. (1976). Changes in the distribution of the dentate gyrus associational system following unilateral or bilateral entorhinal lesion in the adult rat. *Brain Res. 11*: 57-71.

Lynch, G. S., Matthews, D. A., Mosko, S., Parks, T., and Cotman, C. W. (1972). Induced acetylcholineserase-rich layer in the rat dentate gyrus following entorhinal lesions. *Brain Res. 42*: 311-318.

Lynch, G. S., Mosko, S., Parks, T., and Cotman, C. W. (1973). Relocation and hyperdevelopment of the dentate gyrus commissural system after entorhinal lesions in immature rats. *Brain Res. 50*: 174-178.

Matthews, D. A., Cotman, C. W., and Lynch, G. (1976). An electron microscopic study of lesion induced synaptogenesis in the dentate gyrus of the adult rat. I. Magnitude and time course of degeneration. *Brain Res. 115*: 1-21.

McEwen, B. S., Weiss, J. M., and Schwartz, L. S. (1969). Uptake of corticosterone by rat brain and its concentration by certain limbic structures. *Brain Res. 16*: 227-241.

Meibach, R. C., and Siegel, A. (1977). Efferent connections of the septal area in the rat: An analysis utilizing retrograde transport methods. *Brain Res. 1*: 1-20.

Moore, R. Y., and Bloom, F. F. (1979). Central catecholamine neuron systems: Anatomy abd physiology of the norepinephrine and epinephrine systems. *Ann. Rev. Neurosci. 2*: 113-168.

Moore, R. Y., Bjorklund, A., and Stenevi, U. (1971). Plastic changes in the adrenergic innervation of the rat septal area in response to denervation. *Brain Res. 33*: 13-35.

Moore, R. Y., Bjorklund, A., and Stenevi, U. (1974). Growth and Plasticity of adrenergic neurons. In *The Neurosciences: Third Study Program*, F. O. Schmidt and F. G. Worden (Eds.). MIT Press, Cambridge, Mass.

Mosko, S., Lynch, G. S., and Cotman, C. W. (1973). Developmental differences in post-lesion axonal growth in the hippocampus. *Brain Res. 59*: 155-168.

Nadler, J. V., Paoletti, C., Cotman, C. W., and Lynch, G. (1977). Histochemical evidence of altered development of cholinergic fibers in the rat dentate gyrus following lesions. II. Effects of Partial entorhinal and simultaneous multiple lesions. *J. Comp. Neurol. 171*: 589-604.

Pfaff, D. W., Gerlach, J. L., McEwen, B. S., Ferin, M., Carmel, P., and Zimmerman, E. A. (1976). Autographic localization of hormone-concentrating cells in the brain of the female rhesus monkey. *J. Comp. Neurol. 170*: 279-294.

Raisman, G., Cowan, W. M., and Powell, T. P. S. (1965). The extrinsic afferent, commissural and associational fibers of the hippocampus. *Brain 88*: 963-966.

Ramon y Cajal, S. (1911). Histologie du systeme nervoueous de l'homme et des vertebres. A. Moline, Paris.

Reis, D. J., Ross, R. A., Gilad, G., and Joh, T. H. (1978). Reaction of central catecholaminergic neurons to injury: Model systems for studying the neurogiology of central regeneration and sprouting. In *Neuronal Plasticity*, C. W. Cotman (Ed.). Raven Press, New York, pp. 197-226.

Riegle, G. D., and Hess, G. D. (1972). Chronic and acute dexamethasone suppression of stress activation of the adrenal cortex in young and aged rats. *J. Neuroendo. 9*: 175-187.

Scheff, S. W., Benardo, L. S., and Cotman, C. W. (1977). Progressive brain damage accelerates axon sprouting in the adult rat. *Science 197*: 795-797.

Scheff, S. W., Benardo, L. S., and Cotman, C. W. (1978a). Decrease in adrenergic axon sprouting in the senescent rat. *Science 202*: 775-778.

Scheff, S. W., Benardo, L. S., and Cotman, C. W. (1978b). Effect of serial lesions on sprouting in the dentate gyrus: Onset and decline of the catalytic effect. *Brain Res. 150*: 45-53.

Scheff, S. W. Benardo, L. S., and Cotman, C. W. (1980a). Hydrocortisone administration retards axon sprouting in the rat dentate gyrus. *Exp. Neurol. 68*: 195-201.

Scheff, S. W., Benardo, L. S., and Cotman, C. W. (1980b). Decline in reactive fiber growth in the dentate gyrus of aged rats compared to young adult rats following entorhinal cortex removal. *Brain Res. 199*: 21-38.

Scheff, S. W., and Cotman, C. W. (1982). Chronic glucocorticoid therapy alters axon sprouting in the hippocampal dentate gyrus. *Exp. Neurol. 76*: 644-654.

Segal, M., and Landis, S. (1974). Afferents to the hippocampus of the rat studied with the method of retrograde transport of horseradish peroxidase. *Brain Res. 78*: 1-15.

Stenevi, U., and Bjorklund, A. (1978). A pitfall in brain lesion studies: Growth of vascular sympathetic axons into the hippocampus after fimbral lesions. *Neurosci. Lett. 7*: 219-224.

Storm-Mathisen, J. (1974). Choline acetyltransferase and acetylcholinesterase in fascia dentate following lesion of the entorhinal afferents. *Brain Res. 80*: 181-197.

Stumpf, W. E. (1971). Autoradiographic techniques and the localization of estrogen, androgen and glucocorticoids in the pituitary and brain. *Am. Zool. 11*: 725-739.

Swanson, L. W., and Cowan, W. M. (1977). An autoradiographic study of the organization of the efferent connections of the hippocampal formation in the rat. *J. Comp. Neurol. 172*: 49-84.

Swanson, L. W., Wyss, J. N., and Cowan, W. N. (1978). An autoradiographic study of the organization of intrahippocampal association pathway in the rat. *J. Comp. Neurol. 181*: 681-716.

Tang, G., and Phillips, R. (1978). Some age-related changes in pituitary-adrenal function in the male laboratory rat. *J. Gerontol. 33*: 377-382.

Unsicker, K., Krisch, B., Otten, U., and Thoenen, H. (1978). Nerve growth factor-induced fiber outgrowth from isolated rat adrenal chromaffin cells: Impairment by glucocorticoids. *Proc. Natl. Acad. Sci. USA 75*: 3498-3502.

West, J. R., Deadwyler, S. A., Cotman, C. W., and Lynch, G. S. (1975). Time-dependent changes in commissural field potentials in the dentate gyrus following lesions of the entorhinal cortex in adult rats. *Brain Res. 97*: 215-233.

Zimmer, J. (1971). Ipsilateral afferents to the commissural zone of the fascia dentate demonstrated in decommissurated rats by silver inpregnation. *J. Comp. Neurol. 142*: 393-416.

12
Rodent Models of Learning and Memory in Aging Research

Gary Thompson* / *Duke University Medical Center, Durham, North Carolina*

INTRODUCTION

Whereas there is some inconsistency in reports on the nature of the behavioral deficits seen in aging animals (which may reflect the use of dissimilar approaches), there is sufficient evidence to argue that rodent models may be quite useful for the study of behavioral change and, as such, should prove to be a useful tool for investigating the basic neural mechanisms involved in behavioral change with age, as well as various treatments aimed at intervention.

The identification of specific neurochemical changes that correlate with age-dependent alterations in behavior is of obvious importance, since it not only provides insight into our understanding of CNS aging but also contributes to the task of establishing effective remedial measures of importance in reversing or at least ameliorating some of the deficits frequently observed in aged subjects. Of special relevance to the concept of intervention are studies investigating the role that some pituitary hormones have on memory processes. These studies suggest that acquisition and/or retention of information may be modulated by these neuropeptides.

The present chapter will focus on adrenocorticotropic (ACTH) and vasopressin-related neuropeptides and the potential role of these agents on behavior in aged organisms. These substances, in addition to exerting their usual endocrine effects, have been shown to facilitate behavioral responses in a number of different

---

*Present affiliation: Sister Kenny Institute, Minneapolis, Minnesota

experimental paradigms. The independence of the behavioral from the endocrine effects of these neuropeptides has also been established. Given the similarities between some of the behavioral functions that have been shown to decline with age and the behaviors affected by neuropeptides, there is a clear need for research investigating the effects of neuropeptides on behavioral functions in old animals.

AGE-RELATED CHANGES IN LEARNING AND MEMORY

Methodological Issues

Researchers investigating age-related behavioral changes are faced with a number of problems beyond those usually encountered in studies that use young-adult animals. For example, in studies that use appetitively motivated tasks, the question arises as to whether young and old animals are equally motivated by a given amount of reinforcement. Factors such as type and/or complexity of task, sex, drug dosage, activity level, previous exposure to other experimental manipulations, group vs. individual housing, perceptual changes, and general health of the animal may also be confounding variables in aging research. The way in which alterations in the pituitary-adrenal axis may be influenced by housing conditions and how such changes may in turn affect behavior has been shown by Lovely et al. (1972). When young-adult rats were individually housed for 30 or 50 days, they showed higher basal levels of corticosterone than rats that were housed in groups. Shuttle-box acquisition and extinction were facilitated in the individually housed rats. Hatch et al. (1965) also noted that housing conditions may affect behavior via the pituitary-adrenal axis. They assigned weaning rats to either individual or community cages for 13 weeks. The individually caged rats subsequently showed numerous physiological changes. Decreases were evident in body weight, liver glycogen, adrenal cholesterol, splenic, thymic, and ovarian weights, and number of ovarian follicles, while increases were seen in hemoglobin, adrenal, thyroid, and pituitary gland weights, circulating corticosteroids, and production of corticosteroids in response to ACTH. Thus, housing conditions may influence behavior, and this may confound or be a part of the behavior difference noted in the old rat.

The difficulties encountered in attempting to equate motivation levels in animals of different ages led many researchers to use aversively motivated tasks such as active and passive avoidance conditioning. Some confidence in this approach was derived from studies that directly assessed the adequacy of electric shock as a motivational stimulus. Both young and old rats have been used to investigate possible age-associated differences in the detection of and response to electric footshock. (Campbell (1967) showed that young rats of various ages (23, 38, 54, and 100 days) did not differ in their response to shock at low and intermediate intensities. Likewise, when young (40-90 days) and middle-aged (354 days) rats (Paré, 1969) or young (90-150 days) and old (780 days) rats (Jensen et al., 1980) were compared on measures of nociception, flinch, and jump thresholds in response to electric shock, no significant age-related differences were found when adequate controls for sex and body weight were utilized. Therefore, it appears that when appropriate controls are employed, findings obtained using shock as a motivating stimulus are not likely to be confounded by age-related differences in the motivational level generated by a specified amount of electrical current.

The results obtained by Ray and Barrett (1973) point out some difficulties that may be encountered when active avoidance is used as a behavioral measure. Using rats that ranged in age from 45 to 360 days, these investigators demonstrated that age-related differences in performance were evident when the number of avoidances was used as the behavioral measure in a discriminated avoidance task. However, no such differences were seen when the actual number of initial correct discriminations served as the behavioral measure. Ray and Barrett (1973) concluded that performance (nonlearning) factors rather than age accounted for the observed differences. However, this interpretation was not supported by the results of Thompson and Fitzsimons (1976). When rats aged 3, 7, 12, and 24 months were tested on a shock-motivated light-dark discrimination similar to that used by Ray and Barrett (1973), clear age-related deficits in the number of correct initial responses were observed. Taken together, these two studies illustrate the importance of the age variable in aging studies with rats. The 1-year-old rats used by Ray and Barrett would be most appropriately characterized as middle-aged. Linear age-related trends may be obscured if the ages of the rats do not exceed or at least fall at the upper end of the 1.5 to 2-year range.

The rate at which animals extinguish a learned response after the reinforcer is no longer present has often served as a measure of retention. Sprott and Stavnes (1975) point out that problems exist in the interpretation of extinction scores since it is difficult to distinguish between extinction and acquisition of a new, different response. Nevertheless, the results of some recent experiments that used extinction scores as a primary behavioral measure; for example, Smotherman and Levine (1978) and Cooper et al. (1980a) have provided additional insight into the effects of ACTH and vasopressin-related peptides on learning and memory. The findings of these experiments suggest that extinction scores may be used as a reliable index of "strength of aversion," and, thus, the effects of ACTH and vasopressin on strength of aversion can be studied.

Whereas control for many confounding variables in aging research can only be approximated, awareness of the numerous variables that may influence test results and development of novel approaches for controlling them is essential.

Behavioral Studies

This section will deal primarily with studies that have investigated behavioral changes with age, using either appetitively motivated maze learning or shock-motivated active and passive avoidance tasks. Such tasks have been widely used to investigate age-related changes in learning and memory.

Studies that have used maze learning tasks of varying difficulty have generally demonstrated that few significant age differences are apparent with simple mazes, whereas substantial age-related differences are frequently seen with more complex mazes. Maze complexity is generally determined by the number of choice points. When only one or two choice points is used (Botwinick et al., 1962; Birren, 1962; Goodrick, 1972), age-related differences in performance are rarely seen among young (3-4 months), middle-aged (6-15 months), and old (20-27 months) rats. With mazes containing four choice points (Botwinick et al., 1963; Goodrick, 1972), small though significant age-related differences are observed. Large differences in age-related performance levels are seen with mazes having 14 choice points (Goodrick, 1972, 1973). Goodrick (1973) demonstrated that massed practice (four trials per day) on a 14-choice-point maze improved the performance of old rats (26 months) but impaired that of young rats (6 months). Based on the high frequency of perseverative errors among the old rats, Goodrick concluded that behavioral rigidity was a general characteristic of the performance of the old animals. It would be interesting, in this context, to observe the effects of massed practice on the functioning of the pituitary-adrenal system. That is, might not the enhanced performance seen in the old animals given massed practice be associated with increased levels of ACTH?

A recent study by Wallace et al. (1980) investigated the performance of young (6 months) and old (26 months) rats on an eight-armed radial maze. Spatial memory was reported to decline with age, whereas short-term memory (indicated by retention of recent previous choices in the maze and performance on a discriminative delayed response task) did not show an age-related decline. The results obtained in this study are somewhat similar to those observed in aged human subjects. Significant deficits in spatial memory with little change in primary memory have been reported (Perlmutter et al., 1981; Craik, 1977). Spatial memory in rats (ages 10-16 months and 28-34 months) was also studied by Barnes (1979). The animals were placed on a circular platform and allowed to learn the location of the rewarded place based on spatial cues. Old rats were inferior to young ones in performing this task.

Many studies of animal aging have used shock-motivated avoidance tasks. In general, such tasks involve either active or passive avoidance. When active avoidance is required, the animal must move from one location to another in order to avoid or escape electric footshock. On each trial a warning signal, usually a light or a buzzer, is given prior to the onset of the electric shock. Movement to the appropriate location after the warning signal begins, but before the onset of the shock, constitutes an avoidance response. Several learning sessions, each involving numerous trials, are usually given. Extinction of the response is studied by discontinuing the use of footshock and observing the gradual decline of the number of responses made by the animal. In passive avoidance procedures the ability of an animal to withhold a response is assessed. A rat is placed in a well-lighted area in which there is a hole leading to a darkened compartment. Since a rat has a natural tendency to prefer darkness, it will usually enter the dark compartment within a few seconds. Immediately after the rat enters the dark compartment, a brief footshock is given and the animal is removed from the apparatus. Following a retention interval of hours, days, or weeks, the rat is again placed in the lighted area and the time taken to enter the dark compartment is recorded.

Early studies of age-related changes in avoidance performance primarily used active avoidance procedures. Results obtained by Doty (1966a,b) demonstrated that old (22-25 months) rats showed impaired performance relative to young (1-5 months) rats on a delayed discrimination avoidance task, but not on a simple avoidance task or a discrimination avoidance without delay. As was found with maze learning tasks, age-related impairment in avoidance performance appears to be task specific and to depend on task difficulty. Manipulation of intertrial interval with young (1-5 months) and old (20-25 months) rats on simple (Doty and Doty, 1964; Doty, 1966a) and discriminated (Doty, 1966b) avoidance showed that old rats were more impaired than the young at the shorter intervals (i.e., 10 sec and 1 hr). These findings differ from those in maze learning studies discussed previously in that massed practice was found to be disruptive rather than beneficial for old animals when aversive conditioning was used. Doty (1966a) interpreted her results to be suggestive of a defect in attention or immediate memory.

Several studies investigating age-related drug effects in shockmotivated avoidance procedures have shown that old rats tend to be more sensitive than the young to the facilitatory or disruptive effects of certain drugs. For example, Doty and Doty (1964) showed that whereas young rats (4, 9, and 12 months) were impaired when chlorpromazine was injected 10 sec after each trial on a single avoidance task, old (20 months) animals were impaired when the trial injection interval was 10 sec, 30 min, 1 hr, or 2 hr. With regard to facilitatory effects, amphetamine (Doty and Doty, 1966), physostigmine (Doty and Johnson, 1966), and diphenylhydantoin (Gordon et al., 1968) have all been shown to have greater enhancing effects for old than for young rats. There is evidence to suggest that the facilitatory effects of amphetamine and physostigmine are mediated by their effect on ACTH and/or vasopressin. Physostigmine stimulates the release of ACTH (Smelik, 1977) and vasopressin (Sladek and Knigge, 1977). Although systemically administered amphetamine stimulates the release of ACTH, direct intracerebral injection of amphetamine does not alter ACTH release (Martinez et al., 1980). This apparent inconsistency may be explained by the following observations. Vasopressin has been shown to stimulate the release of ACTH (Yates et al., 1971; Baertschi et al., 1980). Consequently, the behavioral effect of amphetamine may result from its stimulation of the central release of ACTH. This chain of events might adequately explain the failure of centrally administered amphetamine to result in behavioral facilitation.

Passive avoidance tasks have received more attention in recent investigations of behavioral changes with age. These tasks avoid many of the methodological problems encountered with active avoidance. Since the animal does not have to move in order to avoid footshock, possible decreased activity level in old animals is not likely to significantly influence performance. Also, only one learning trial is necessary in a passive avoidance task (although some versions use several learning trials). Therefore, retention testing is less contaminated by learning over multiple trials.

Age-related differences in passive avoidance performance have been obtained in numerous studies. Gold and McGaugh (1975) tested 2-, 12-, and 24-month-old rats on a one-trial passive avoidance task and examined retention performance at intervals of 1 day, 1 week, 3 weeks, and 6 weeks. The 2-month-old rats showed good retention for 3 weeks and began to show significant decline at the 6-week retest interval. One-year-old rats showed good retention at 1 day, substantial decline at 1 week, and poor retention at 3 weeks. Two-year-old rats showed significantly decreased retention latencies even at the 1-day retention interval. At the 1-week retest interval these old rats showed little evidence of memory for the passive avoidance response. Subsequent testing of the old rats, either 2 or 6 hr after the initial passive avoidance trial, indicated that these animals showed good retention at 2 hr, but not at 6 hr. Therefore, it appears that the passive avoidance response is acquired, but is forgotten by the old animals in relatively short periods of time. Whereas these results might be explained by a retrieval deficit in the old rats, other interpretations are also possible. For example, the same findings could result if the association between shock and the dark compartment was not as strong in the old animals as in the young. Such associations are influenced by the pituitary-adrenal system (Levine and Jones, 1965). Tang and Phillips (1978) reported that the function of this system shows age-related changes in some respects. That is, the amount of ACTH released in response to stress decreases with age. Based on these findings, ACTH administered prior to the acquisition of a passive avoidance response might be expected to selectively benefit old animals.

Age-related changes in passive avoidance responding have been reported by many researchers (McNamara et al., 1977; Ordy et al., 1978; Thompson and Cooper, 1979; Bartus et al., 1980; Jensen et al., 1980). The consistency of the findings in these studies suggests that the passive avoidance procedure may be very useful in investigations designed to examine the relationship of age-related behavioral changes to the neurochemical profile of the central nervous system. Indeed, much of the research investigating neuropeptide influences on young animals has used passive avoidance procedures.

As a prelude to more detailed discussion of ACTH in the next session, it is important to reemphasize one of the primary goals of intervention in the aging process, namely, the demonstration of the means by which age-related declines in behavioral functioning may be delayed or reversed. It is interesting to note that much of the animal research that has demonstrated the presence of declines in performance with age has utilized the same procedures on which the behavioral effects of ACTH (and vasopressin) can be seen.

ACTH AND RELATED PEPTIDES

ACTH is an anterior pituitary hormone that stimulates the release of glucocortico-steroids from the adrenal cortex. The pituitary-adrenal system is actively involved in the adaptation of the organism to stress, influencing such functions as blood pressure and energy metabolism. In addition to these peripheral endocrine functions, ACTH has central nervous system effects on behavior. The results of a study by De Wied (1969) showed that removal of the pituitary gland (i.e., hypophysectomy) resulted in impaired shuttlebox avoidance acquisition and accelerated extinction. ACTH replacement after hypophysectomy with subcutaneous administration of a long-acting ACTH preparation restored shuttlebox performance toward normal levels (De Wied, 1964). ACTH fragments devoid of peripheral endocrine effects (i.e., $ACTH_{4-10}$ and $ACTH_{1-10}$) also returned shuttlebox performance to normal (De Wied, 1969).

ACTH and related peptides have been demonstrated, in numerous experimental situations, to exert influences on the acquisition and maintenance of new behavior patterns in intact rats. Levine and Jones (1965) demonstrated that ACTH was effective in enhancing acquisition of a passive avoidance response (inhibition of a stabilized bar-pressing response for water following the presentation of two electric shocks) when subcutaneous administration was begun 3 days prior to the initial shock trial and continued for 12 daily injections. These researchers state that the resumption of bar-pressing after electric shock is similar to the extinction of an avoidance response and, consequently, that their results are consistent with those of Murphy and Miller (1955), which suggested that ACTH had no significant effect on acquisition of an active avoidance response, but significantly retarded the extinction of that response. Anderson et al. (1968) successfully replicated the results of Levine and Jones (1965) using hypophysectomized rats.

Delay of extinction mediated by ACTH or ACTH-related peptides has been demonstrated in aversively motivated procedures using active avoidance (De Wied, 1966; Bohus et al., 1968), passive avoidance (Ader et al., 1972; Levine and Jones, 1965; Lissak and Bohus, 1972; De Wied, 1974), and conditioned taste aversion (Rigter and Popping, 1976; Smotherman and Levine, 1978).

Behavioral effects of ACTH-related peptides are also seen with procedures that use appetitive reinforcement. For example, Guth et al. (1971) trained and extinguished water-deprived rats on a lever-press response for water. When stringent control over extraneous noise and motivation was used, subcutaneous injection of ACTH (10 IU) 0.5 hr before the acquisition sessions resulted in a highly significant increase in the number of lever presses per session late in training. ACTH-related peptides ($ACTH_{1-39}$, synthetic $ACTH_{1-24}$, and $ACTH_{4-10}$) delayed the extinction of a food-rewarded response in food-deprived rats trained to run down an alley for reinforcement (Garrus et al., 1974). $ACTH_{4-10}$ also delayed the extinction of a sexually motivated response on a task in which rats were trained to reach an estrogen-primed female in the goal box of a runway (Bohus et al., 1975). This effect was seen only in rats that were rewarded during the acquisition period, thus suggesting that the effect of the peptide was to preserve the arousal state related to learning rather than to affect sexual arousal per se.

Antiamnesic effects of ACTH-related peptides have also been observed. These peptides typically are not found to be effective in preventing amnesia when injected prior to the amnesia-inducing treatment (Rigter et al., 1974; Lande et al., 1972). However, the reversal of amnesia by ACTH-related peptides has been demonstrated. $ACTH_{4-10}$ reverses CO_2-induced amnesia when injected 1 hr before the retention test in a passive avoidance procedure, but not when injected 1 hr before the acquisition trial (Rigter et al., 1974). Reversal of amnesia by $ACTH_{4-10}$ for a thirst-motivated response was obtained by Rigter and Van Riezen (1975). In this study, water-deprived rats that received a CO_2 treatment after having access to water showed evidence of amnesia for that access on a retrieval test given 24 hr later. This amnesia was not present in CO_2-treated rats that were injected with $ACTH_{4-10}$ 1 hr prior to the retrieval test.

AGE-DEPENDENT CHANGES IN THE PITUITARY-ADRENAL AXIS

Several studies that have investigated age-related changes in the pituitary-adrenal axis have not found a significant decline with age in basal corticosterone levels (Adelman, 1975; Hess and Reigle, 1970; Lewis and Wexler, 1974; Tang and Phillips, 1978). Thus, aged rats appear to have no difficulty in maintaining nonstressed corticosteroid levels.

The results of Tang and Phillips (1978) indicate that basal secretion of ACTH may actually increase with age. However, these investigators also demonstrate that old animals are impaired with respect to the young in their ability to respond to stress with increased secretion of ACTH. They suggest that this may result from decreased ability of the pituitary to synthesize and/or secrete ACTH or a deline in corticotropin-releasing factor secretion in response to stress. Since many animal studies investigating behavioral change with age involved the use of stress-inducing situations (i.e., shock-motivated avoidance, food-deprivation, and conditioned flavor aversion), artificially increasing the amount of ACTH released in response to stress should have some potential for selectively enhancing behavioral performance in old animals.

Rigter and Crabbe (1979) cite an unpublished study by Rigter that investigated age-related differences in the effect of the ACTH 4-9 analogue, Org 2766. Young (2 months) and old (25 months) male rats were trained on a complex maze for food reward. Two trials per day were given during acquisition, with a 4 to 5-hr interval between trials. The acquisition criterion was no more than one error during two consecutive trials. One week after reaching criterion, a one-day session of four trials was given with 10 min between each trial. No injections were given during acquisition, but either Org 2766 (0.1 µg/rat) or saline was injected 1 hr before the beginning of the 1-week retest session. Young (2 months) and old (27 months) rats did not differ with regard to trials to criterion or errors. However, more errors were made by the old rats during the retest. Org 2766 appeared to facilitate the performance of both young and old animals, but this effect reached statistical significance only for the old. Rigter points out that although these results suggested that Org 2766 may have influenced memory retrieval, old animals performed as well as the young on the first retention trial, making most of their errors on subsequent trials.

Although ACTH-related peptides may affect behavioral performance in old animals, it is difficult to determine the nature of these effects. Even if two groups of animals demonstrate relatively equivalent performance during the acquisition of a task, this does not necessarily mean that they have learned the response to the same degree, or that differences in subsequent performance during retention testing indicate the presence of retrieval deficits. For example, if the level of ACTH present during acquisition modulates the extent to which a response is learned and subsequently retrieved from memory, the levels necessary for acquisition and retention of a response may be different. Consequently, a lowered level of ACTH may not appear to affect acquisition performance, whereas it may nevertheless subsequently allow the expression of deficits during retention testing. Given the complex role that neuropeptides may play in behavioral performance, more effective means of differentiating between acquisition and retrieval deficits are needed. One approach to this problem would be to use a design similar to that of Rigter et al. (1974). Young and old animals could be exposed to one of four experimental conditions on a one-trial passive avoidance task: (1) ACTH injection prior to acquisition (ACQ) and saline injection prior to retention (RET) testing; (2) saline prior to ACQ and ACTH prior to RET; (3) ACTH prior to ACQ and RET; and (4) saline prior to ACQ and RET. Predictions of outcomes based on the hypothesized presence of acquisition as opposed to retrieval deficits could then be compared with the obtained results.

VASOPRESSIN-RELATED PEPTIDES

Vasopressin is a posterior pituitary peptide which also acts as an antidiuretic hormone in mammals. It is synthesized in the supraoptic and paraventricular nuclei of the hypothalamus, and then transported to the posterior pituitary for storage and subsequent release. Arginine vasopressin (AVP) is the naturally occurring form of vasopressin in most mammals, whereas lysine vasopressin (LVP) is found in pig pituitaries.

The primary endocrine function of vasopressin involves water retention. Vasopressin acts on the kidney to promote reabsorption of water, thus causing the excretion of concentrated urine. Elevation of blood pressure in mammals by vasopressin has been demonstrated; however, the amount of vasopressin required for this effect exceeds that which is normally released by the posterior pituitary (Turner and Bagnara, 1976).

The involvement of vasopressin in behavioral processes was demonstrated in early studies by De Wied (1965) and De Wied and Bohus (1966). Posterior lobectomy including removal of the intermediate lobe of the pituitary was demonstrated to result in decreased resistance to extinction of a conditioned avoidance response (CAR) in rats. Pitressin, a crude extract derived from posterior and intermediate lobes of the pituitary, was effective in returning the rate of extinction to the level of that seen in sham-operated controls. Whereas a long-acting effect was obtained with pitressin (i.e., significant retention of the CAR was still evident 3-5 weeks after discontinuation of treatment with pitressin), melanocyte-stimulating hormone, an ACTH-related peptide, was effective in inhibiting extinction only while animals were being treated with this peptide.

De Wied (1971), using a pole-jumping avoidance response, demonstrated that vasopressin was the peptide in pitressin responsible for the long-term delay of extinction effect. In order to determine the critical time period for the effect of LVP on the maintenance of the avoidance response, rats were injected immediately, 1 or 6 hr after the last trial of the first extinction session. Injection within 1 hr was necessary to obtain relatively complete inhibition of extinction. Various other peptides including oxytocin, angiotension II, insulin, and growth hormone were without apparent effect on maintenance of the avoidance response.

Findings consistent with those obtained with active avoidance procedures are also found with passive avoidance. Subcutaneous injection of LVP 1 hr before the first retention trial (24 hr after the last learning trial) significantly increased avoidance latency (Ader and De Wied, 1972; Bohus et al., 1972).

The effects of vasopressin on resistance to extinction can also be demonstrated with tasks that use appetitive rather than aversive motivation. Hostetter et al. (1977) trained rats on a food-reinforced black-white discrimination T-maze task. Vasopressin injections (0.4 IU) given during the extinction phase prolonged extinction in rats that were reinforced for choosing the black arm of the T maze. No effects were seen with rats that received vasopressin and were rewarded in the white T-maze arm or with rats that received saline injections. Two measures of activity used in this study (running speed and open-field activity) did not reveal any differences between groups. Therefore, it is unlikely that the effects of vasopressin on extinction scores were secondary to possible effects of activity. Bohus (1977) demonstrated that vasopressin could delay extinction of a sexually motivated learning task in male rats.

Vasopressin-related peptides have been demonstrated to have potent anti-amnesic effects. These peptides can reverse the amnesia induced by a variety of agents including puromycin (Lande et al., 1972; Flexner et al., 1978), CO_2 (Rigter et al., 1974, 1975), pentylenetetrazol (Bookin and Pfeifer, 1977), electroconvulsive shock (Pfeifer and Bookin, 1978), and diethyldithiocarbamate (Adin, 1980). These studies cited above in which puromycin was the amnesic agent investigated retention of right-left discrimination in a Y maze. All of the remaining studies used a passive avoidance task with vasopressin injections usually given 1 hr before the acquisition trial(s) and/or 1 hr before the retention trial. In two of the five studies using passive avoidance, antiamnesic effects were obtained when vasopressin injections were given either before acquisition or before retention. Results obtained in the two remaining studies demonstrated antiamnesic effects only when vasopressin was injected prior to retention. Thus, decreased resistance to extinction and reversal of induced amnesia are two areas in which vasopressin has been shown to exert significant effects in young animals. As will be discussed in the next session, old animals clearly show decreased resistance to extinction and memory deficits on certain behavioral tasks. Therefore, there is obvious potential for therapeutic intervention using vasopressin with old animals.

VASOPRESSIN AND AGE

Age-related decline in posterior pituitary hormones is well documented. Dunihue (1965) measured the amount of neurosecretory material in this region in young (10 months) and old (30 months) rats and reported moderate-to-severe reductions. Dunihue concluded that his finding along with available physiological and biochemical data suggested a decrease in the synthesis and storage of neurohypophyseal peptides with age. Additional support for this view comes from a more recent study by Turkington and Everitt (1976). Among other parameters, these investigators measured urinary excretion and plasma levels of vasopressin in rats of four ages (200, 400, 700, and 900 days). Significant age-related decreases were observed in daily urinary secretion and baseline plasma levels of vasopressin.

Since vasopressin has facilitatory effects on passive avoidance performance in young and old animals, and old animals show impairment on passive avoidance, the question arises as to the possible relationship between decreased vasopressin levels with age and impaired performance on tasks on which aging animals tend to show deficits. Recent studies reported by Thompson and Cooper (1979) and Cooper et al. (1980b) suggest that performance deficits on passive avoidance and conditioned taste aversion in old animals can be reversed by vasopressin.

In the study by Thompson and Cooper (1979), young (5-7 months) and old (24-30 months) rats were trained on a simple one-trial passive avoidance task. The retention task for each animal was given after 1 week. One hour prior to the retention test each rat received subcutaneous injection of either LVP (0.5 μg/kg) or saline. Maximal (300 sec) median retention latencies by the saline-treated young rats precluded the possibility of demonstrating a facilitative effect of LVP in this age group. However, old rats that were injected with saline showed impaired performance on the retention test whereas old rats injected with LVP had retention latencies equal to those demonstrated by young rats.

A series of studies by Cooper et al. (1980a) investigated age-related changes in conditioned taste aversion. First, 19-month-old rats were demonstrated to show significantly faster extinction of a conditioned taste aversion than rats aged 3, 6, or 10 months (McNamara and Cooper, 1979). This difference in extinction rate between young and old rats was not due to age differences in the ability of the animals to taste saccharin since 3- and 19-month-old rats showed relatively equal preference for five different saccharin concentrations (0.01, 0.1, 0.2, 1.0, and 5% solutions), and since both age groups showed the highest preference for the 0.1% concentration. Young (3 months) and old (19 months) rats were then subjected to a conditioned taste aversion procedure (three saccharin-amphetamine pairings) in which either subcutaneous LVP (1 μg/kg) or water injections were given to rats 1 hr before the daily two-bottle (i.e., saccharine or water) choice test every fourth day of the extinction phase of the experiment. Vasopressin significantly delayed the rate of extinction in both young and old rats. The old rats appeared to benefit somewhat more than the young from the vasopressin treatments since the preference scores were similar in young and old animals on vasopressin treatment days, but were higher for old rats on the days that preceded each of the first three vasopressin treatment days. Thus, with vasopressin treatments the extinction rates of the old animals were comparable with those of the young. This effect was no longer evident after the fourth vasopressin treatment day. To test the hypothesis that old rats simply forget learned information rapidly, old animals were divided into two groups. Using the same aversive conditioning procedure described above, half of the animals were given a daily two-bottle choice test beginning 24 hr after the last saccharin-amphetamine pairing. The other animals were given water only (30 min per day) for 8 days, followed by a daily two-bottle choice test beginning on the ninth day. The saccharin preference scores of these two groups were essentially identical, and the course of extinction was approximately parallel. Thus, rapid forgetting in old animals does not appear to adequately explain the age differences observed with the conditioned flavor-aversion procedure.

An alternative explanation is that age differences in extinction scores are the result of differences in strength of aversion. To test this, young and old rats were given a single 0.1% saccharin-amphetamine pairing and were provided with a two-bottle choice test beginning 24 hr later. The extinction rate of the old rats was significantly faster than that of the young. This suggests that the age difference in extinction rate probably reflects a difference in the initial strength of association that developed in response to the aversive stimulus. Subcutaneous injection of vasopressin (1 mg/kg) 1 hr prior to the two-bottle choice test significantly reduced the saccharin intake by old rats during the recovery period (Cooper et al., 1980b).

Cooper et al. (1980b) conclude that their results support the hypothesis that age-dependent changes in behavior result in part from age-related changes in the availability of vasopressin. Furthermore, it is suggested that with the conditioned taste-aversion procedure, the primary influence of vasopressin is associated with the initial strength of aversion.

CONCLUSION

Although there are relatively few animal studies which have directly addressed the issue of age-related changes in the ability of neuropeptides to influence behavioral performance, the research reviewed above suggests that the use of animal models can make a valuable contribution with regard to defining the conditions under which successful intervention in the aging process may occur. Results obtained from studies using young-adult animals suggest that future research along these lines could prove most useful in: (1) characterizing the mechanisms responsible for the decline in behavioral performance associated with increasing age, and (2) developing effective therapeutic strategies for delaying or reversing these age-associated impairments.

Whereas there is still a lack of consistency among various reports of age-related changes in behavior, some generalizations appear to be evident. First, numerous studies using various experimental procedures have demonstrated that ACTH and vasopressin-related neuropeptides can enhance behavioral performance under certain conditions, both in young and old animals. Second, old animals, in some cases, show selective improvement, suggesting that these neuropeptides may be compensating for some age-related loss of function. The precise mechanisms by which performance is enhanced are not known. Regardless of whether neuropeptides exert their effects on strength of aversion, memory retrieval, or some other mechanism, it seems clear that these substances may be of use as tools for successfully altering the onset and/or progression of behavioral deficits that accompany the aging process.

The similarity between the tasks on which old rats show behavioral deficits and those on which ACTH and vasopressin exert their facilitatory effects is quite striking. Also, an increasing number of studies are providing evidence for the role of specific neurotransmitters in age-related behavioral deficits. Recent studies by Bartus and his colleagues (Bartus, 1979, 1980; Bartus et al., 1980) suggest that cholinergic mechanisms are associated with age-related changes in memory. Complex interactions between vasopressin and catecholaminergic neurotransmitters have also been reported. Vasopressin appears to alter brain levels, turnover, and disappearance of norepinephrine and/or dopamine in various brain regions (Kovàcs et al., 1979a,b). Ramaekers et al. (1977) suggest that vasopressin also affects serotoninergic neurotransmission.

Since more information is accumulating regarding the tasks on which old animals consistently show behavioral deficits, additional knowledge about the generality of neuropeptide behavioral effects will undoubtedly follow. For example, Wallace et al. (1980) demonstrated the presence of spatial memory deficits in old rats showing intact short-term memory. Given the similarity of these findings to those reported with human subjects (Perlmutter et al., 1981), it would be interesting to investigate the effects of neuropeptides on spatial memory in rats.

The extensive amount of research on neuropeptides using animal models and the subsequent interest in the investigation of the effects of neuropeptides in human subjects illustrates the important role that animal models play in generating information that may be useful in effectively addressing problems with humans in clinical settings. Given the extent of concern among researchers and clinicians regarding memory impairment in elderly individuals, the need for more animal studies investigating age-related changes in learning and memory, and the influence of neuropeptides, neurotransmitters, and other CNS substances on these changes cannot be overemphasized.

REFERENCES

Adelman, R. C. (1975). Impaired hormonal regulation of enzyme activity during aging. *Fed. Proc. 34*: 179-182.

Ader, R., and De Wied, D. (1972). Effects of vasopressin on active and passive avoidance learning. *Psychon. Sci. 29*: 46-48.

Ader, R., Weijnen, J. A., and Moleman, P. (1972). Retention of passive avoidance response as a function of the intensity and duration of electric shock. *Psychon. Sci. 26*: 125-128.

Adin, K. E. (1980). Lysine vasopressin attenuation of diethyldithiocarbamate-induced amnesia. *Pharm. Biochem. Behav. 12*: 343-346.

Anderson, D. C., Winn, W., and Tam, T. (1968). Adrenocorticotrophic hormone and acquisition of a passive avoidance response: a replication and extension. *J. Comp. Physiol. Psychol. 66*: 497-499.

Baertschi, A. J., Vallet, P., Bauman, J. B., and Girard, J. (1980). Neural lobe of pituitary modulates corticotropin release in the rat. *Endocrinology 106*: 878-882.

Barnes, C. A. (1979). Memory deficits associated with senescence: a neurophysiological and behavioral study in the rat. *J. Comp. Physiol. Psychol. 93*: 74-104.

Bartus, R. T. (1979). Physostigmine and recent memory: effects in young and aged non-human primates. *Science 206*: 1087-1089.

Bartus, R. T. (1980). Cholinergic drug effects on memory and cognition in animals. In *Aging in the 1980s*, L. Poon (Ed.). APA Press, Washington, D.C., pp. 163-180.

Bartus, R. T., Dean, R. L., Goas, A. J., and Lippa, A. S. (1980). Age-related changes in passive avoidance retention: modulation with dietary choline. *Science 209*: 301-303.

Birren, J. E. (1962). Age differences in learning a two choice water maze by rats. *J. Gerontol. 17*: 207-213.

Bohus, B. (1977). Effects of desglycinamide-lysine vasopressin (DG-LVP) on sexually motivated T-maze behavior of the male rat. *Horm. Behav. 8*: 52-63.

Bohus, B., Ader, R., and De Wied, D. (1972). Effect of vasopressin on active and passive avoidance behavior. *Horm. Behav. 3*: 191-197.

Bohus, B., Hendrick, H., Van Kolfschoten, A. A., and Krediet, T. G. (1975). The effect of ACTH4-10 on copulatory and sexually motivated approach behavior in the male rat. In *Sexual Behavior: Pharmacology and Biochemistry*, M. Sandler and G. L. Gessa (Eds.). Raven Press, New York, pp. 269-275.

Bohus, B., Nyakas, C. S., and Endroczi, E. (1968). Effects of adrenocorticotrophic hormone on avoidance behavior of intact and adrenalectomized rats. *Int. J. Neuropharm. 7*: 307-314.

Bookin, H. B., and Pfeifer, W. D. (1977). Effect of lysine vasopressin on pentylenetetrazol-induced retrograde amnesia in rats. *Pharm. Biochem. Behav. 7*: 51-54.

Botwinick, J., Brinley, J. F., and Robbin, J. S. (1962). Learning a position discrimination and position reversal by Sprague-Dawley rats of different ages. *J. Gerontol. 17*: 315-319.

Botwinick, J. Brinley, J. F., and Robbin, J. S. (1963). Learning and reversing a four choice multiple Y-maze by rats of three ages. *J. Gerontol. 18*: 279-282.

Campbell, B. A. (1967). Developmental studies of learning and motivation in infraprimate mammals. In *Early Behavior: Comparative and Developmental Approaches*, J. Stevenson, H. Hess, and H. Rheingold (Eds.). Wiley, New York, pp. 43-71.

Cooper, R. L., McNamara, M. C., Thompson, W. G., and Marsh, G. R. (1980a). Vasopressin modulation of learning and memory in the rat. In *Aging in the 1980s*, L. Poon (Ed.). APA Press, Washington, D.C., pp. 201-211.

Cooper, R. L., McNamara, M. C., and Thompson, W. G. (1980b). Vasopressin and conditioned flavor aversion in aged rats. *Neurobiol. Aging 1*: 53-57.

Craik, F. (1977). Age differences in human memory. In *Handbook of the Psychology of Aging*, J. E. Birren and K. W. Schaie (Eds.). Van Nostrand Reinhold, New York, pp. 671-684.

De Wied, D. (1964). Influence of anterior pituitary on avoidance learning and escape behavior. *Am. J. Physiol. 207*: 255-259.

De Wied, D. (1965). The influence of posterior and intermediate lobe of the pituitary and pituitary peptides on the maintenance of a conditioned avoidance response. *Int. J. Neuropharm. 4*: 157-167.

De Wied, D. (1966). Inhibitory effect of ACTH and related peptides on extinction of conditioned avoidance behavior in rats. *Proc. Soc. Exp. Biol. Med. 122*: 28-32.

De Wied, D. (1969). Effects of peptide hormones on behavior. In *Frontiers in Neuroendocrinology*, W. Ganong and L. Martini (Eds.). Oxford University Press, New York, pp. 97-140.

De Wied, D. (1971). Long term effect of vasopressin on the maintenance of a conditioned avoidance response in rats. *Nature 232*: 58-60.

De Wied, D. (1974). Pituitary-adrenal system hormones and behavior. In *The Neurosciences, Third Study Program*, F. O. Schmitt and F. G. Worden (Eds.). MIT Press, Cambridge, Mass., pp. 653-666.

De Wied, D., and Bohus, B. (1966). Long term and short term effects on retention of a conditioned avoidance response in rats by treatment with long acting pitressin and a-MSH. *Nature 212*: 1484-1486.

Doty, B. A. (1966a). Age and avoidance conditioning in rats. *J. Gerontol. 21*: 287-290.

Doty, B. A. (1966b). Age differences in avoidance conditioning as a function of distribution of trials and task difficulty. *J. Genet. Psychol. 109*: 249-254.

Doty, B. A., and Doty, L. A. (1964). Effect of age and chlorpromazine on memory consolidation. *J. Comp. Physiol. Psychol. 57*: 331-334.

Doty, B. A., and Doty, L. A. (1966). Facilitative effects of amphetamine on avoidance conditioning in relation to age and prolem difficulty. *Psychopharmacologia 9*: 234-241.

Doty, B. A., and Johnson, M. M. (1966). Effects of post-trial eserine administration, age and task difficulty on avoidance conditioning in rats. *Psychon. Sci. 6*: 101-102.

Dunihue, F. W. (1965). Reduced juxtaglomerular cell granularity, pituitary neurosecretory material, and width of the zona glomerulosa in aging rats. *Endocrinology 77*: 948-951.

Flexner, J. B., Flexner, L. B., Walter, R., and Hoffman, P. L. (1978). ADH and related peptides: effect of pre- or post-training treatment on puromycin amnesia.
Pharm. Biochem. Behav. 8: 93-95.

Garrud, P., Gray, J. A., and De Wied, D. (1974). Pituitary-adrenal hormones and
extinction of rewarded behavior in the rat. *Physiol. Behav. 12*: 109-119.

Gold, P. E., and McGaugh, J. L. (1975). Changes in learning and memory during
aging. In *Neurobiology of Aging*, J. M. Ordy and K. R. Brizzee (Eds.). Plenum,
New York, pp. 145-158.

Goodrick, C. L. (1972). Learning by mature-young and aged Wistar albino rats as
a function of test complexity. *J. Gerontol. 27*: 353-357.

Goodrick, C. L. (1973). Maze learning of mature-young and aged rats as a function
of distribution of practice. *J. Exp. Psychol. 98*: 344-349.

Gordon, P., Tobin, S. S., Doty, B. A., and Nash, M. (1968). Drug effects on behavior in aged animals and man: diphenylhydantoin and procainamide. *J.
Gerontol. 23*: 434-444.

Guth, S., Seward, J. P., and Levine, S. (1971). Differential manipulation of passive avoidance by exogenous ACTH. *Horm. Behav. 2*: 127-138.

Hatch, A. M., Wiberg, G. S., Zawidzka, Z., Cann, M., Airth, J. M., and Grice, H.
C. (1965). Isolation syndrome in the rat. *Toxicol. Appl. Pharm. 7*: 737-745.

Hess, G. D., and Reigle, G. D. (1970). Adrenocortical responsiveness to stress and
ACTH in aging rats. *J. Gerontol. 25*: 354-358.

Hostetter, G., Jubb, S. L., and Kozlowski, G. P. (1977). Vasopressin affects the
behavior of rats in a positively-rewarded discrimination task. *Life Sci. 21*:
1323-1328.

Jensen, R. A., Martinez, J. L., McGaugh, J. L., Messing, R. B., and Vasquez, B. J.
(1980). The psychobiology of aging. In *The Aging Nervous System*, F. J.
Pirozzolo and G. L. Maletta (Eds.). Praeger, New York, pp. 110-125.

Kovàcs, G. L., Bohus, B., and Versteeg, D. H. G. (1979a). The effects of vasopressin on memory processes: the role of noradrenergic neurotransmission.
Neuroscience 4: 1529-1537.

Kovàcs, G. L., Bohus, B., Versteeg, D., De Kloet, E. R., and De Wied, D. (1979b).
Effect of oxytocin and vasopressin on memory consolidation: sites of action
and catecholaminergic correlates after local microinjection into limbic-midbrain structures. *Brain Res. 175*: 303-314.

Lande, S., Flexner, J. B., and Flexner, L. B. (1972). Effect of corticotrophin and
desglycinamide lysine vasopressin on suppression of memory by puromycin.
Proc. Natl. Acad. Sci. USA 69: 558-560.

Levine, S., and Jones, L. W. (1965). Adrenocorticotropic hormone (ACTH) and
passive avoidance learning. *J. Comp. Physiol. Psychol. 59*: 357-360.

Lewis, B. K., and Wexler, B. C. (1974). Serum insulin changes in male rats associated with age and reproductive activity. *J. Gerontol. 29*: 139-144.

Lissak, K., and Bohus, B. (1972). Pituitary hormones and avoidance behavior of
the rats. *Int. J. Psychobiol. 2*: 103-115.

Lovely, R. H., Pagano, R. R., and Paolino, R. M. (1972). Shuttle-box-avoidance performance and basal corticosterone levels as a function of duration of individual housing in rats. *J. Comp. Physiol. Psychol. 81*: 331-335.

McNamara, M. C., and Cooper, R. L. (1979). Age differences in conditioned taste aversion: possible role of vasopressin. Paper presented at the meeting of the Society for Neuroscience, Atlanta, Georgia.

McNamara, M. C., Benignus, G., Benignus, V. A., and Miller, A. T., Jr. (1977). Active and passive avoidance in rats as a function of age. *Exp. Aging Res. 3*: 3-16.

Martinez, J. L., Jensen, R. A., Messing, R. B., Vasquez, B. J., Soumireu-Mourat, B., Geddes, D., Liang, K. C., and McGaugh, J. L. (1980). Central and peripheral actions of amphetamines on memory storage. *Brain Res. 182*: 157-166.

Murphy, J. V., and Miller, R. E. (1955). The effect of adrenocorticotrophic hormone (ACTH) on avoidance conditioning in the rat. *J. Comp. Physiol. Psychol. 48*: 47-49.

Ordy, J. M., Brizzee, K. R., Kaack, B., and Hansche, J. (1978). Age differences in short-term memory and cell loss in the cortex of the rat. *Gerontologia 24*: 276-285.

Perlmutter, M., Metzger, R., Nezworski, T., and Miller, K. (1981). Spatial and temporal memory in 20 and 60 year olds. *J. Gerontol. 36*: 59-65.

Pfeifer, W. D., and Bookin, H. B. (1978). Vasopressin antagonizes retrograde amnesia in rats following electroconvulsive shock. *Pharm. Biochem. Behav. 9*: 261-263.

Ramaekers, F., Rigter, H., and Leonard, B. E. (1977). Parallel changes in behavior and hippocampal serotonin metabolism in rats following treatment with desglycinamide lysine vasopressin. *Brain Res. 120*: 485-492.

Ray, O. S., and Barrett, R. J. (1973). Interaction of learning and memory with age in the rat. In *Psychopharmacology and Aging*, C. E. Eisdorfer and W. E. Fann (Eds.). Plenum, New York, pp. 17-40.

Rigter, H., and Crabbe, J. C. (1979). Modulation of memory by pituitary hormones and related peptides. *Vitam. Horm. 37*: 153-241.

Rigter, H., and Popping, A. (1976). Hormonal influences on the extinction of conditioned taste aversion. *Psychopharmacologia 46*: 255-261.

Rigter, H., and Van Riezen, H. (1975). The antiamnesic effect of $ACTH_{4-10}$: its independence of the nature of the amnesic agent and the behavioral test. *Physiol. Behav. 14*: 563-566.

Rigter, H., Elbertse, R., and Ban Riezen, H. (1975). Time-dependent antiamnesic effects of $ACTH_{4-10}$ and desglycinamide-lysine vasopressin. *Prog. Brain Res. 42*: 164-171.

Rigter, H., Van Riezen, H., and De Wied, D. (1974). The effects of ACTH and vasopressin analogues on CO_2-induced retrograde amnesia in rats. *Physiol. Behav. 13*: 381-388.

Sladek, C. D., and Knigge, K. M. (1977). Cholinergic stimulation of vasopressin release from the rat hypothalamo-neurohypophyseal system in organ culture. *Endocrinology 101*: 411-420.

Smelik, P. G. (1977). Neurotransmitter control of ACTH release. In *Endocrinology*, V. H. T. James (Ed.). Oxford, Amsterdam, pp. 158-162.

Smotherman, W. P., and Levine, S. (1978). ACTH and $ACTH_{4-10}$ modification of neophobia and taste aversion responses in the rat. *J. Comp. Physiol. Psychol. 92*: 22-33.

Sprott, R. L., and Stavnes, K. (1975). Avoidance learning, behavior genetics, and aging: a critical review and comment on methodology. *Exp. Aging Res. 1*: 145-168.

Tang, F., and Phillips, J. G. (1978). Some age-related changes in pituitary-adrenal function in the male laboratory rat. *J. Gerontol. 33*: 377-382.

Thompson, W. G., and Cooper, R. L. (1979). The effects of age and vasopressin on passive avoidance responding in rats. Paper presented at the meeting of the Gerontological Society, Washington, D.C.

Thompson, C. I., and Fitzsimons, T. R. (1976). Age differences in aversively motivated visual discrimination learning and retention in male Sprague-Dawley rats. *J. Gerontol. 31*: 47-52.

Turkington, M. R., and Everitt, A. V. (1976). The neurohypophysis and aging, with special reference to the antidiuretic hormone. In *Hypothalamus, Pituitary, and Aging*, A. V. Everitt and J. A. Burgess (Eds.). Charles C Thomas, Springfield, Ill., pp. 123-136.

Turner, C. D., and Bagnara, J. T. (1976). *General Endocrinology*, Sanders, Philadelphia.

Wallace, J. E., Krauter, E. E., and Campbell, B. A. (1980). Animal models of declining memory in the aged: short-term and spatial memory in the aged rat. *J. Gerontol. 35*: 355-363.

Yates, F. E., Russell, S. M., Dallman, M. F., Hedge, G. A., McCann, S. M., and Dhariwal, P. S. (1971). Potentiation by vasopressin of corticotropin-releasing factors. *Endocrinology 88*: 3-15.

13

Drug Effects in an Animal Model of Memory Deficits in the Aged: Implications for Future Clinical Trials

Reginald L. Dean, III, Costas C. Loullis, and Raymond T. Bartus /
*Medical Research Division of American Cyanamid Co., Lederle Laboratories,
Pearl River, New York*

INTRODUCTION

Among the many behavioral impairments that develop with old age (i.e., disturbances in cognition, affect, psychomotor function, sleep, and sexual function), loss of cognitive functions is generally recognized as the most debilitating (Weinberg, 1980). It has been particularly difficult, however, to accurately quantify the specific behavioral mechanisms impaired in the aged human subject, in part because of intertask differences, motivational factors, and other methodological problems which often plague gerontological research. Defining the etiology has also been difficult because of technical and moral restrictions which limit the type of neurological, biochemical, and pharmacological tests that can be conducted in humans.

Over the last several years, we have developed a nonhuman primate, behavioral test procedure which seems sensitive to many of the cognitive changes observed in aged humans (Bartus, 1979a). Early tests with this procedure comparing performance between young and aged monkeys revealed that one of the most severe and consistently observed deficits was decreased memory for recent (but not immediate) stimulus events (Fig. 1). That is, a selective impairment was seen only when information had to be remembered temporarily for a duration of several seconds to a few minutes. This age-related deficit in recent memory has been observed both in new world and old-world monkeys (Bartus et al., 1978; Bartus et al., 1980; Medin,

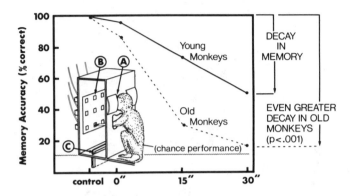

Memory Condition (retention interval)

Figure 1 Differences in performance of young (3-4 years) and aged (18-21 years)
rhesus monkeys on automated, delayed-response procedure (used to assess recent
memory). Inset drawing is of the Automated General Experimental Device (AGED)
with its features: (a) Stimulus observation window; (b) stimulus response panels;
and (c) one-way viewing screen. (From Bartus, 1979b.)

1969), as well as in mice and rats of different strains (Dean et al., 1981; Kubanis
et al., 1981; Lippa et al., 1980; Ordy and Schjeide, 1973).

Other behavioral impairments observed in the aged nonhuman primate included an increased sensitivity to interfering stimuli (Bartus and Dean, 1979) and
increased perseveration or an inability to change behavioral habits (Bartus et al.,
1979). However, in this subject-paced task procedure, the ability to learn two-
choice discrimination problems as well as encode and respond to simple sensory
stimuli appeared to remain relatively unimpaired. Collectively, these behavioral
studies demonstrated that: (1) some degree of specificity for age-related behavioral
deficits exists, for not all behaviors measured were impaired, nor to the same degree; and (2) reasonable similarity exists between the most serious age-related
deficits in both human and nonhuman primates. On this basis it was suggested
that the nonhuman primate may provide a valid and reliable means of assessing
drugs ultimately intended to treat geriatric cognitive deficits.

Use of this primate model to study aging processes offers several important
benefits. The usual advantages of using animal subjects in behavioral research (such
as providing more specific test procedures and greater control and regimentation
of the test and nontest environment) become particularly apparent when dealing
with aged subjects, which may confound accurate test measurements because of
increased variability, decreased motivation, and so forth. Another advantage of
this model is that the effects of many nonbiological variables which may confound
an accurate estimate of cognitive capacities in aged humans (i.e., difficulties in ad-
justing to the test environment, failure to understand completely the test direc-

tions or procedures, various social or cultural influences, and so forth) are eliminated or greatly minimized by use of nonhuman primates which have been fully adapted to the laboratory and the routine of daily testing. The use of this nonhuman primate model of aging has an additional advantage in that the behavioral repertoire of the nonhuman primate is sufficiently sophisticated to allow the study and measurement of many behaviors which are interesting and relevant to human aging (e.g., attention, reaction time, learning and memory, and so forth). Thus, comparisons with human behavioral functions should be more meaningful and perhaps less hazardous than when alternative classes of animals are used.

Finally, recent evidence comparing brains from aged monkeys and humans has revealed certain similarities in age-related alterations in morphology, neurophysiology, and neurochemistry. These similarities suggest that the neurological and neurochemical changes observed may play common roles in similar behavioral deficits observed in aged humans and nonhuman primates. Thus, the possibility of obtaining valid and predictive information regarding the effects of drugs to reduce age-related memory loss by using nonhuman primates seemed well founded.

This chapter describes the use of a nonhuman primate model in psychopharmacological studies of aging. It is based on our recent efforts to improve performance of the memory task in aged monkeys using several different pharmacological approaches.

METHODS FOR PRIMATE BEHAVIORAL AND PSYCHOPHARMACO-LOGICAL STUDIES

All testing was conducted in the Automated General Experimental Device (AGED) (Fig. 1). The AGED and its application to geriatric research have been discussed in detail previously (Bartus, 1979a), and only a brief description of the apparatus and test procedure will be provided here.

Apparatus

One of AGED's main features is that it is totally automated and computer controlled. Thus, potential experimenter bias during the experimental procedure, problems of experimenter-subject interactions, and the need for extensive pre-experimental taming procedures required of manual procedures are all eliminated or greatly minimized with an automated procedure. Furthermore, the degree of experimental control, accuracy, and specificity is increased substantially, as is the overall efficiency of the test.

Another important feature is that all trials are subject-paced. The self-pacing procedure is critical to an objective evaluation of performance in the aged, for many investigators have shown that experimenter-paced tasks produce spuriously low estimates of the aged subject's capacities. To initiate a trial, the monkey places its head in the stimulus observation window which separates the monkey from the stimulus-response (S-R) matrix. This window is equipped with a photo-cell and an infrared light source to detect when the monkey's head is oriented toward the stimulus, thus increasing the likelihood that the monkey will begin to process the stimulus at the start of each trial.

Another feature is the precise experimental control and manipulation of the S-R matrix. An automatically controlled one-way viewing screen is between the S-R matrix and the monkey. When the raised screen is backlit, it allows the monkey to view but not respond to the S-R panels; when it is not backlit, it is opaque and visually isolates the S-R matrix from the monkey. The monkey is allowed to respond only when the screen is lowered. The use of nine individual panels in the S-R matrix is intended to increase the sensitivity of the testing procedure by increasing the range of possible above-chance scores (chance = one-ninth or 11.1%). The nine S-R panels are arranged in the form of a relatively small 3 X 3 matrix (measuring 9 X 9 in.) to minimize the problems of monkeys using overt body orientation (instead of covert memory mechanisms) when delayed-response procedures are used.

Because the AGED apparatus is flexible, it has the advantage of allowing multiple behavioral paradigms to be used. Almost limitless variations of stimuli can be used since any color or pattern which can be photographed can be projected onto the S-R panel. Further, with relatively subtle changes in the computer program, rather large variations are achieved in the types of behavior measured (e.g., memory vs. visual perception). Thus, the animal does not have to learn or adjust to totally new test paradigms, making direct comparisons of the effects of drugs on different types of behavior less hazardous.

The final prominent feature of this apparatus is that the stimulus cue, response manipulanda, and reinforcement well are spatially contiguous, thereby facilitating drug and gerontological testing. Because of this configuration, naive animals learn to operate the apparatus for food reinforcement very quickly, and relatively little effort is required on the part of a test-sophisticated monkey to perform in the apparatus for extended periods of time. This feature is important in evaluation and comparison of specific behavioral functions in aged subjects who may suffer from decreased motivation, attention, physical stamina, psychomotor coordination, and other noncognitive impairments.

General Behavioral Procedure

For all of the drug studies reviewed here, an indirect delayed-response procedure was used to measure memory for recent stimulus events. Each trial was initiated when the monkey placed its face into the stimulus observation window. When this occurred, the backlights came on, allowing the S-R matrix to be viewed, and a green light flashed on one of the nine S-R panels. Following the stimulus presentation, the backlights and the stimulus remained off and either the one-way viewing screen was immediately lowered (0-sec control conditions) or a retention interval was initiated. When the retention interval expired, the one-way viewing screen was lowered, the backlight came on, and the monkey could respond by pushing one of the nine panels. If a correct response was made, the stimulus was reilluminated on the correct panel, a conditioned tone sounded, and a reinforcement pellet was delivered to the exposed reinforcement well. If a response was incorrect, a buzzer sounded, the screen was quickly raised to prevent further responding, and the apparatus was set up for the next trial. The 0-sec control condition was assumed to require relatively little memory for the stimulus location, whereas the longer retention conditions presumably required the stimulus information to be remembered for the duration of the retention interval before the choice response was made.

General Dosing Procedure

Unless specified, all drugs were injected intramuscularly, 30 min prior to the behavioral session. The doses for each drug were selected on the basis of published animal and clinical data (if available) and from previous dose-range studies in our own laboratory. All doses were given in a quasi-random fashion. A maximum of two doses was given per week to each monkey with a minimum of 2 nondrug days separating each drug administration.

Drug and saline control scores were directly compared by computing a nondrug statistical confidence limit for each monkey, which was based on that monkey's own baseline control scores. In this way, it was possible to determine whether a change in performance under any single dose of drug reflected a significant and statistically reliable change from the particular monkey's normal baseline performance.

PHARMACOLOGICAL APPROACHES TO REDUCING AGE-RELATED COGNITIVE IMPAIRMENTS

Historically, many different pharmacological approaches have been used to treat cognitive deficits in elderly and demented patients. Whereas some of these are no longer considered viable therapeutic alternatives, no single approach has yet gained the consensus as the treatment of choice, and the efficacy of all remains controversial. The remainder of this chapter briefly reviews the current rationale of several of these approaches and describes the results of tests performed with the nonhuman primate model just discussed. This review of pharmacological effects in aged monkeys, however, is not intended to provide evidence as to which is the superior approach, for this question can only be answered by testing humans. Rather, these data are presented as one means of objectively selecting from among alternative approaches, to provide direction for further, intensive investigations in humans.

CNS Stimulants

CNS stimulants have historically been used for the therapeutic management of the aged. It has been assumed by clinicians that through their euphoric, mood-lifting, or general energizing effects, CNS stimulants might counteract age-related problems involving fatigue, inattention, learning and memory, motivation, depression, motor dysfunctions, and so forth. Despite this early popularity, the efficacy of such treatments has never been satisfactorily established, and is widely questioned (for review, see Ban, 1980; Crook, 1979; Jarvik et al., 1972). In an attempt to help clarify this issue and provide a basis for direct comparison of the effects of various CNS stimulants with other pharmacological agents, we directly compared four different CNS stimulants (methylphenidate, magnesium pemoline, pentylenetetrazole-niacin mixture, and caffeine) over a range of doses, for their ability to enhance recent memory performance in impaired, aged (19-23 years) and younger, unimpaired rhesus monkeys (5-6 years) on this test procedure outlined earlier (Bartus, 1979c). The first three drugs were selected because of the contemporary claims of possible efficacy in geriatric behavioral disorders, whereas caffeine was tested as a relevant CNS stimulant for purposes of comparison.

This comparison demonstrated that none of four CNS stimulants significantly improved (but often impaired) performance in this memory task. Methylphenidate and caffeine impaired the performance of both age groups, even at relatively low doses. In contrast, magnesium pemoline produced fewer adverse effects and even demonstrated some improvement in performance, although not quite statistically significant ($p < 0.06$). The pentylenetetrazole-niacin mixture resulted in different effects in the two age groups. The young group's responses to this drug followed a typical, progressive dose-response function, with a suggestion of improvement (but not significant, $p > 0.05$) at the lowest dose and a significant impairment at the highest dose. The aged monkeys responded differently to this drug mixture, following an inverted U-shaped function. Significant impairment was seen at the lowest dose, relatively little change in performance at the next two higher doses, and, finally, significant impairment at the highest dose.

These data are consistent with the majority of human clinical literature, which indicates that CNS stimulants generally do not improve and very often impair performance of tasks involving recent memory (Ban, 1980; Crook et al., 1977; Prien, 1973). CNS stimulants also have numerous adverse side effects, such as cardiac stimulation, increased irritability, decreased appetite, rapid development of tolerance, and so forth. To the degree to which conclusions from animal research can be generalized to humans, these data offer little support for the idea that general CNS stimulation represents an effective approach for the treatment of *cognitive* impairments that accompany old age.

Enhancement of Cholinergic Activity

The idea that central cholinergic mechanisms are intimately involved with general learning/memory phenomena was first popularized by Deutsch and colleagues

(1971). Drachman and Leavitt (1974) later proposed that an age-related dysfunction in the cholinergic system might be responsible for the specific memory loss observed in elderly and senile dementia patients. In the last several years, abundant pharmacological, neurochemical, and electrophysiological evidence has accumulated to support a possible cholinergic involvement in age-related memory disorders (for a recent comprehensive review, see Bartus et al., 1982b).

Three separate avenues have been used to enhance cholinergic activity in the elderly. The earliest attempt used was physostigmine, a drug which inhibits acetylcholinesterase activity. Inhibition of this enzyme results in a slower breakdown of acetylcholine in the synapse, thus allowing acetylcholine to remain active for longer periods of time, presumably increasing the degree of stimulation of cholinergic receptors.

Physostigmine has been tested in young adults, with limited improvement found at a single dose and impaired performance at higher doses (Davis et al., 1976, 1978). In aged subjects, relatively little improvement was observed, but only a single dose had been tested (Drachman, 1978; Smith and Swash, 1979). More recently, we evaluated the effect of physostigmine on recent memory in young (5-7 years) and memory-impaired, aged rhesus monkeys (over 18 years), systematically evaluating several doses on all subjects (Bartus, 1979b). The performance of the young monkeys treated with physostigmine was similar to that reported for young humans—no effect at low doses (< 0.01 mg/kg), some improvement at a restricted range of doses (0.01-0.02 mg/kg), and deficits at the highest dose (0.04 mg/kg). Although the aged monkeys also improved at the same general doses, their overall response as a group was much more variable than that for the younger subjects. That is, the performance of some aged monkeys was impaired at low doses which did not affect young monkeys and continued improvement was observed in a few aged monkeys at the highest dose, which typically impaired young monkeys. Since this study, similar effects have been achieved in the elderly humans (Christie et al., 1981; Davis et al., 1979).

In another study using aged Cebus monkeys (over 18 years) very similar results were obtained (Bartus et al., 1980). For example, large intrasubject variability in response to different doses of physostigmine was again observed in the aged monkeys (Fig. 2). That is, certain monkeys were substantially improved by certain doses of physostigmine, whereas other were improved or not affected at all. Thus, as a group, there was little consistency between aged subjects within any single dose. A follow-up study retesting the best dose per individual monkey demonstrated that five out of six monkeys again exhibited a reliable improvement from baseline, with the sixth monkey responding positively at one dose level above the previous best dose (Fig. 3). The results of this "best-dose" paradigm demonstrated that the increased variability of physostigmine in aged subjects was indeed a valid and reliable phenomena. Similar effects have also been reported in elderly humans (Davis et al., 1979).

Another means of enhancing cholinergic activity may be through dietary manipulation of precursors to the cholinergic system. Numerous studies have

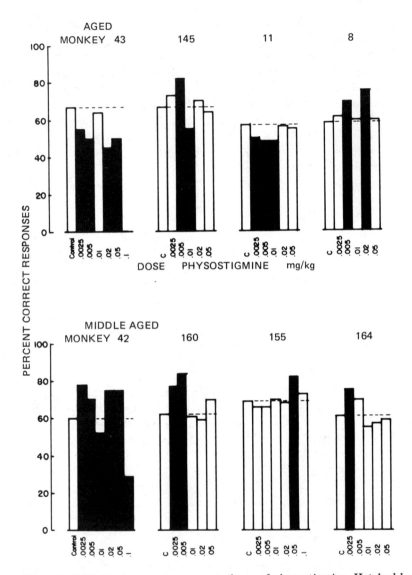

Figure 2 Individual responses to acute doses of physostigmine. Hatched bars indicate drug scores which exceed that aged Cebus monkey's (over 18 years) normal range of baseline control scores (defined on the basis of p = 0.01 confidence limit of all control sessions). (From Bartus et al., 1980.)

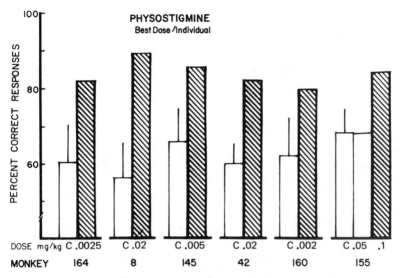

Figure 3 Effects of retesting best dose of physostigmine for each individual aged Cebus monkey, based on dose-response effects obtained in previous study (Fig. 2). (From Bartus et al., 1980.)

demonstrated that dietary or systemic manipulation of choline, the precursor for synthesis of acetylcholine, or lecithin, the normal dietary source of choline, increases central cholinergic activity (reviewed in Haubrich et al., 1979). In addition to the somewhat controversial findings that acetylcholine levels are altered by precursor manipulation, significant increases have also been observed in: (1) the activity of the synthesizing enzyme choline acetyltransferase, (2) the number of nicotinic receptors, and (3) transsynaptic, cholinergically stimulated dopamine activity (for review see Bartus et al., 1983). These biochemical studies, when considered with the cholinergic model for memory deterioration in old age, logically suggest that geriatric cognition might be improved by providing abundant amounts of choline or lecithin. Unfortunately, attempts to treat cognitively impaired elderly with cholinergic precursors have failed to demonstrate reliable or therapeutically relevant effects (Bartus et al., 1982b).

Consistent with these failures in elderly and demented humans, recent tests in our nonhuman primate model revealed that acute choline administration exerted no measurable effects on performance at any dose when tested (Bartus et al., 1980) on the basis of several long-term human clinical trials (Christie et al., 1979; Etienne et al., 1981) and the present monkey data involving a wide range of ineffective doses; it seems doubtful that any dose of choline could be expected to produce consistent effects in aged subjects on cognitive tests. Further neurochemical research is required in order to ascertain whether choline loading necessarily leads to functionally relevant increases in acetylcholine at the *synapse*, as opposed to increases in presynaptic acetylcholine levels which might not be related to neurotransmission. Methodologically, studies which directly measure release, preferably in vivo, are the clear choice.

A third possible means of increasing cholinergic activity is through direct stimulation of the cholinergic receptors by muscarinic agonists (thereby mimicking acetylcholine at the receptor sites). One such potent muscarinic agonist is arecoline. Although arecoline had been reported to improve memory in young subjects (Sitaram et al., 1978), no reports on elderly subjects yet existed. When tested in our aged monkey model, arecoline produced significant improvement over baseline performance (Bartus et al., 1980). Moreover, it differed from physostigmine in that consistent effects across subjects and doses were observed (Fig. 4). These results with aged monkeys have recently been independently corroborated in Alzheimer patients (Christie et al., 1981).

In summary, the general finding of these cholinergic studies is that our results with aged nonhuman primates are similar to the limited data available from the geriatric clinic. That is, similar intrasubject variability in response to physostigmine and repeatability with the best-dose paradigm have been observed in both aged humans and monkeys. Further, choline has generally failed to improve geriatric memory in humans and failed to enhance performance in the aged monkeys. Finally, the consistent improvement across subjects and doses with arecoline that we observed in aged monkeys has also been reported in Alzheimer patients.

Collectively, these results offer a possible (albeit tentative) direction for future clinical testing and drug development. Certainly, the differences found with physostigmine, arecoline, and choline could be due to many factors, including differences in bioavailability, degree of side effects, or other unknown or lesser recognized pharmacological effects of the drugs. However, one possibility suggested by this systematic comparison is that the closer one gets to directly stimulating the muscarinic receptor, the more effective and consistent are the facilitative effects on memory performance of aged subjects.

Enhancement of Catecholamine Activity

There is considerable evidence that catecholamines may be involved in the modulation of learning and memory. In general, the animal literature suggests that in young subjects catecholamine antagonists impair whereas catecholamine agonists will facilitate certain forms of learning and memory (Zornetzer, 1978). Further, numerous age-related changes in catecholamines of the CNS have been reported in several mammalian species (for a recent review, see Kubanis and Zornetzer, 1981). For example, significant decreases in catecholamine levels, turnover rate, and reuptake have been observed in several brain regions in old subjects. Tyrosine hydroxylase. the rate-limiting enzyme in catecholamine synthesis, has also been

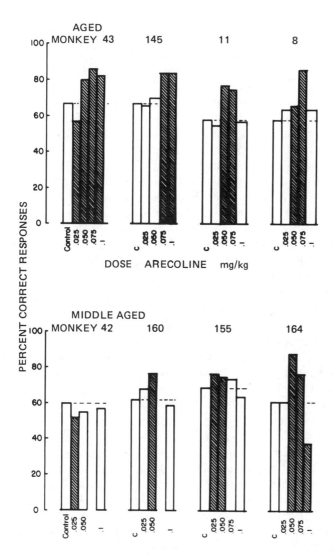

Figure 4 Effects of arecoline, a muscarinic agonist, on memory performance in aged Cebus monkeys. Contrary to the wide variation in the effective dose for each monkey observed with physostigmine (Fig. 2 and text), a more consistent dose-response function between subjects was observed, with 0.05 and 0.075 mg/kg producing reliable improvement in performance. (From Bartus et al., 1980.)

reported to decline with age. Further, neurochemical studies have also demonstrated decreases in catecholamine receptor binding and catecholamine-stimulated cyclic adenosine monophosphate (cAMP) activity in the aged brain. However, a clear relationship between age-related changes in the catecholamine system and the specific memory loss that occurs with age has not been established, and little has yet been done to investigate the role of catecholamine-potentiating drugs on learning and memory in aged mammals. Although several CNS stimulants possess catecholamine-stimulating effects, they fail to significantly improve age-related dysfunctions in cognition both in the clinic and in our model (see previous section). However, this lack of specificity of CNS stimulants and the prominent, adverse side effects associated with stimulants may interfere with their therapeutic effects. We, therefore, tested two other, more selective catecholamine-enhancing drugs, L-dopa (the dopamine precursor) and apomorphine (a dopamine agonist), in aged Cebus monkeys (over 18 years). Contrary to the positive effects obtained with the cholinergic enhancers (physostigmine and arecoline) in this test procedure, neither the dopaminergic agonist nor the precursor was able to induce reliable facilitation in performance. These results are in agreement with several human clinical trials using L-dopa (Gershon, 1980; Kristensin et al., 1977; Parkes et al., 1974; Van Woert et al., 1970). This lack of significant improvement in aged subjects, via catecholaminergic stimulation, is consistent with the inability of catecholamine antagonists to *induce* specific memory *impairments* in *young* subjects. Both haloperidol, a dopamine-receptor blocker (Bartus, 1978), and propranolol, a beta-adrenergic blocker (Bartus, 1980), failed to mimic the specific impairments on memory for recent events observed naturally with aging and pharmacologically with the anticholinergic, scopolamine (Bartus and Johnson, 1976).

Whereas the catecholamine system apparently plays some role in general learning and memory performance, no evidence yet exists that pharmacological disruption of this system can induce the specific memory loss observed in the elderly, nor has stimulation of the system convincingly produced improvement of age-related memory loss. Thus, the role of age-related catecholamine changes in memory performance remains unclear, as well as the potentially beneficial effects of catecholamine stimulation. It is possible that stimulation of the catecholamine system may only improve memory in the elderly that have a functionally intact cholinergic system, or that combining catecholaminergic agents with other drugs may produce particularly beneficial effects. However, to date, no clear empirical evidence exists for their use in treating geriatric memory loss.

Anticoagulants (Antisludging Therapy)

Many theories dealing with the cognitive decline in human aging emphasize the role of cerebral vascular factors, suggesting age-related alterations in the circulatory system contribute to the cognitive impairments of the aged by reducing cerebral blood flow and brain energy metabolism. One postulated alteration is blood sludging, which involves the intravascular adhesion or clumping of red blood cells and is known to occur as a natural consequence of disease or physical trauma. It has been suggested that sludged blood also increases with age and dementia, and may impair brain function through a number of factors, including decreased oxygen availability to the brain as well as alterations in the blood-brain barrier (Bicher et al., 1971; Cullen and Swank, 1954).

Indeed, controversial clinical evidence suggests that sludged blood may play an important role in the etiology of senility. Walsh (1969a,b) reported dramatic behavioral effects resulting from long-term anticoagulant therapy in geriatric patients, and suggested that pharmacological treatment with anticoagulants may reverse and even protect against the resulting age-related behavioral deficits (Walsh and Walsh, 1972). However, as with many clinical studies involving critically ill patients, the studies were not well-controlled by most laboratory standards. As such, the results cannot be considered conclusive and are open to several alternate interpretations.

Relatively little animal data are available on the effects of experimentally increased blood sludging on behavior. Malcolm et al. (1972) reported an impairment in performance on a delayed-discrimination task with chemically induced sludged blood in healthy adult rats. Since an impairment was found only under the delayed condition, and not under the immediate discrimination condition, their data suggested that sludged blood may preferentially impair recent memory and, therefore, could conceivably play an important role in the age-related memory loss. We attempted to evaluate this possibility in greater detail to determine the empirical validity of this approach.

In this study, two interrelated, logical approaches were used (Marriott et al., 1979). In the first, sludged blood was artificially (chemically) induced in younger subjects and their behavior was evaluated for effects on memory performance. The rationale of this approach was that if sludged blood is primarily responsible for age-related decline in recent memory, then induced sludged blood in young, healthy animals should result in behavioral deficits qualitatively similar to those observed in old age. The second approach involved evaluating the blood from young and aged monkeys to determine whether those monkeys with severe memory impairments have increased sludged blood.

In the first procedure, blood sludging was induced in young rats (3 months) with intravenous injections of high-molecular-weight dextran. Previous studies revealed that a 300 mg/kg dose produced a 10-fold increase in the erythrocyte sedimentation rate, a quantification measure of the degree of blood sludging. The performance of the dextran-treated rats on a delayed, spatial alteration task was measured at various delay intervals (15-120 sec) and compared with the nondextran control scores.

The date demonstrated that the accuracy of performance on the delayed alteration procedure was not reduced after the dextran treatment. The only obvious behavioral effect of dextran was a significant drop in the number of trials completed during the session. Further studies revealed that dextran suppressed responding in a dose-dependent manner.

In the second procedure, the blood from young (5-8 years) and aged (18-24 years) rhesus monkeys, who differ significantly in their recent memory ability, was examined to compare the degree of blood sludging in each group and to determine if sludging was correlated with performance on our memory task. Although the aged animals showed a trend toward a higher erythrocyte sedimentation rate, no statistically significant differences were found between the two age groups, and considerable overlap existed between age groups for the degree of sludging. Because a similar overlap does not exist in the memory ability of the two age groups, blood sludging does not appear to be a prominent or consistent feature in the physiological changes seen with aging in rhesus monkeys and does not seem to be well correlated with the memory deficits observed on this task. Whereas claims of the clinical efficacy of anticoagulant therapy in some senile patients require further replication and study to explain such effects, our results offer no support for increased blood sludging as an adequate explanation for age-related impairments in memory, and cannot be used to support further efforts to attempt to treat these impairments with anticoagulation therapy.

Nootropics

Nootropic compounds are a relatively new class of drugs which purportedly exert no sedative or stimulant effects, and have been claimed to improve learning and memory in a number of behavioral paradigms. Four nootropiclike drugs which currently claim controversial efficacy for improving geriatric cognition are piracetam, vincamine, dihydroergotoxine, and centrophenoxine. Whereas their chemical structures are quite different and their specific mechanism(s) of action still unknown, they share some common features (recently reviewed in Bartus and Dean, 1981; Loew, 1980; Scott, 1979).

Biochemically, all are claimed, to some extent, to enhance cerebral energy metabolism as measured by changes in adenosine triphosphate (ATP) turnover, adenylate kinase activity, anaerobic glycolysis, oxygen utilization, glucose utilization, or pCO_2. Interestingly, recent biochemical evaluations of brains from aged subjects have demonstrated that differences in energy metabolism occur as aging progresses, which may contribute to some of the cognitive decline (Gibson, 1982; Gibson et al., 1981).

Pharmacologically, these drugs are most effective under conditions of metabolic stress, such as electroconvulsive shock, hypoxia, or ligated/perfused circulatory systems. Under these conditions, these drugs are reported to preserve EEG or facilitate recovery of EEG, protect or reverse the amnestic effects on learning tasks, and increase survival. As a whole, these studies suggest that these drugs might improve energy metabolism or oxygen/glucose utilization in the aged brain and that these effects might be partly responsible for the positive effects of the drugs in the geriatric clinic.

Because the very efficacy of these drugs is still open to question, representative nootropic drugs were administered to aged monkeys in our model. In the first study, piracetam, vincamine, and dihydroergotoxine were administered to aged rhesus monkeys (over 18 years) chronically in a counterbalanced manner for a minimum of 9 consecutive days (P.O., b.i.d.) (Bartus and Dean, 1981). A washout period of a minimum of 1 week occurred between drugs. The results demonstrated that all three drugs produced some improvement in performance in the aged monkey (Fig. 5). Not all monkeys demonstrated the same qualitative response, for some exhibited clear improvement, others showed no change, and still a few isolated cases showed mild impairments compared with the nondrug control scores. These effects agree with the general findings of many clinical trials (Ban, 1980).

Recently, we compared the effects of chronic administration of piracetam and centrophenoxine in aged Cebus monkeys (over 18 years) and very similar effects were obtained (Bartus and Dean, 1981). Again, certain monkeys exhibited reliable increases in performance, whereas other showed no apparent improvement. The fact that reliable positive effects were obtained with certain memory-impaired subjects, but not others, provides an objective reason to be encouraged that the nonhuman primate may be useful for determining why some elderly patients respond favorably to some of these agents, while others do not. One possibility is that the memory loss seen in aging is the result of a complex, multifaceted etiology and, thus, only a subpopulation of geriatric patients will respond to this type of treatment. Further characterization of this subpopulation to determine possible differences in the behavioral and neurochemical deficits should provide invaluable information to increase our understanding of this problem and to develop effective therapy.

Neuropeptides

In recent years, evidence has accumulated suggesting that neuropeptides of hypothalamic and pituitary origins may influence behavior, independent of their neuroendocrine effects. These extraendocrine effects appear to occur by directly influencing the CNS and are long-lasting, despite the short half-lives of neuropeptides (Kastin et al., 1979).

One current hypothesis is that neuropeptides stimulate their target cells in the brain through receptor-coupled second messenger systems (Wiegant et al., 1981). The action of the second messenger system (i.e., cAMP, cGMP, calmodulin) is the modulation of protein kinase activities, which govern the production and degradation of phosphoproteins. These phosphoproteins then specify the effector cell's response. Thus, neuropeptides function as either neurotransmitters or modulators of neurotransmitters, resulting in a long-lasting neurochemical change (i.e., modulation of nucleic acids and proteins) which is reflected in subsequent behavior.

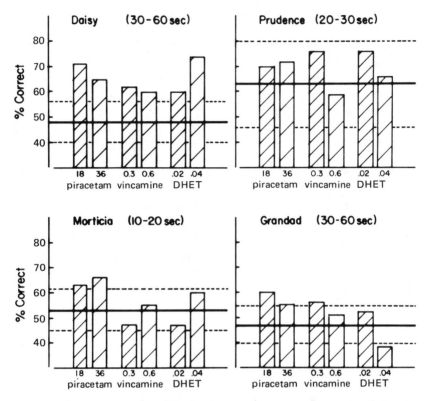

Figure 5 Effects of piracetam, vincamine, and dihydroergotoxine (DHET) on memory performance in aged rhesus monkeys. Heavy horizontal line illustrates the mean of several saline control days and area between dashed lines depicts range of baseline control performance (defined by p < 0.01 confidence limits). Duration of retention interval for each monkey is in parenthesis. (From Bartus and Dean, 1981).

Behaviorally, it has been demonstrated repeatedly that many neuropeptides, particularly vasopressin and adrenocorticotropic hormone (ACTH), affect measures of attention, anxiety, and learning and memory in several mammalian species (for a thorough review, see Rigter and Crabbe, 1979). Interestingly, these are the same behaviors which have been commonly reported in the geriatric literature to be significantly altered with age. Unfortunately, most studies with the cognitively impaired (i.e., mild impairments due to age, dementia, stroke, head injuries, and so forth) have generally failed to show significant improvement with neuropeptides on memory tasks which measure recent memory (for a review of their effects on various forms of cognitive dysfunction, see Ferris et al., 1980; Rigter and Crabbe, 1979).

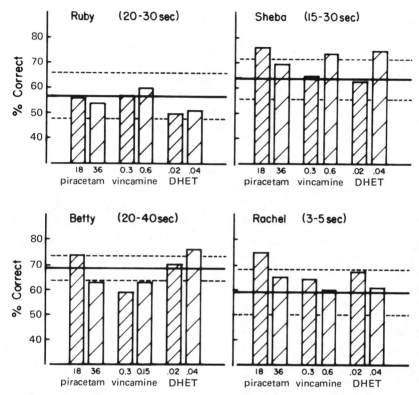

Figure 5   (continued)

To further evaluate the effects of these and other neuropeptides on age-related memory impairments under controlled laboratory conditions, we tested ACTH$_{4\text{-}10}$, lysine vasopressin, arginine vasopressin, oxytocin, and somatostatin in our model (using s.c. injections) (Bartus et al., 1982a). ACTH$_{4\text{-}10}$, the behaviorally active amino acid sequence of the anterior pituitary adrenocorticotropin hormone (ACTH$_{1\text{-}39}$), is devoid of endocrine effects and has been shown to influence learning and memory (De Wied, 1980). Vasopressin, also known as antidiuretic hormone, has two forms. One is lysine vasopressin, which is unique to porcine, but is the form used in several of the earlier clinical trials involving memory. The other is arginine vasopressin and is common to most mammals, including human and nonhuman primates. Oxytocin, which like vasopressin is secreted from the posterior pituitary, has been shown to impair memory in young rats and humans (Bohus et al., 1978a,b; Ferrier et al., 1980). Finally, somatostatin, a hypothalamic hormone which inhibits the release of growth hormones, has been observed to decrease significantly in the brains of Alzheimer patients (Davies and Terry 1981; Rossor et al., 1980) and aged rodents (Hoffman and Sladek, 1980).

None of the neuropeptides produced sufficiently consistent effects across subjects to be reflected by changes in group means. Evaluations of each individual subject against its own baseline performance ($p = 0.001$ confidence limits of all nondrug control days) revealed that all five neuropeptides produced some minimal improvement, but only three of the five did so with any consistency (both forms of vasopressin and $ACTH_{4-10}$). In no case were clear, dose-response functions obtained, even within individual subjects.

Arginine vasopressin appeared to produce the best overall effects, as is depicted in Figure 6, with three of the five monkeys exhibiting significant improvement in performance. The same three monkeys who responded to arginine vasopressin also responded to the lysine form. Once again, the two monkeys who failed to improve with the arginine form of vasopressin also showed no improvement with the lysine form. Although not directly compared, the effects of the arginine form appeared to be somewhat more consistent and robust than those obtained under the lysine form. It may be relevant to these results that the arginine form, but not the lysine form of vasopressin, exists naturally in human and nonhuman primates. Three of the six aged monkeys also performed better under $ACTH_{4-10}$ compared with baseline. However, in two of these cases only a single dose was effective, whereas the third improved significantly on five of six tests (two tests for each of three doses). Very little improvement in performance was observed under any dose of somatostatin or oxytocin.

These data demonstrate that reliable changes in performance on a memory task with aged primates can be achieved, suggesting that certain neuropeptides may indeed play some role in the expression or mediation of memory for recent events. In this vein, the data reported here are somewhat unique in that they eliminate a popular criticism of the current literature that the data have depended too heavily on the testing of *rodents* in *shock*-motivated tasks. Additionally, the improvements observed in this study involve a behavior that is naturally impaired by age and one which has many operational similarities and some empirical relevance to measures of recent memory in humans (Bartus et al., 1983). At the same time, however, even the best effects obtained must be considered quantitatively subtle. In no case were consistent group effects obtained with any single dose of any neuropeptide tested. By comparison, the behavioral results reported by others with rodents in certain shock-motivated tasks appear much more reliable between subjects and more robust in absolute terms (Rigter and Crabbe, 1979). A question of certain importance, therefore, concerns what significance these data from aged monkeys may have. To the extent to which this animal model accurately predicts clinical reality, these limitations on overall improvement seriously question the therapeutic utility of the presently research neuropeptides for treatment of age-related cognitive dysfunctions. At the same time, a consistent finding emerging

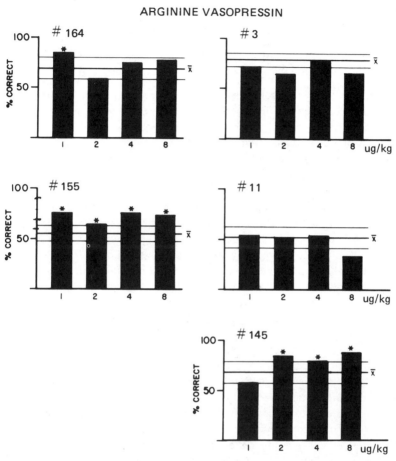

Figure 6 Effect of four doses of arginine vasopressin on performance of a memory task in each of five differently aged monkeys. The mean performance of all non-drug and saline sessions is shown for each individual monkey. Doses of neuropeptides which produced performance exceeding the upper limit of the control scores were considered effective if performance again exceeded the control scores a second, consecutive time. These doses are indicated by the asterisk. Note the wide variation between individual monkeys, with reliable improvement observed in certain monkeys, and no measurable effects in others. (From Bartus et al., 1982.)

from many of the studies in aged monkeys is that certain subpopulation of subjects exist which may respond favorably to several potentially useful therapeutic approaches. However, the current state of the art is such that only subtle improvement can be expected with existing drugs and only in (yet undefined) subpopulations of subjects. Whether the small improvement observed in certain aged monkeys here is indicative of a pharmacological effect that can be related to meaningful clinical improvement in elderly humans remains to be seen.

SYNTHESIS AND DISCUSSION

Earlier research using aged monkeys in this test procedure focused on the spectrum of behavioral changes which occur in learning and memory situations. The profile of changes observed by these studies bore a striking resemblance to the major behavioral deficits observed in elderly and demented humans. They also suggested that aged primates tested in this procedure may provide a valid and reliable model for providing preliminary information on potential geriatric drugs. The series of studies reviewed in this paper were intended to further explore this possibility, and from these studies several conclusions can be drawn.

First, these studies suggest that it is indeed possible to develop procedures with animals to obtain valid information about drugs for treatment of human geriatric memory problems. Not only were certain classes of drugs found to induce modest but reliable improvement in memory in aged monkeys, but the similarity of the results obtained with these series of studies is strikingly similar to the consensus developed from recent clinical studies in humans. In these monkey studies various CNS stimulants, choline, apomorphine, and somatostatin were not effective in improving performance in aged monkeys. The human data have shown that these compounds, with the exception of somatostatin (which has not yet been tested in geriatric humans), also have been generally unsuccessful in improving cognitive dysfunctions. On the other hand, physotigmine, arecoline, several nootropics, and neuropeptides were shown to produce reliable (albeit modest) improvement in aged monkeys tested in this procedure. Once more, similar, modest, positive results have been published with elderly and demented humans. The similarity of these effects in aged monkeys and humans suggests that valid animal models may be used to facilitate the search for therapeutically useful drugs.

In fact, the studies reviewed here may already provide some initial information for this purpose. For example, it is clear that even though statistically reliable improvement can be obtained with certain drugs, wide variance in the most effective dose and high variability within subjects must be taken into account in testing the efficacy of new drugs or in attempting to treat a population of patients which has too often been assumed to be homogenous. More recent successes in aged humans with physotigmine (Davis et al., 1979), using protocols based on prior animal work (Bartus, 1979b), supports this optimistic viewpoint.

These studies with aged monkeys also provide some tentative directions for future studies in geriatric humans. For example, one hypothesis that has emerged from our studies with manipulations of the cholinergic system is that the closer one gets to stimulating the muscarinic receptor, the more effective and consistent are the facilitative effects on memory of aged subjects. Certainly, it will require more than a single study to effectively evaluate this hypothesis. However, if supported with additional data, involving other drugs and replicated in human studies, it may provide a clearer idea of where to look for neurochemical changes which may be responsible for the cognitive impairments and how to effectively reduce the dysfunction by the pharmacological manipulation of the cholinergic system.

Other potentially interesting possibilities involve the use of neuropeptides and so-called nootropics. Although neither class of drug produced remarkable improvement, each, nevertheless, were shown to produce reliable effects within certain subjects tested. These results, therefore, serve to corroborate the weak and controversial effects previously reported in the clinic and encourage continued investigation of certain representative drugs within each of these two classes. In addition to possibly identifying a subpopulation of patients that may be substantially improved, it is plausible that information gained during these studies will ultimately aid in the discovery and development of second-generation drugs which produce even greater effects in a wider range of subjects. The data reported in this paper demonstrate that continued use of valid animal models should facilitate these efforts.

One important advantage of using aged nonhuman primates, particularly in this test situation, is that the individual subject's response to a number of different drugs can be directly compared with individual differences objectively measured and accounted for. Further, variations in response functions eventually can be correlated with several neurochemical parameters, as well as to the degree of memory impairment. This comparison will provide yet additional information to aid in the search for effective drugs. By systematically incorporating the information obtained from animal models into the design of clinical protocols in humans, the goal of achieving truly successful treatments would seem to be a bit more easy.

REFERENCES

Ban, T. A. (1980). *Psychopharmacology for the Aged*. Karger, New York.

Bartus, R. T. (1978). Short-term memory in the rhesus monkey: Effects of dopamine blockade via acute haloperidol administration. *Pharmacol. Biochem. Behav. 9*: 353-357.

Bartus, R. T. (1979a). Effects of aging on visual memory, sensory processing and discrimination learning in the non-human primate. In *Aging, Vol. 10: Sensory Systems and Communication in the Elderly*, J. M. Ordy and K. Brizzee (Eds.). Raven Press, New York, pp. 85-114.

Bartus, R. T. (1979b). Physotigmine and recent memory: Effects in young and aged non-human primates. *Science 206*: 1087-1089.

Bartus, R. T. (1979c). Four stimulants of the central nervous system: Effects on short-term memory in young versus aged monkeys. *J. Am. Geriatr. Soc. 27*: 289-297.

Bartus, R. T. (1980). Cholinergic drug effects on memory and cognition in animals. In *Aging in the 1980's: Psychological Issues*, L. W. Poon, (Ed.). American Psychological Association, Washington, D.C., pp. 163-180.

Bartus, R. T., and Dean, R. L. (1979). Recent memory in aged non-human primates: Hypersensitivity to visual interference during retention. *Exp. Aging Res.* 5: 385-400.

Bartus, R. T., and Dean, R. L. (1981). Age-related memory loss and drug therapy: Possible directions based on animal models in aging, *Aging, Vol. 17: Brain Neurotransmitters and Receptors in Aging and Age-Related Disorders*, S. J. Enna, T. Samorajski, and B. Beer (Eds.). Raven Press, New York, pp. 209-223.

Bartus, R. T., and Johnson, H. R. (1976). Short-term memory in the rhesus monkey: Disruption from the anti-cholinergic scopolamine. *Pharmacol. Biochem. Behav.* 5: 39-40.

Bartus, R. T., Beer, B., and Dean, R. L. (1983). Logical principles in the development of animal models of age-related memory loss. In: *Clinical and Preclinical Assessment in Geriatric Psychopharmacology*, T. Crook, S. Ferris, and R. T. Bartus (Eds.). Mark Powley Assoc., New Canann, Conn., in press.

Bartus, R. T., Dean, R. L., and Beer, B. (1980). Memory deficits in aged cebus monkeys and facilitation with central cholinomimetics. *Neurobiol. Aging 1*: 145-152.

Bartus, R. T., Dean, R. L., and Beer, B. (1982a). Neuropeptide effects on memory in aged monkeys. *Neurobiol. Aging 3*: 40-45.

Bartus, R. T., Dean, R. L., Beer, B., and Lippa, A. S. (1982b). The cholinergic hypothesis of geriatric memory dysfunction: A critical review. *Science 217*: 408-417.

Bartus, R. T., Dean, R. L., and Fleming, D. (1979). Aging in the rhesus monkey: Effects on visual discrimination learning and reversal learning. *J. Gerontol. 34*: 209-219.

Bartus, R. T., Fleming, D., and Johnson, H. R. (1978). Aging in the rhesus monkey: Effects on short-term memory. *J. Gerontol. 33*: 858-871.

Bicher, H. I., Bruley, D., Knisely, M. H., and Reneau, D. D. (1971). Effect of microcirculation changes on brain tissue oxygenation. *J. Physiol. 217*: 689-707.

Bohus, B., Kovacs, G. L., and DeWied, D. (1978a). Oxytocin, vasopressin, and memory: Opposite effects on consolidation and retrieval processes. *Brain Res. 157*: 414-417.

Bohus, B., Urban, I., Van Wimersma Greidanus, T. B., and DeWied, D. (1978b). Opposite effects of oxytocin and vasopressin on avoidance behavior and hippocampal theta rhythm in the rat. *Neuropharmacology 17*: 239-247.

Christie, J. E., Blackburn, I. M., Glen, A. I. M., Zeisel, S., Shering, A., and Yates, C. M. (1979). Effects of choline and lecithin on CSF choline levels and on cognitive function in patients with presenile dementia of the Alzheimer type. In *Nutrition and the Brain, Vol. 5: Choline and Lecithin in Brain Disorders*, A. Barbeau, J. H. Growdon, and R. J. Wurtman (Eds.). Raven Press, New York, pp. 377-387.

Christie, J. E., Shering, A., Ferguson, J., and Glen, A. I. M. (1981). Physostigmine and arecoline: Effects of intravenous infusions in Alzheimer presenile dementia. *Brit. J. Psychiatr. 138*: 46-50.

Crook, T. (1979). Central nervous system stimulants: Appraisal of use in geropsychiatric patients. *J. Am. Geriatr. Soc. 27*: 476-477.

Crook, T., Ferris, S., Sathananthan, G., Raskin, A., and Gershon, S. (1977). The effect of methylphenidate on test performance in the cognitively impaired aged. *Psychopharmacology 52*: 251-255.

Cullen, C. F., and Swank, R. L. (1954). Intravascular aggregation and adhesiveness of the blood elements associated with alimentary lipemia and injections of large molecular substances. *Circulation 9*: 335-346.

Davies, P., and Terry, R. D. (1981). Cortical somatostatin-like immunoreactivity in cases of Alzheimer's disease and senile dementia of the Alzheimer type. *Neurobiol. Aging 2*: 9-14.

Davis, K. L., Hollister, L. E., Overall, J., Johnson, A., and Train, K. (1979). Physostigmine: Effects on cognition and affect in normal subjects. *Psychopharmacology 51*: 23-27.

Davis, K. L., Mohs, R. C., and Tinklenberg, J. R. (1979). Enhancement of memory by physostigmine. *N. Engl. J. Med. 301*: 946.

Davis, K. L., Mohs, R. C., Tinklenberg, J. R., Pfefferbaum, A., Hollister, L. E., and Kopell, B. S. (1978). Physostigmine: Improvement of long-term memory processes in normal humans. *Science 201*: 272-274.

Dean, R. L., Scozzafava, J., Goas, J. A., Regan, B., Beer, B. and Bartus, R. T. (1981). Age-related differences in behavior across the life span of the C57B1/6j mouse. *Exp. Aging Res. 7*: 427-451.

Deutsch, J. A. (1971). The cholinergic synapse and the site of memory. *Science 175*: 788-794.

De Wied, D. (1980). Behavioral actions of neurohypophysial peptides. *Proc. R. Soc. Lond. (B) 210*: 183-195.

Drachman, D. (1978). Central cholinergic system and memory. In *Psychopharmacology: A Generation of Progress*, M. Lipton, A. DiMascio, and K. Killam (Eds.). Raven Press, New York, pp. 651-662.

Drachman, D., and Leavitt, J. (1974). Human memory and the cholinergic system: A relationship to aging? *Arch. Neurol. 30*: 113-121.

Drachman, D. A., and Sahakian, B. J. (1980). Memory and cognitive function in the elderly: A preliminary trial of physostigmine. *Arch. Neurol. 37*: 674-675.

Etienne, P., Dastoor, D., Gauthier, S., Ludwick, R., and Collier, B. (1981). Alzheimer disease: Lack of effect of lecithin treatment for 3 months. *Neurology 31*: 1552-1554.

Ferrier, B. M., Kennett, D. J., and Devlin, M. C. (1980). Influence of oxytocin on human memory processes. *Life Sci. 27*: 2311-2317.

Ferris, S. H., Reisberg, B., and Gershon, S. (1980). Neuropeptide modulation of cognition and memory in humans. In *Aging in the 1980's: Psychological Issues*, L. W. Poon (Ed.). American Psychological Association, Washington, D.C., pp. 212-220.

Gershon, S. (1980). Psychopharmacology of neurotransmitter systems in aging. *Psychopharm. Bull. 16*: 76-77.

Gibson, G. E. (1982). Metabolic assessment of drug effects in aged animals. In *Assessment for Geriatric Psychopharmacology*, T. Crook, S. Ferris, and R. T. Bartus (Eds.). M. Powley Assoc., New Canaan, Conn., in press.

Gibson, G. E., Peterson, C., and Sansone, J. (1981). Neurotransmitter and carbohydrate metabolism during aging and mild hypoxia. *Neurobiol. Aging 2*: 165-172.

Haubrich, D. R., Gerber, N. H., and Pflueger, A. B. (1979): Choline availability and the synthesis of acetylcholine. In: *Nutrition and the Brain, Vol. 5: Choline and Lecithin in Brain Disorders*, A. Barbeau, J. H. Growdon, and R. J. Wurtman (Eds.). Raven Press, New York, pp. 57-71.

Hoffman, G. E., and Sladek, J. R. (1980). Age-related changes in dopamine, LHRH and somatostatin in the rat hypothalamus. *Neurobiol. Aging 1*: 27-38.

Jarvik, M. E., Gritz, E. R., and Schneider, N. G. (1972). Drugs and memory disorders in human aging. *Behav. Biol. 7*: 643-668.

Kastin, A. J., Olson, R. D., Schally, A. V., and Coy, D. H. (1979). CNS effects of peripherally administered brain peptides. *Life Sci. 25*: 401-414.

Kristensin, V., Olsen, M., and Theilgaard, A., (1977). Levodopa treatment of presenile dementia. *Acta. Psychiatr. Scand. 55*: 41-51.

Kubanis, P., and Zornetzer, S. F. (1981). Age-related behavioral and neurobiological changes: a review with an emphasis on memory. *Behav. Neural Biol. 31*: 115-172.

Kubanis, P., Gobbel, G., and Zornetzer, S. F. (1981). Age-related memory deficits in Swiss mice. *Behav. Neurol. Biol. 32*: 241-247.

Lippa, A. S., Pelham, R. W., Beer, B., Critchett, D. J., Dean, R. L., and Bartus, R. T. (1980). Brain cholinergic dysfunction and memory in aged rats. *Neurobiol. Aging 1*: 13-19.

Loew, D. M. (1980). Pharmacologic approaches to the treatment of senile dementia. In *Aging, Vol. 13: Aging of the Brain and Dementia*, L. Amaducci, A. N. Davidson, and P. Antuono (Eds.). Raven Press, New York, pp. 287-294.

Malcolm, R., Bicher, H. I., Duncan, R. C., and Knisely, M. H. (1972). Behavioral effects of erythrocyte aggregation. *Microvasc. Res. 4*: 94-97.

Marriott, J. G., Bartus, R. T., Moyer, C., and Voigtman, R. E. (1979). The effects of blood sludging upon short-term memory in rats and rhesus monkeys: An evaluation of its role in age-related cognitive declines. *Physiol. Beh. 22*: 715-722.

Medin, D. L. (1969). Form perception and pattern reproduction by monkeys. *J. Comp. Physiol. Psychol. 68*: 412-419.

Ordy, J. M., and Schjeide, O. A. (1973). Univariate and multivariate models for evaluating long-term changes in neurobiological development, maturity and aging. In *Progress in Brain Research, Vol. 40: Neurobiological Aspects of Maturation and Aging*, D. H. Ford (Ed.). Elsevier, New York, pp. 25-52.

Parkes, J. D., Marsden, C. D., Rees, J. E., Curzon, G., Kantamaneni, B. D., Knill-Jones, R., Akbar, A., Das, S., and Kataria, M. (1974). Parkinson's disease, cerebral arteriosclerosis and senile dementia: Clinical features in response to levodopa. *Q.J. Med. 43*: 49-61.

Prien, R. F. (1973). Chemotherapy in chronic brain syndrome: A review of the literature. *Psychopharmacol. Bull. 9*: 5-8.

Rigter, H., and Crabbe, J. C. (1979). Modulation of memory by pituitary hormones and related peptides. *Vit. Horm. 337*: 153-241.

Rossor, M. M., Emson, P. C., Mountjoy, C. O., Roth, M., and Iversen, L. L. (1980). Reduced amounts of immunoreactive somatostatin in the temporal cortex in senile dementia of Alzheimer type. *Neurosci. Lett. 20*: 373-377.

Scott, F. L., (1979). A review of some current drugs used in the pharmacotherapy of organic brain syndrome. In *Aging, Vol. 8: Physiology and Cell Biology of Aging*, A. Cherkin, C. E. Finch, N. Kharasch, T. Makinodan, F. L. Scott, and B. S. Strehler (Eds.). Raven Press, New York, pp. 151-184.

Sitaram, N., Weingartner, H., and Gillin, J. C. (1978). Human serial learning: Enhancement with arecoline and choline and impairment with scopolamine. *Science 201*: 274-276.

Smith, C. M., and Swash, M. (1979). Physostigmine in Alzheimer's disease. *Lancet 1*: 42.

Van Woert, M. H., Heninger, G., Rathey, U., and Bowers, M. B. (1970). L-dopa in senile dementia. *Lancet 1*: 573-574.

Walsh, A. C. (1969a). Arterial insufficiency of the brain: Progression prevented by long-term anticoagulant therapy in eleven patients. *J. Am. Geriatr. Soc. 17*: 93-104.

Walsh, A. C. (1969b). Prevention of senile and presenile dementia by bishydroxy-coumarin (Dicumarol) therapy. *J. Am. Geriatr. Soc. 17*: 477-487.

Walsh, A. C., and Walsh, B. H. (1972). Senile and presenile dementia: further observations on the benefits of a dicumarol-psychotherapy regimen. *J. Am. Geriatr. Soc. 29*: 127-131.

Weinberg, J., (1980). Geriatric psychiatry. In *Comprehensive Textbook of Psychiatry Vol. III*, H. I. Kaplan, A. M. Freedman, and B. J. Sadock (Eds.). Williams & Wilkins, Baltimore, pp. 3024-3024.

Wiegant, V. M., Zwiers, H., and Gispen, W. H. (1981). Neuropeptides and brain cAMP and phosphoproteins. *Pharmacol. Ther. 12*: 463-490.

Zornetzer, S. F. (1978). Neurotransmitter modulation and memory: A new neuropharmacological phrenology? In *Psychopharmacology: A Generation of Progress*, M. A. Lipton, A. Dimascio, and K. F. Killam (Eds.). Raven Press, New York, pp. 637-649.

14

Psychopharmacology, Neurotransmitter Systems, and Cognition in the Elderly

Richard C. Mohs and Kenneth L. Davis / *Veterans Administration Medical Center, Bronx, New York, and Mount Sinai School of Medicine, New York, New York*

INTRODUCTION

Currently, it is not possible to treat most cases of cognitive impairment in the elderly effectively. Although a considerable amount of information is available on the neuropathological changes associated with dementing illnesses, this information has not yet led to the development of effective treatments for most dementing illnesses. Recently, investigators have made some progress in understanding the neurotransmitter abnormalities associated with dementing illnesses. It appears that Alzheimer's disease, which is the most common cause of dementia in elderly people, is associated with a specific loss of cholinergic function. Other data suggest that the dementia observed in some cases of Parkinson's disease and the dementia of Korsakoff's syndrome may also be associated with specific neurotransmitter abnormalities. These findings have raised the possibility that some dementias could be treated by administering drugs that help restore normal levels of neurotransmitter activity.

The purpose of this chapter is to review what is known about the neurotransmitter abnormalities in dementia and to summarize recent psychopharmacological studies investigating the cognitive effects of drugs that affect specific neurotransmitter systems. In the sections that follow, we will first review in some detail recent psychopharmacological and neurochemical studies implicating a cholinergic deficit in Alzheimer's disease, and we will discuss the prospects for treating

Alzheimer patients with drugs that increase cholinergic activity. Later we will present evidence for other neurotransmitter deficits in Alzheimer's disease and will mention what is known about the neurotransmitter abnormalities responsible for the cognitive deficits observed in some patients with Parkinson's disease and Korsakoff's syndrome.

CHOLINERGIC DRUGS AND MEMORY

Much of the recent biological work on dementia in the elderly has been concerned with studies of the neurotransmitter acetylcholine. Psychopharmacological and neurochemical studies suggest that this neurotransmitter plays a critical role in normal memory functioning and that a deficit in cholinergic function may be responsible for a large percentage of age-related dementias. Before we review these studies, it will be useful to describe briefly the functioning of cholinergic neurons. Acetylcholine is synthesized in presynaptic nerve terminals from two precursors, choline and acetyl-coenzyme A, in a reaction catalyzed by the enzyme choline acetyl-transferase (CAT). A variety of evidence suggests that the rate-limiting step in acetylcholine synthesis is the transport of choline into cholinergic terminals by a high-affinity uptake system (Jenden, 1979; Simon and Kuhar, 1975). Acetylcholine released into the synaptic cleft is eventually inactivated by the enzyme acetylcholinesterase.

Anticholinergic Amnesia

Many studies have demonstrated that drugs such as atropine, scopolamine, and ditran, which block cholinergic receptors, also cause memory impairments (Drachman and Leavitt, 1974; Ghoneim and Mewaldt, 1975; Ketchum et al., 1973; Peterson, 1977). On tasks that assess the capacity of short-term memory such as the digit span (Atkinson and Shiffrin, 1971), performance is not impaired by anticholinergics (Drachman and Leavitt, 1974; Ghoneim and Mewaldt, 1975; Mohs et al., 1981). However, when subjects must learn new material that exceeds the capacity of short-term memory, performance is substantially impaired by anticholinergics (Drachman and Leavitt, 1974; Ghoneim and Mewaldt, 1975; Mohs et al., 1981). The distinction between short- and long-term memory is fundamental to many current theories of memory (Atkinson and Shiffrin, 1971). Essentially, these theories hold that short-term memory is a limited capacity store used to hold small amounts of information for short periods of time, whereas long-term memory is a more permanent store of unlimited capacity. Studies of patients with hippocampal lesions demonstrate that this structure is necessary for storage of new information in long-term memory (Milner, 1970). Anticholinergic drugs usually do not impair the ability to retrieve information learned prior to drug administration (Drachman and Leavitt, 1974; Ghoneim and Mewaldt, 1975). Stated another way, it appears that the ability to store new information in long-term memory is the aspect of memory most easily disrupted by a decrease in cholinergic activity. The fact that the hippocampus has a high concentration of cholinergic neurons suggests that the amnesic effects of cholinergic drugs are largely mediated by neurons in this brain area (Lewis and Shute, 1978).

In an interesting and provocative series of studies, Drachman and Leavitt (1974) were able to demonstrate that the memory impairments produced by cholinergic blockade in healthy young adults are quite similar to those observed in elderly people showing an age-related memory loss. In elderly people, as well as following cholinergic blockade, there is a diminished ability to store new material in long-term memory, along with a relative sparing of short-term memory capacity and the ability to retrieve material already stored in memory (Drachman and Leavitt, 1974). In other experiments, Drachman (1977) demonstrated that the amnesic effects of anticholinergic drugs are specifically related to the effects of these drugs at cholinergic synapses and are not a result of their sedative properties. Amphetamine, which increases activity at catecholaminergic synapses and produces increased arousal, was not able to reverse the memory impairment produced by scopolamine and, in fact, enhanced the drug's amnesic effects (Drachman, 1977). Physotigmine, on the other hand, which temporarily inhibits cholinesterase and thereby slows the inactivation of acetylcholine, readily reverses the sedative and the amnesic effects of anticholinergic drugs (Drachman, 1977; Grenacher and Baldesserini, 1975).

Cholinergic Deficit in Alzheimer's Disease

Alzheimer's disease is the most common cause of dementia among people over age 55 and may occur in some younger people as well. Most studies indicate that this disorder accounts for between 40 and 60% of all dementias among elderly people (Hachinski et al., 1974; Tomlinson et al., 1970). It has been estimated that this disease afflicts between 600,000 and 1.5 million people in the United States and that it is the fourth or fifth leading cause of death (Katzman, 1976). Neurohistologically, Alzheimer's disease is characterized by large numbers of senile plaques and neurofibrillary tangles, particularly in the hippocampus and in the neocortex (Tomlinson et al., 1970). The earliest and most prominent behavioral symptom associated with this disorder is an impaired ability to store new information in long-term memory, a symptom referred to in the clinical literature as a loss of memory for recent events (Mohs et al., 1982; Roth and Hopkins, 1953; Sim and Sussman, 1962). As the disease progresses, disturbances in the ability to use language and in the ability to execute learned movements usually develop along with other psychiatric and neurological disturbances (Mohs et al., 1982; Sim and Sussman, 1962). The life expectancy for patients who develop dementia of the Alzheimer type is considerably less that the life expectancy for age-matched controls (Go et al., 1978; Roth, 1955).

A major factor in the recent surge of interest in geriatric psychopharmacology was the discovery, first reported in 1976 (Bowen et al., 1976; Davies and Maloney, 1976), that Alzheimer's disease is associated with what appears to be a specific cholinergic deficit. Patients dying with Alzheimer's disease were found to have levels of choline acetyltransferase (CAT) in the hippocampus and cortex that were only 20% of the levels found in age-matched controls. CAT is thought to be located only in presynaptic cholinergic terminals and, thus, is regarded as a marker for intact cholinergic neurons (Kuhar, 1976). Preliminary analyses of enzymes associated with other neurotransmitters, including γ-aminobutyric acid (GABA), dopamine, noradrenaline, and serotonin, revealed that these enzymes were unaffected or were reduced to a much lesser extent (Davies, 1979).

Other reports confirming and extending these findings appeared quickly. It was found that the loss of CAT activity is specifically associated with the neuropathological changes of Alzheimer's disease and does not accompany the vascular changes of multi-infarct dementia (Perry et al., 1977; White et al., 1977). In patients who had been given mental status examinations prior to death, it was found that the loss of CAT activity correlated both with memory loss and with the numbers of senile plaques and neurofibrillary tangles (Perry et al., 1978). These correlations were also found when neurochemical and neurohistological measures were taken from biopsy rather than autopsy material (Sims et al., 1980). A finding of potentially great importance from a psychopharmacological perspective is that receptors for acetylcholine were found to be normal (Perry et al., 1977; White et al., 1977) or only slightly reduced (Reisine et al., 1978). Thus, it is likely that enough cholinergic receptors are present in Alzheimer patients to enable near-normal postsynaptic activity if an appropriate agonist were present.

Enhancement of Memory by Cholinomimetics

An obvious implication of the results discussed above is that drugs which enhance activity at cholinergic synapses might alleviate some of the cognitive deficits in patients with Alzheimer's disease and also possibly enhance memory in normal people. Much of our own work has been devoted to determining whether this is true. Our studies began before the cholinergic deficit in Alzheimer's disease had been reported, and were based primarily on the well-documented amnesic effects of anticholinergic drugs and on the fact that physostigmine, a short-acting cholinesterase inhibitor, reverses these amnesic effects (Grenacher and Baldesserini, 1975).

Physostigmine in Normal Subjects

Our first study was an attempt to determine whether physostigmine could enhance memory in normal subjects. Placebo and either 2 or 3 mg IV physostigmine, doses based on previous clinical studies of physostigmine given to manic patients (Janowski et al., 1973) and patients with movement disorders (Davis and Berger, 1978), were given on separate days (Davis et al., 1976). Contrary to what we had expected, these doses of physostigmine impaired all aspects of memory and produced a generalized stress response accompanied by nausea and neuroendocrine changes (Davis and Davis, 1979). In an effort to avoid the nonspecific stress-related effects of high-dose physostigmine, we subsequently tested the cognitive effects of 1 mg of physostigmine given intravenously over a 1-hr period (Davis et al., 1978). In comparison with placebo, this dose of physostigmine significantly enhanced performance on a learning task that involved storage of information in long-term memory, marginally enhanced retrieval from long-term memory, and had no effect on short-term memory. Thus, physostigmine was most effective in enhancing that aspect of memory that is most impaired by anticholinergics and that is first to be impaired by Alzheimer's disease. Similar enhancement of learning was also demonstrated following the administration of low doses of arecoline, a muscarinic agonist, to healthy young adults (Sitaram et al., 1978).

Studies with Precursors

Efforts to find a safe, long-acting cholinomimetic have been concerned primarily with choline, a precursor to acetylcholine that must be obtained in the diet. Large amounts of choline can safely be given to humans, and data obtained by Wurtman and colleagues (Cohen and Wurtman, 1976; Ulus and Wurtman, 1976) and others (Haubrich et al., 1975) demonstrate that increases in dietary choline or phosphatidylcholine (lecithin) are followed by increases in brain acetylcholine levels. However, clinical studies in which several different doses of choline or lecithin were given to healthy young adults (Davis et al., 1980; Mohs and Davis, 1980), nondemented elderly people (Mohs et al., 1979, 1980) or patients with Alzheimer's disease (Boyd et al., 1977; Etienne et al., 1978) failed to demonstrate any effect of these substances on memory. Preclinical studies have not yet determined whether, and to what extent, choline actually enhances cholinergic activity (Hanin, 1979; Krnjevic and Reinhardt, 1979). Nevertheless, there is evidence that choline's effects might be enhanced under conditions that cause cholinergic neurons to release more acetylcholine. For example, precursor loading with choline prevents the decrease in brain acetylcholine concentration that normally occurs when cholinergic receptors are blocked by atropine (Wecker and Schmidt, 1980; Wecker et al., 1978). A recent clinical study in young adults (Mohs et al., 1981) found that choline also caused a partial reversal of the amnesic effects of scopolamine. In a preliminary study, the combination of lecithin plus piracetam, a drug that may release acetylcholine (Wurtman et al., 1981), was found to produce a global improvement in some Alzheimer patients (Friedman et al., 1981). These results suggest that precursors to acetylcholine might be useful therapeutically if given in combination with other drugs that increase the release of acetylcholine.

Agonists and Cholinesterase Inhibitors in Alzheimer's Disease

Attempts to treat Alzheimer patients, either with cholinergic agonists or with cholinesterase inhibitors, have been limited because few of these drugs are approved for use in humans. An additional difficulty is that physostigmine and arecoline, the most readily available cholinesterase inhibitor and cholinergic agonist, respectively, both have half-lives of less than 1 hr; consequently, they are not easy to administer chronically. What evidence is available, however, indicates that drugs in these classes would be of some benefit to patients with Alzheimer's disease. We tested memory functions in 10 Alzheimer patients after placebo and after three different doses of physostigmine. All patients demonstrated some enhancement of memory storage while receiving one of the physostigmine doses, and this enhancement was subsequently replicated in a double-blind, crossover study comparing placebo with the dose that maximally enhanced each patient's memory (Davis and Mohs, 1983; Davis et al., 1979). Similar results with physostigmine have been reported by a group of British investigators who also found some enhancement of memory in Alzheimer patients given low doses of arecoline (Christie et al., 1981). These studies, together with numerous reports of improvement in individual patients (Muramoto et al., 1979; Peters and Levin, 1979; Smith and Swash, 1979), appear to establish the ability of physostigmine to improve memory in Alzheimer patients. Since the obtained effects have been transient and rather small, an assessment of the clinical utility of cholinesterase inhibitors and cholinergic agonists must await the testing of longer-acting drugs. One potentially useful drug in this regard may be tetrahydroamino acridine (THA), a cholinesterase inhibitor that is clinically active for 6-12 hr in man (Summers et al., 1980). In a preliminary, nonblind study, this drug was reported to improve some aspects of behavior and cognition in a group of Alzheimer patients (Summers et al., 1981).

EFFECTS OF NONCHOLINERGIC DRUGS

Alzheimer's Disease

Although the evidence for a specific cholinergic deficit in Alzheimer's disease is quite compelling, evidence of underactivity in other neurotransmitter systems has also been obtained. In some studies, brains of Alzheimer patients have been reported to have reduced levels of dopamine (Adolfsson et al., 1979), norepinephrine, and serotonin (Mann et al., 1980). The deficits observed in these systems are usually not as great as those reported for the cholinergic system and, in fact, are not observed in all series (Yates et al., 1979).

From a psychopharmacological perspective, few attempts have been made to exploit these noncholinergic abnormalities in Alzheimer's disease and, of the studies conducted, none has demonstrated a significant improvement. Levodopa had no effect on any aspect of cognition or behavior when given to Alzheimer patients over several weeks (Kristensen et al., 1977). Similarly, Alzheimer patients given a combination of tyrosine, 5-hydroxytryptophan (5-HTP), and carbidopa showed no improvement in any aspect of cognition (Meyer et al., 1977). Methylphenidate, a stimulant that increases catecholaminergic activity, also had no effect on memory when given in several different doses to a fairly heterogeneous group of elderly people, some of whom probably had Alzheimer's disease (Crook et al., 1977). These studies, although not conclusive, do not support the notion that the cognitive dysfunction of Alzheimer's disease can be alleviated by enhancing the activity of neurotransmitters other than acetylcholine.

Parkinson's Disease and Korsakoff's Syndrome

Among the many conditions besides Alzheimer's disease that can cause dementia, two are of interest because the cognitive impairment in these conditions may result from specific neurotransmitter deficits. In addition to the motor impairment that is characteristic of the disease, many patients with Parkinson's disease have cognitive impairments that become quite severe in some individuals (Sweet et al., 1976). Early studies indicated that cognitive test performance improved along with motor control when patients were treated with drugs that enhance dopaminergic activity (Meier and Martin, 1970; Sweet et al., 1976). Unfortunately, these studies never convincingly demonstrated that the improved cognitive test performance reflected a direct effect on cognition rather than an effect secondary to improved motor control and motivation. More recent studies indicate that a high percentage of parkinsonian patients have neuronal changes characteristic of Alzheimer's disease when examined at autopsy (Hakim and Mathieson, 1979). These data raise the possibility that the severe forms of parkinsonian dementia are a result of concurrent Alzheimer's disease and, thus, are predominantly a reflection of an Alzheimer cholinergic deficit rather than of the parkinsonian dopaminergic deficit. Future studies will be necessary to determine whether this is true.

Recent studies in patients with Korsakoff's syndrome raise the possibility that a noradrenergic deficit may be responsible for the memory loss associated with this condition. One study found that lowered levels of 3-methoxy-4-hydroxyphenylglycol (MHPG), the primary metabolite of noradrenaline (measured in CSF), were correlated with the degree of memory impairment in patients with Korsakoff's syndrome (McEntee and Nair, 1978). A subsequent study found that clonidine, an alpha-adrenergic agonist, enhanced memory in Korsakoff patients whereas methysergide, a serotonin reuptake blocker, did not (McEntee and Nair, 1980). These results are of particular interest in light of the fact that cholinergic activity in the hippocampus is modulated by noradrenergic inputs (Ladinsky et al., 1980). Thus, one could speculate that the memory deficits of Korsakoff's syndrome and Alzheimer's disease, which are similar in some respects, might both be due to abnormalities in hippocampal neurotransmitter activity; these abnormalities could result from a defect in either noradrenergic or cholinergic neurons for Korsakoff and Alzheimer patients, respectively. Further neurochemical and psychopharmacological studies will be needed to determine the extent to which this speculation is correct.

CONCLUSIONS

Recent work on the neurochemical changes associated with dementing illnesses has raised the possibility that some of these conditions might be treated with drugs that increase neurotransmitter activity. A deficit in cholinergic activity has been established as an important cause of dementia in Alzheimer's disease, and psychopharmacological studies indicate that cholinomimetic drugs can alleviate some symptoms of Alzheimer's disease for brief periods. No satisfactory chronic treatment for this disease has yet been developed. It is not yet clear whether parkinsonian dementia reflects a loss of dopaminergic neurons necessary for normal cognition or whether it is due to the concurrent development of Alzheimer's disease in a high percentage of parkinsonian patients. Studies implicating a noradrenergic deficit in Korsakoff's syndrome may lead to an increased understanding of the interactions between cholinergic and noradrenergic systems necessary for normal cognitive function.

ACKNOWLEDGMENT

The authors' research is supported by United States Public Health Service grant AG-02219 from the National Institute on Aging and by the Medical Research Service of the Veterans Administration.

REFERENCES

Adolfsson, R., Gottfries, C. G., Roos, B. E., and Winblad, B. (1979). Changes in the brain catecholamines in patients with dementia of the Alzheimer type. *Br. J. Psychiatry 135*: 216-223.

Atkinson, R. C., and Shiffrin, R. M. (1971). The control of short-term memory. *Sci. Am. 225*: 82-90.

Bowen, D. M., Smith, C. B., White, P., and Davison, A. N. (1976). Neurotransmitter-related enzymes and indices of hypoxia in senile dementia and other abiotrophies. *Brain 99*: 459-496.

Boyd, W. D., Graham-White, J., Blackwood, G., Glen, I., and McQueen, J. (1977). Clinical effects of choline in Alzheimer senile dementia. *Lancet 2*: 711.

Christie, J. E., Shering, A., Ferguson, J., and Glen, A. I. M. (1981). Physostigmine and arecoline: Effects of intravenous infusions in Alzheimer presenile dementia. *Br. J. Psychiatry 138*: 46-50.

Cohen, E. L., and Wurtman, R. J. (1976). Brain acetylcholine: Control by dietary choline. *Science 191*: 561-562.

Crook, T., Ferris, S., Sathananthan, G., Raskin, A., and Gershon, S. (1977). The effect of methylphenidate on test performance in the cognitively impaired aged. *Psychopharmacology 52*: 251-255.

Davies, P. (1979). Neurotransmitter-related enzymes in senile dementia of the Alzheimer type. *Brain Res. 171*: 319-329.

Davies, P., and Maloney, A. J. F. (1976). Selective loss of central cholinergic neurons in Alzheimer's disease. *Lancet 2*: 1403.

Davis, B. M., and Davis, K. L. (1979). Acetylcholine and anterior pituitary hormone secretion. In *Brain Acetylcholine and Neuropsychiatric Disease*, K. L. Davis and P. A. Berger (Eds.). Plenum, New York, pp. 445-458.

Davis, K. L., and Berger, P. A. (1978). Pharmacological investigations of the cholinergic imbalance hypothesis of movement disorders and psychosis. *Biol. Psychiatry 13*: 23-49.

Davis, K. L., and Mohs, R. C. (1983). Multiple dose intravenous physostigmine in Alzheimer's disease: Enhancement of memory processes. *Am. J. Psychiatry 139*: 1421-1424.

Davis, K. L., Hollister, L. E., Overall, J., Johnson, A., and Train, K. (1976). Physostigmine: Effects on cognition and affect in normal subjects. *Psychopharmacology 51*: 23-27.

Davis, K. L., Mohs, R. C., Tinklenberg, J. R., Hollister, L. E., Pfefferbaum, A., and Kopell, B. S. (1978). Physostigmine: Improvement of long-term memory processes in normal humans. *Science 201*: 272-274.

Davis, K. L., Mohs, R. C., and Tinklenberg, J. R. (1979). Enhancement of memory by physostigmine. *N. Engl. J. Med. 301*: 946.

Davis, K. L., Mohs, R. C., Tinklenberg, J. R. Hollister, L. E., Pfefferbaum, A., and Kopell, B. S. (1980). Cholinomimetics and memory: The effect of choline chloride. *Arch. Nerol. 37*: 49-52.

Drachman, D. A. (1977). Memory and cognitive function in man: Does the cholinergic system have a specific role? *Neurology 27*: 783-790.

Drachman, D. A., and Leavitt, J. (1974). Human memory and the cholinergic system. *Arch. Neurol. 30*: 113-121.

Etienne, P., Gauthier, S., Johnson, G., Collier, B., Mendis, T., Dastoor, D., Cole, M., and Muller, H. F. (1978). Clinical effects of choline in Alzheimer's disease. *Lancet 1*: 508-509.

Friedman, E., Sherman, K. A., Ferris, S. H., Reisberg, B., Bartus, R., and Schneck, M. K. (1981). Clinical response to choline plus piracetam in senile dementia: Relation to red cell choline levels. *N. Engl. J. Med. 304*: 1490-1491.

Ghoneim, M. M., and Mewaldt, S. P. (1975). Effects of diazepam and scopolamine on storage, retrieval and organizational processes in memory. *Psychopharmacologia (Berl.) 44*: 257-262.

Go, R. C. P., Todorov, A. B., Elston, R. C., and Constantinidis, J. (1978). The malignancy of dementias. *Ann. Neurol. 3*: 559-561.

Grenacher, R. P., and Baldesserini, R. J. (1975). Physostigmine: Its use in acute anticholinergic syndrome and with antidepressant and antiparkinson drugs. *Arch. Gen. Psychiatry 32*: 375-380.

Hachinski, V. C., Lassen, N. A., and Marshall, J. (1974). Multi-infarct dementia: A cause of mental deterioration in the elderly. *Lancet 2*: 207-210.

Hakim, A. M., and Mathieson, G. (1979). Dementia in Parkinson disease: A neuropathologic study. *Neurology 29*: 1209-1214.

Hanin, I. (1979). Choline and lecithin in the treatment of neurologic disorders. *N. Engl. J. Med. 300*: 1113.

Haubrich, D. R., Wang, P. F. L., Clody, D. E., and Wedeking, P. W. (1975). Increase in rat brain acetylcholine induced by choline or deanol. *Life Sci. 17*: 975-980.

Janowski, D. S., El-Yousef, M. K., Davis, J. M., and Sekerke, H. J. (1973). Parasympathetic suppression of manic symptoms by physistigmine. *Arch. Gen. Psychiatry 28*: 542-547.

Jenden, D. J. (1979). The neurochemical basis of acetylcholine precursor loading as a therapeutic strategy. In *Brain Acetylcholine and Neuropsychiatric Disease*, K. L. Davis and P. A. Berger (Eds.). Plenum, New York, pp. 483-514.

Katzman, R. (1976). The prevalence and malignancy of Alzheimer disease. *Arch. Neurol. 33*: 217-218.

Ketchum, J. S., Sidell, F. R., Crowell, E. B., Aghajanian, G. K., and Hayes, A. H. (1973). Atropine, scopolamine, and ditran: Comparative pharmacology and antagonists in man. *Psychopharmacologia (Berl.) 28*: 121-145.

Kristensen, V., Olsen, M., and Theilgaard, A. (1977). Levodopa treatment of presenile dementia. *Acta Psychiatry Scand. 55*: 41-51.

Krnjevic, K., and Reinhardt, W. (1979). Choline excites cortical neurons. *Science 206*: 1321-1323.

Kuhar, M. (1976). The anatomy of cholinergic neurons. In *Biology of Cholinergic Function*, A. M. Goldberg and I. Hanin (Eds.). Raven Press, New York, pp. 3-27.

Ladinsky, H., Consolo, S., Tirelli, A. S., and Forloni, G. L. (1980). Evidence for noradrenergic mediation of the oxotremorine-induced increase in acetylcholine content in rat hippocampus. *Brain Res. 187*: 494-498.

Lewis, P. R., and Shute, C. C. D. (1978). Cholinergic pathways in CNS. In *Handbook of Psychopharmacology. Chemical Pathways in the Brain*, L. L. Iversen, S. D. Iversen, and S. H. Snyder (Eds.). Plenum, New York, pp. 315-356.

Mann, D. M. A., Lincoln, J., Yates, P. O., Stamp, J. E., and Toper, S. (1980). Changes in the monoamine containing neurons of the human CNS in senile dementia. *Br. J. Psychiatry 136*: 533-541.

McEntee, W. J., and Nair, R. G. (1978). Memory impairment in Korsakoff's psychosis: A correlation with brain noradrenergic activity. *Science 202*: 905-907.

McEntee, W. J., and Nair, R. G. (1980). Memory enhancement in Korsakoff's psychosis by clonidine: Further evidence for a noradrenergic deficit. *Ann. Neurol. 7*: 466-470.

Meier, M. J., and Martin, W. E. (1970). Intellectual changes associated with Levodopa therapy. *JAMA 213*: 465-466.

Meyer, J. S., Welch, K. M. A., Deshmukh, V. D., Perez, F. I., Jacob, R. H., Haufrect, D. B., Mathew, N. T., and Morrell, R. M. (1977). Neurotransmitter precursor amino acids in the treatment of multi-infarct dementia and Alzheimer's disease. *J. Am. Geriatr. Soc. 25*: 289-298.

Milner, B. (1970). Memory and the medial temporal regions of the brain. In *Biology of Memory*, K. H. Pribram and D. E. Broadbent (Eds.). Academic Press, New York, pp. 29-50.

Mohs, R. C., and Davis, K. L. (1980). Choline chloride effects on memory: Correlation with the effects of physostigmine. *Psychiatr. Res. 2*: 149-156.

Mohs, R. C., Davis, K. L., Tinklenberg, J. R., Hollister, L. E., Yesavage, J. A., and Kopell, B. S. (1979). Treatment of memory deficits in the elderly with choline chloride. *Am. J. Psychiatry 136*: 1275-1277.

Mohs, R. C., Davis, K. L., Tinklenberg, J. R., and Hollister, L. E. (1980). Choline chloride effects on memory in the elderly. *Neurobiol. Aging 1*: 21-25.

Mohs, R. C., Davis, K. L., and Levy, M. I. (1981). Partial reversal of anticholinergic amnesia by choline chloride. *Life Sci. 29*: 1317-1323.

Mohs, R. C., Rosen, W. G., and Davis, K. L. (1982). Defining treatment efficacy in patients with Alzheimer's disease. In *Alzheimer's Disease: A Report of Progress in Research*, S. Corkin, K. L. Davis, J. H. Growden, E. Usdin, and R. J. Wurtman (Eds.). Raven Press, New York, pp. 351-356.

Muramoto, O., Sugishita, M., Sugita, H., and Toyokura, Y. (1979). Effect of physostigmine on constructional and memory tasks in Alzheimer's disease. *Arch. Neurol. 36*: 501-503.

Perry, E. K., Perry, R. H., Blessed, G., and Tomlinson, B. E. (1977). Necropsy evidence of central cholinergic deficits in senile dementia. *Lancet 1*: 189.

Perry, E. K., Tomlinson, B. E., Blessed, G., Bergmann, K., Gibson, P. H., and Perry, R. H. (1978). Correlation of cholinergic abnormalities with senile plaques and mental test scores in senile dementia. *Br. Med. J. 2*: 1457-1459.

Peters, B. H., and Levin, H. S. (1979). Effects of physostigmine and lecithin on memory in Alzheimer disease. *Ann. Neurol. 6*: 219-221.

Peterson, R. C. (1977). Scopolamine induced learning failures in man. *Psychopharmacology 52*: 283-289.

Reisine, T. D., Yamamura, H. I., Bird, E. D., Spokes, E., and Enna, S. J. (1978). Pre- and post-synaptic neurochemical alterations in Alzheimer's disease. *Brain Res. 159*: 477-481.

Roth, M. (1955). The natural history of mental disorder in old age. *J. Ment. Sci. 101*: 281-301.

Roth, M., and Hopkins, B. (1953). Psychological test performance in patients over sixty. I. Senile psychosis and the affective disorders of old age. *J. Ment. Sci. 99*: 439-450.

Sim, M., and Sussman, I. (1962). Alzheimer's disease: Its natural history and differential diagnosis. *J. Nerv. Ment. Dis. 135*: 489-499.

Simon, J. R., and Kuhar, M. J. (1975). Impulse-flow regulation of high affinity choline uptake in brain cholinergic nerve terminals. *Nature 255*: 162-163.

Sims, N. R., Bowen, D. M., Smith, C. C. T., Flack, R. H. A., Davison, A. N., Snowden, J. S., and Neary, D. (1980). Glucose metabolism and acetylcholine synthesis in relation to neuronal activity in Alzheimer's disease. *Lancet 1*: 333-336.

Sitaram, N., Weingartner, H., and Gillin, J. C. (1978). Human serial learning: Enhancement with arecoline and impairment with scopolamine correlated with performance on placebo. *Science 201*: 274-276.

Smith, C. M., and Swash, M. (1979). Physostigmine in Alzheimer's disease. *Lancet 1*: 42.

Summers, W. K., Kaufman, K. R., Altman, F., and Fisher, J. M. (1980). THA-A review of the literature and its use in treatment of five overdose patients. *Clin. Toxicol. 16*: 269-281.

Summers, W. K., Viesselman, J. O., Marsh, G. M., and Candelora, K. (1981). Use of THA in treatment of Alzheimer-like dementia: Pilot study in twelve patients. *Biol. Psychiatry 16*: 145-153.

Sweet, R. D., McDowell, F. H., Feigenson, J. S., Loranger, A. W., and Goodell, H.

(1976). Mental symptoms in Parkinson's disease during chronic treatment with levodopa. *Neurology 26*: 305-310.

Tomlinson, B. E., Blessed, G., and Roth, M. (1970). Observations on the brains of demented old people. *J. Neurol. Sci. 11*: 205-242.

Ulus, I. H., and Wurtman, R. J. (1976). Choline administration: Activation of tyrosine hydroxylase in dopaminergic neurons of rat brain. *Science 194*: 1060-1061.

Wecker, L., and Schmidt, D. E. (1980). Neuropharmacological consequences of choline administration. *Brain Res. 184*: 234-238.

Wecker, L., Dettbarn, W., and Schmidt, D. E. (1978). Choline administration: Modification of the central actions of atropine. *Science 199*: 86-87.

White, P., Hiley, C. R., Goodhardt, J. J., Currasco, L. H., Keet, J. P., Williams, I. E. I., and Bowen, D. M. (1977). Neocortical cholinergic neurons in elderly people. *Lancet 1*: 668-671.

Wurtman, R. J., Magil, S. G., and Reinstein, D. K. (1981). Piracetam diminishes acetylcholine levels in rats. *Life Sci. 28*: 1091-1093.

Yates, C. M., Allison, Y., Sampson, J., Maloney, A. J. F., and Gordon, A. (1979). Dopamine in Alzheimer's disease and senile dementia. *Lancet 2*: 851-852.

15

Vasopressin and Memory During Aging in the Human

Jean-Jacques Legros, Patricia Gilot, and Martine Timsit-Berthier /
University of Liege-Sart-Tilman, Liege, Belgium

Maurice W. M. Bruwier / *Hôpital Geriatrique du Val D'Or, Liege, Belgium*

INTRODUCTION

The concept of neurosecretion, which suggests that neurons secrete peptide-like substances into the circulatory system, emerged from the work of Scharrer and Scharrer in the early 1950s. The first hormones recognized as neuropeptides were vasopressin and oxytocin, which are secreted from neurons terminating in the neurohypophysis. However, later studies showed that many other cells, including those situated outside the CNS (e.g., in the gut), also display neurosecretory properties. In fact, at the present time there are more than 40 different neuropeptides fitting the amine peptide uptake decarboxylation (APUD) concept of A. G. E. Pearse. The early studies on neuropeptides focused on the peripheral (including hypophyseal) actions of these hormones, whereas more recent studies have clearly demonstrated central effects (e.g., vasopressin, angiotensin, TRH, LH-RH, and so forth). Studies on the more recently discovered opioids have simultaneously investigated both types of action. Hence, in the last 15 years, the concept of a peptidergic action on the CNS (and consequently behavior), previously claimed by a few neuropharmacologists and neurophysiologists, has become widely accepted. This chapter will deal primarily with the central influence of one of the first discovered neuropeptides, vasopressin, as it affects memory during aging in man.

Vasopressin is a nonapeptide secreted by the neurohypophysis and synthesized in magnocellular neurons of the supraoptic and paraventricular nuclei, as well as

317

the parvocellular neurosecretory neurons of the suprachiasmatic nucleus. In all species investigated so far, vasopressin and its associated neurophysin are synthesized in neurons separated from those producing oxytocin. The dissociation of these two neuropeptides was demonstrated by Burford et al., (1971) and Sunde and Sokol (1975), who showed biochemically, the absence of vasopressin, but not oxytocin neurophysin, in the brain of Brattleboro rats that are homozygous for diabetes insipidus (i.e., lacking the genetic capability to synthesize vasopressin) (see review in Legros, 1979). Vasopressin neurons are situated in the ventral part of the supraoptic nucleus and the medial part of the paraventricular nucleus, whereas the oxytocin neurons are found in the dorsal part of the supraoptic and lateral part of the paraventricular nucleus (Scharrer and Scharrer, 1954). Gainer et al. (1977) showed that vasopressin and its respective neurophysin are manufactured from a common precursor, a glycopeptide with a molecular weight of 20,000.

The mechanism by which neurohypophyseal hormones are released has been a subject of controversy for some time. Some authors held that the hormones were released by dissociation of the nonapeptide from its carrier (neurophysin) and then discharged into the bloodstream by virtue of their low molecular weight. Based on morphological evidence, others argued that release was mediated by exocytosis (emiocytosis, inverse pinocytosis), during which the whole contents of the neurosecretory granule were emptied into the capillary. According to the first hypothesis, the neurophysins, which are of greater molecular weight and nondiffusible, remain in the cell where they are broken down. The second hypothesis requires that neurophysins be present in the blood and their levels be raised under conditions of neurohypophyseal activation.

In 1968, Ginsburg and his group (Ginsburg, 1968; Ginsberg and Jayasena, 1968) extracted a substance that was immunologically related to the neurophysins from pig blood. Also in 1968, Fawcett, Powell and Sachs demonstrated that a substance with a molecular weight close to that of the neurophysins was released after hemorrhage induced in dogs given a hypothalamic perfusion of labeled cystine. In 1969, we developed a radioimmunoassay for human neurophysins (Legros et al., 1969) and showed that serum levels of these carrier proteins change under different physiopathological conditions, pregnancy, and in response to the injection of estrogens (Legros and Franchimont, 1970). Furthermore, we have shown that when isolated rat neurohypophyses are electrically stimulated (Nordmann et al., 1971) or exposed to increased extracellular potassium concentration (Matthews et al., 1973), there is a concomitant release of neurophysins and biologically active hormones. This simultaneous release of neurophysins and hormones has been confirmed in vivo by several investigators during hemorrhage in goats (McNeilly et al., 1972) or pigs (Dax et al., 1977), after administration of estrogens in the rat (Legros and Grau, 1973), and after inhalation of cigarette smoke in humans (Robinson, 1975). Once they have been released, the hormones apparently dissociate from the neurophysins. They might be bound to one or more plasma proteins; however, these hypothetical complexes have not been isolated nor have their characteristics been described.

In man, besides the hypothalamopituitary tract, vasopressin- and neurophysin-containing fibers from magnocellular neurons also project via the stria terminalis to the central amygdala. Descending fibers are distributed to the solitary nucleus in the medulla oblongata, the central gray and lateral parts of the spinal cord. In addition, vasopressin fibers originating in the parvocellular neurons of the suprachiasmatic nucleus are directed to the lateral septum, posterior hypothalamus, interpeduncular nucleus, mediodorsal thalamus, lateral habenula, and preventricular gray of the brain stem. In addition, fine fibers are present in the medial amygdala and the ventral hippocampus (Weindl and Sofroniew, 1979). The wide distribution of vasopressin fibers in the brain and their connection with the limbic system strongly suggest that vasopressin may have important neuromodulatory and behavioral effects in mammals. Indeed, a great deal of evidence has accumulated supporting a role of vasopressin in learning and memory in rats (van Wimmersma-Greidanus and Versteeg, 1980). De Wied was the first to report that the extinction of a conditioned avoidance response in rats is markedly accelerated after the removal of the posterior pituitary lobe. Subsequent studies have shown that treatment with a posterior pituitary extract or vasopressin restores the posterior lobectomized animal's extinction score to control values (De Wied, 1965; De Wied et al., 1976). The implication that vasopressin is involved in memory processes is further supported by the finding that *intraventricular* administration of vasopressin antiserum, after a learning trial, leads to a deficit in passive avoidance retention, whereas *peripheral* administration of the antiserum has no effect on behavior (Van Wimmersma-Greidanus and Versteeg, 1980).

CLINICAL STUDIES IN THE ELDERLY

In light of the animal studies and the fact that neurophysin levels decrease between the ages of 50 and 60 in man (Legros, 1975), we assessed the effect of vasopressin on memory function during aging. The results of these two studies are summarized in Tables 1-5.

The first study was a double-blind study in 23 male patients (aged 50-65 years) who were free from metabolic, cardiovascular, and psychiatric diseases. Twelve randomly selected men received 16 IU of lysine vasopressin (LVP) per day intranasally (divided in three doses), and 11 men received placebo for 3 days. In addition to clinical (i.e., weight, pulse rate, blood pressure) and biological (i.e., urinary volume, serum and urine osmolarity, blood urea nitrogen, proteins, and sodium plasma levels) measurements, psychological measures were also made, including evaluation of mood, attention (KT, WAIS: digit symbol), and memory (PRM, 15 words, 30 figures, complex figures of Rey). All measurements were made before and after the 3-day treatment period with LVP or placebo. No statistically significant changes were noted in the clinical, biological, and mood evaluations. However, the psychometric tests revealed statistically significant differences (median-Tests-21 statistics) between the two groups of subjects. The subjects

Table 1 Major Characteristics of Two Clinical Studies on the Effect of Exogenous Vasopressin on Memory Function During Aging

Study 1		
Placebo: n = 13	Nasal spray	Clinical, biological, and endocrinogical data at days 0 and +3
Age = 60 ± 5		
LVP: n = 12	3 days	Psychological testing at days 0 and + 3 (KT, WAIS, PRM, BENTON, 15 words, 30 figures, complex figure, BS, BS', LH, LH', LV)
Age = 59 ± 6	7 a.m., 2 p.m., and 9 p.m. (± 16 IU per day)	
Study 2		
Placebo: n = 8	Nasal spray	Clinical, biological, and endocrinological data at days, 0, +7, and +14
Age = 80 ± 4		
LVP: n = 12	14 days	Psychological testing at days 0 and +14 (PRM, BENTON, complex figure)
Age: 79 ± 8	7 a.m., 2 p.m., and 9 p.m. (± 16 IU per day)	

Table 2 Summary of the Clinical Data Obtained Before and After LVP Treatment (Mean ± S.D.) in Two Studies on the Effect of Vasopressin on Memory During Aging

	Study 1 (age = 60; 3 days)			Study 2 (age = 80; 14 days)		
	Before	After	p	Before	After	p
Weight	76.1 ± 8.9	75.8 ± 9.1	NS	58.4 ± 10.9	57.6 ± 11.1	NS
Pulse rate	82 ± 8	81 ± 8	NS	82 ± 4	81 ± 4	NS
BP (systolic)	12 ± 1	12 ± 1	NS	12 ± 1	13 ± 2	NS
BP (diastolic)	8 ± 1	7 ± 1	NS	7 ± 1	8 ± 1	< 0.05
ECG	Not recorded			No significant change		

Table 3 Summary of the Biological Data Obtained Before and After LVP Treatment (Mean ± S.D.) in Two Studies on the Effect of Vasopressin on Memory During Aging

	Study 1 (age = 60; 3 days)			Study 2 (age = 80; 14 days)		
	Before	After	p	Before	After	p
Serum urea	39.1 ± 6.2	42.1 ± 3.4	(< 0.1)	35 ± 12.4	38 ± 8.5	(< 0.1)
Serum proteins	6.4 ± 2.6	6.4 ± 4.7	NS	7.2 ± 0.5	6.9 ± 0.4	(< 0.1)
Hemoglobin	–	–	–	13.3 ± 0.9	12.6 ± 1.3	(< 0.005)
Plasma Na	145.1 ± 2.9	142.7 ± 4.9	NS	142.6 ± 3.4	142.1 ± 3.2	NS
Serum osmolality	289.3 ± 5.6	290.1 ± 4.7	NS	290.5 ± 11.1	290.4 ± 11.8	NS

receiving LVP performed better in tests of attention, concentration, and motor rapidity (KT Attention Test and WAIS Digit Symbol Test), and in memory tests using visual graphic material for the measurement of visual retention (30 figures of Rey) and recognition (subtests 2,5,3, and 4 of the PRM and complex figures of Rey). Using audio-verbal material, it was found that LVP improved attention and immediate memory (WAIS Digit Span) as well as learning and recognition (15 words of Rey) (Legros et al., 1978).

Table 4 Summary of Some Psychometric Data Obtained Before and After LVP Treatment (Mean ± S.D.) in Two Studies on the Effect of Vasopressin on Memory During Aging

	Study 1 (age = 60; 3 days)			Study 2 (age = 80; 14 days)		
	Before	After	p	Before	After	p
PRM						
2	12 ± 3	15 ± 3	<0.01	9 ± 4	8 ± 3	NS
3	14 ± 3	15 ± 3	NS	5 ± 5	4 ± 3	NS
4	12 ± 3	15 ± 2	<0.01	4 ± 4	4 ± 3	NS
5	15 ± 4	19 ± 2	NS	9 ± 5	8 ± 5	NS
6	12 ± 3	15 ± 2	<0.01	7 ± 3	5 ± 4	NS
7	12 ± 2	15 ± 3	<0.05	6 ± 4	5 ± 4	NS

Table 5 Summary of Some Psychometric Data Obtained Before and After LVP Treatment (Mean ± S.D.) in Two Studies on the Effect of Vasopressin on Memory During Aging

	Study 1 (age = 60; 3 days)			Study 2 (age = 80; 14 days)		
	Before	After	p	Before	After	p
Benton total	4 ± 2	6 ± 2	NS	1 ± 1	1 ± (2)	NS
Error	9 ± 4	6 ± 3	NS	20 ± 6	21 ± 8	NS
Complex Figure	19 ± 6	21 ± 5	<0.01	5 ± 4	5 ± 6	NS

The second study was carried out in 20 male inpatients (aged 73-91) hospitalized for minor medical reasons or social problems. Using a double-blind procedure, 8 subjects received placebo whereas 12 received LVP for 14 days. In this study, we were particularly interested in the possible side effects of the longer LVP treatment period and factors which could influence the response to LVP treatment. Therefore, in addition to the usual biological and clinical data, we also recorded one electrocardiogram (ECG) before treatment, and at 7 and 14 days after treatment was initiated. The ECGs were analyzed by a cardiologist unaware of the treatment each patient received. Further, since in the first study some patients on LVP claimed to be improved, while no positive changes were noticed in the objective psychometric tests, a blind clinical evaluation was performed by nurses after 2 weeks of treatment. Patients were rated as 0, no significant improvement; +, slight improvement; and ++, definite improvement with an increase in social contacts which in *all cases* was noted from the third to fifth day of treatment.

Basal psychometric scores were very low with no significant improvement noticed after the 2 weeks of therapy. In contrast, the nurse's rating revealed that 5 of 12 patients receiving LVP showed a ++ improvement. This improvement was not noticed in any subjects in the placebo group (Table 6). Upon considering the various psychological scores and clinical and biological data which could differentiate the responder (R) from the nonresponder (NR) in the LVP treatment group, we saw two major differences. The responders had a lower basal (before treatment) neurophysin level (IRN) and higher blood pressures than the nonresponders (Table 7).

Apart from our own data in the elderly, some preliminary results suggest that vasopressin may be useful for treating incipiens mental retardation due to Alzheimer's type of senile dementia (Delwaide et al., 1980; Weingartner et al., 1981). However, negative results have also been obtained by Tinklenberg and Berger (1981) in seven men aged 47-60 (four alcoholic, three presenile dementia) using Des-Amino-Des-Arginine Vasopressin, (DDAVP;Minrin) for 3-8 days. In this study, however, a slight improvement was noted in three of the less impaired patients. Tinklenberg and Berger (1981) concluded that "any effectiveness of DDAVP may be restricted to clinical populations with minor cognitive impairments and that dosages greater than what are customarily used in endocrinology are required for behavioral effects."

ENDOGENOUS NEUROPITUITARY FUNCTION AND MEMORY IN THE HUMAN

As mentioned earlier, a number of studies in the rat support the hypothesis that endogenous vasopressin has a physiological role in cognitive function. In this regard, it is of interest to note that certain drugs acting upon the central cholinergic system and improving the consolidation phase of memory (i.e., nicotine, physostigmine, arecholine, and choline) also affect vasopressin release.

To our knowledge, there are no data on neurohypophyseal function in humans suffering from posttraumatic amnesia. On the other hand, a transient (1-8 day) diabetes insipidus, in which vasopressin release and/or synthesis is decreased, often occurs during the decay of posttraumatic coma.

Table 6 Subjective Improvement (Nurse Rating) in 12 Patients Aged 79 ± 8 Receiving LVP for 14 Days and in 8 Patients Aged 80 ± 4 Receiving Placebo for the Same Period (see text for rating score). The Differences Between the two Groups are Significant ($p = 0.05$).

	0	and	+	++
Placebo	4		4	0
LVP	3		4	5

Table 7 Major Clinical and Biological Data in the Patients (aged 79 ± 8 years) Having Received LVP for 14 days. Results are Divided into Two Groups: Responders (R) and Nonresponders (NR)

	R (++) n: 5	NR (0, +) n: 7	
Age	81.6 ± 8.1	77 ± 7.5	NS
Weight	73.4 ± 16.6	58.7 ± 10.7	NS
Basal neurophysin (IRN) (ng/ml)	0.96 ± 0.75	2.36 ± 1.5	<0.05
Osmolality (mOsm/kg)	288 ± 8.5	293.3 ± 12.5	NS
BP before	12.1 ± 1.7	12.7 ± 1.8	NS
	6.6 ± 1.1	6.8 ± 0.9	
BP after	14 ± 2.9	12.4 ± 1.3	NS
	7.6 ± 1.4	6.7 ± 0.7	
	max. p = 0.1	max. p = NS	
	min. p = 0.01	min. p = NS	

Clinical data are also lacking in patients suffering from central diabetes insipidus. In fact, few of these patients may be studied, since the disease often occurs secondary to other organic inflictions or trauma involving other hypothalamic nuclei and endocrine functions. Although not studying memory specifically, Waggoner et al. (1978) noted that treatment with DDAVP in eight children suffering from diabetes insipidus elicited an increase in their "creative capacity." Subsequently, our group (Gilot et al., 1980) studied five patients suffering from a familial central diabetes insipidus which is a rare affliction similar to that found in Brattleboro rats. In these patients, we found that withdrawal of substitutive therapy for 8 days produced low scores on memory tests. Although it was not possible to delineate a specific type of memory disturbance, there was a general improvement in memory noted in the scores of all patients 3 days after resuming therapy. This improvement was observed mainly in those patients whose scores were the lowest during the first session; however, only the Benton test was significantly improved in all five patients. Hence, these results support the hypothesis of a role for endogenous vasopressin in memory in man.

In a study designed to determine the action of exogenous vasopressin in the normal man aged 50-65, we found a relationship (r = 0.47) between the basal levels of neurophysins (IRN) and item 7 of Rey's PRM before any treatment (placebo or vasopressin). No correlation was found with the other items of the test or between item 7 and LH, FSH, GH, prolactin (hPr), testosterone, and 17-β-estradiol levels. Since item 7 of Rey's PRM more specifically explores the consolidation phase of memory, these results are in agreement with the experimental data in the rat concerning the role of vasopressin.

In a second study, we found the same trend although the differences were not significant. However, when all the values were pooled (N = 39), there was a significant relationship between IRN levels and item 7 of Rey's PRM (r = 0.38, p < 0.05) which was not found with the other items of this test (Fig. 1).

It is noteworthy that peripheral hormonal levels give a poor index of the CSF levels. It has been previously demonstrated that there is no relationship between plasma and CSF neurophysins (Robinson and Zimmerman, 1973) or AVP (Jenkins et al., 1980) levels. Thus, the correlation of psychoendocrine measures with blood hormone levels could simply mean that these two parameters have similar temporal changes within a given age group (e.g., 50-60 years). This may be due to the preferential central regulation of neuropituitary release at that age, whereas in older subjects (e.g., 73-91 years) neurophysin blood levels represent more the metabolic and physiological (i.e., kidney function) states of the patients. Indeed,

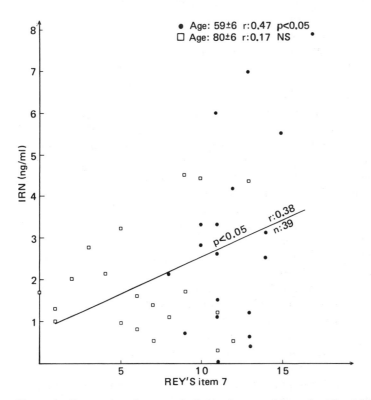

Figure 1 Comparison between individual score of item 7 of Rey's PRM and basal neurophysins (IRN) levels in two different groups of patients: 19 patients aged 59 ± 6 years and 21 patients aged 80 ± 6 years. When all the values are pooled, there is a significant psychoendocrine relationship (r = 0.38, p = 0.05). (From Legros et al., 1980.)

the neurophysin levels are somewhat higher after the age of 70 than between 50 and 70. An explanation for the late increase in neurophysins is that, as suggested by clinical studies, in extreme age tubular defects induce variable responses of AVP release (Legros, 1978; Legros et al., 1980).

MECHANISM OF ACTION OF VASOPRESSIN IN MEMORY

The principal actions of vasopressin on memory function are summarized in Table 8. Although our results obtained from elderly individuals do not rule out the possibility that the subjective improvement resulting from vasopressin treatment is due, in some patients, to general cardiocirculatory effects of the peptide, a number of recent studies demonstrate a CNS action of vasopressin through this hormone's effect on the turnover of monoamines.

It has been shown previously that several limbic structures are involved in the consolidation of memory and in the retrieval of stored information. These include the rostral septal area, the region of the parafascicular nucleus of the thalamus, and the dorsal hippocampus (Van Wimmersma-Greidanus and Versteeg, 1980). In two of these regions, the dorsal septal nucleus and the parafascicular nucleus, norepinephrine (NE) turnover is enhanced by intraventricular vasopressin administration, suggesting that the effect of vasopressin in memory processes is mediated by increased NE turnover in these regions. Data obtained from Brattleboro homozygous rats showed that these rats have altered brain catecholamine turnover in a direction opposite to that induced by intraventricular vasopressin administration (Telegdy and Kovacs, 1979). Furthermore, the intraventricular administration of vasopressin antiserum decreases NE turnover in the dorsal septal nucleus, the parafascicular nucleus, and the rostral part of the solitary nucleus (Van Wimmersma-Greidanus and Versteeg, 1980). Further support for the hypothesis that vasopressin affects memory consolidation through a NE mechanism was provided by the work of Kovacs and co-authors (1979) who showed that the destruction of the ascending dorsal NA bundle with 6-OH-dopamine abolished the effect of vasopressin on memory consolidation in rats.

In humans, noninvasive neurophysiological methods have been used to study the influence of vasopressin on brain function. The most commonly used technique is the spontaneous electroencephalographic (EEG) recording. These records reflect basis bioelectrical states of the brain which can be analyzed by mathematical methods (i.e., Fourier analysis, period analysis). The EEG sometimes contains subtle variations in electrical activity which can be interpreted by these methods. This quantitative EEG approach provides a very precise analysis of the various properties of psychoactive drugs.

Evoked potentials (EP), which directly reflect the arrival of a stimulus at the site of the sensory areas, also furnish important information about brain activity. Slow-evoked potentials, also called event-related potentials, among which are the contingent negative variation (CNV), and the late positivity of the evoked potential

Table 8 Summary of Some Experimental Elements Adduced as Evidence for and Against Certain Possible Modes of Action of Vasopressin on the Central Nervous System, in Particular on the Memory Consolidation Phase

Possible mode of action	For	Against	Experimental elements
Action on water and ion metabolism		X	Effectiveness of DGLVP (des-9-glycinamide-8-lysine-vasopressin) on the memory, whereas this peptide has no action on the water and ion metabolism in animals and man (Flexner et al., 1977)
		X	No action on the water metabolism in normal human beings at dose exerting an effect on the attention and memory (Legros et al., 1978)
Action on paradoxical sleep	X		Increase in hippocampal theta rhythms in rats treated with vasopressin (Urban and de Wied, 1978)
Neuromediator-like action	X	?	Demonstration of recurrent inhibition in the monkey (Vincent and Arnauld, 1975), but this phenomenon is also found in the Brattleboro rat which produces no vasopressin
CRF-like action (corticotropin-releasing factor)		X	Long-lasting psychological action which is different from that of ACTH (de Wied and Gipsen, 1977)
		X	No release of peripheral ACTH in clinically effective doses in man (Audibert, personal communication)
Action on the synthesis of cerebral proteins	X	?	Effectiveness of vasopressin in the case of puromycin-induced amnesia, but puromycin also disturbs the metabolism of cerebral catecholamines in the rat (Flexner and Goodman, 1975)
Action on the cerebral phosphorylases	X		Increase in the activity of the total cerebral phosphorylases in the rabbit under the influence of vasopressin (Constantinescu, 1968)
Action on the turnover of cerebral amines	X		Increase in the turnover of neuronal noradrenaline (Tanaka et al., 1977)
		X	No action on the turnover of dopamine (contrary to what is observed in the case of $ACTH_{4-10}$) in the mouse (Iuvone, et al., 1978)
		X	Increase in serotonin content of hippocampus in the DGLVP-treated rat (Ramaekers et al., 1977)

Source: From Legros, 1979.   **327**

constitute an actual interface between elementary neuronal activities and complex psychological processes. They express the subject's personal option towards the stimulus and experimental situation, although these electrical events have received little investigation.

Quantitative EEG analysis (spectral analysis) of healthy volunteers showed that an intramuscular injection of 10 IU LVP was followed by an increase in delta waves and a decrease in alpha waves. These changes appeared after 1 hr and persisted up to 6 hr after injection. It should be noted that in these healthy volunteers LVP injected intramuscularly provoked paling of the face and discomfort, together with an irresistible feeling of drowsiness. On the other hand, nasal spray administration of 15 IU of LVP did not affect the quantitative EEG measurements (Timsit-Berthier et al., 1978).

Classical visual EEG analysis (i.e., without any mathematical treatment) was also performed in amnesic patients after chronic nasal spray administration of 15 IU of LVP for 15 days. LVP induced spikes and spike and wave forms diffusely over the cortex without generating seizures (Timsit-Berthier et al., 1979). These functional disturbances disappeared quickly after treatment was discontinued.

The *contingent negative variation* (CNV) may be most useful for interpreting the effects of vasopressin on CNS neural activity. To understand its full significance, it is necessary to remember that the CNV develops as a negative shift in the potential recorded during a simple time-reaction task in which a warning stimulus is first presented. The amplitude of the negative wave varies with the arousal level, attention, and motivation of the subject. In control conditions, the subject's interest in the task normally diminishes as time passes, and his successive CNVs decrease in amplitude. This apparent habituation of the negative wave thus develops both short-term (i.e., within the experimental session) and long-term (i.e., between sessions) when the experiment is repeated.

CNV amplitude is always maximal at the beginning of the first recording session. The administration of 15 IU LVP (nasal spray) in young volunteers tends to reduce this spontaneous diminution of the CNV amplitude and to slow down the course of habituation, both short-term (i.e., within hours following a first recording) and long-term (i.e., within weeks following a first recording). More precisely, it has been shown that LVP tended to increase the relative amplitude of CNVs from 0.5-6 hr after nasal spray administration (Timsit-Berthier et al., 1980). Most of these modifications of the CNV are compatible with, but not specific to, an increase in dopaminergic brain function.

The cholinergic system, due to its critical involvement in senile dementia (Perry, 1979) and in memory processes in man (Sitaram et al., 1978), has also received attention. Indeed, septal-hippocampal cholinergic pathways are known to be involved in the storage of memory. In man, the amnesia produced by lesions of the hippocampal complex is characterized not only by the severity of memory storage impairment but also by the isolated occurrence of memory impairment. Furthermore, the pattern of cognitive changes in aging and dementias is similar to that seen after cholinergic blockade (Sitarem et al., 1978); and it is interesting that vasopressin release is, at least partly, under cholinergic control. Last, many of the effects of vasopressin on memory, such as increased attention and increased memory consolidation, resemble those produced by nicotine (see Remond and Isard, 1978, for review).

It is of interest to determine how vasopressin reaches its target sites in the brain. Few studies have been devoted to the passage of vasopressin through the blood-brain barrier. According to Landgraf et al. (1979), experimental data in the rat indicate that vasopressin not only enters the brain but also accumulates in the blood-barrier system. A frequently used route for vasopressin administration in clinical practice is intranasal spray. It is interesting to note that besides a rapid passage in the blood, a slow passage of the substance through the nasal mucosa to the CSF, presumably through a direct transport in the perineural sheath of the olfactory nerves, has been observed (Gopinath et al., 1979).

CONCLUSIONS

The action of vasopressin on the brain in the human is now well established. Although some psychopharmacological and clinical psychological arguments favor the hypothesis of action of the consolidatory phase of memory, wider, less specific actions on attention, arousal, and emotion may also exist, perhaps through peripheral actions of this hormone.

In particular, a specific action on long-term memory and on attention has been described between the ages of 50 and 65, while a less specific action on social integration has been demonstrated after the age of 70 in humans. In the latter group, the beneficial effect could be related to a peripheral action of the peptide on the cardiocirculatory system. In Alzheimer patients, an improvement on memory test was noticed only in patients with the incipiens form of dementia. This suggests that vasopressin might be beneficial if used as soon as the first symptoms or psychological deficits are noted.

The perfection of structural analogues of the neurohypophyseal peptides, which are free from undesirable antidiuretic action, should result in a wider scope for their use in therapy. Furthermore, the identification of better neuropsychological and neuroendocrine parameters could be useful to more accurately predict those individuals responsive to vasopressin treatment. The identification of such parameters would not only provide a means for identifying those patients who would benefit from treatment, but would also help to better understand the mechanism of action of this neuropeptide.

ACKNOWLEDGMENT

The work described in this review was supported by grants from the Belgian FRSM and the Fondation Reine Elisabeth. This text was typed by Miss Monique Foder.

REFERENCES

Burford, G. D., Jones, C. W., and Pickering, B. T. (1971). Tentative identification of a vasopressin-neurophysin and an oxytocin-neurophysin in the rat. *Biochem. J. 124*: 809-813.

Constantinescu, J. (1968). Action de la vasopressine sur la phosphorylase cerebrale. *Rev. Rom. Physiol. 5*: 231-238.

Dax, E. M., Cumming, I. A., Lawson, R. A. S., and Johnston, C. I. (1977). The physiological release of specific individual neurophysins into the circulation of pigs. *Endocrinology 100*: 635-641.

Delwaide, P. J., Devoitille, J. M., and Ylieff, M. (1980). Acute effect of drugs upon memory of patients with senile dementia. *Acta Psychiatr. Belg. 80*: 748-754.

De Wied, D. (1965). The influence of the posterior and intermediate lobe of the pituitary and pituitary peptides on the maintenance of a conditioned avoidance response in rats. *Int. J. Neuropharmacol. 4*: 157-167.

De Wied, D., and Gispen, W. H. (1977). Behavioral effects of peptides. In *Peptides in Neurobiology*, H. Gainer (Ed.). Plenum, New York, pp. 397-448.

Fawcett, C. P., Powell, A. E., and Sachs, H. (1968). Biosynthesis and release of neurophysin. *Endocrinology 83*: 1299-1310.

Flexner, L. B., and Goodman, R. H. (1975). Studies on memory: inhibitions of protein synthesis also inhibit catecholamines synthesis. *Proc. Natl. Acad. Sci. USA 72*: 4660-4663.

Flexner, J. B., Flexner, L. B., Hoffman, P. L., and Walter, R. (1977). Dose-response relationship in attenuation of puromycin-induced amnesia by neurohypophyseal peptides. *Brain Res. 134*: 139-144.

Gainer, H., Sarne, Y., and Brownstein, M. (1977). Neurophysin biosynthesis. Conversion of a putative precursor during axonal transport. *Science 195*: 1354-1356.

Gilot, P., Crabbe, J., Legros, J. J. (1980). Bilan Mnesique de cinq sujets presentant un diabete insipide central idiopathique familial. *Acta Psychiat. Belg. 80*: 755-761.

Ginsburg, M. (1968). Production, release, transportation and elimination of the neurohypophyseal hormones. In *Neurohypophyseal Hormones and Similar Polypeptides*, B. Berde (Ed.). Springer-Verlag, Berlin, pp. 286-298.

Ginsburg, M., and Jayasena, K. (1968). The occurrence of antigen reacting with antibody to porcine neurophysin. *J. Physiol. (Lond.) 197*: 53-63.

Gopinath, P. G., Gopinath, G., and Anand-Kumar, T. C. (1979). Target site of intranasally sprayed substances and their transport across the nasal mucosa: a new insight delivery into the intranasal route of drug delivery. *Curr. Ther. Res. 23*: 596-607.

Iuvone, P. M., Morasco, J., Delanoy, R. J., and Dunn, A. J. (1978). Peptides and the conversion of H^3 tyrosine to catecholamines: effects of ACTH-analogs, melanocyte-stimulating hormones and lysine-vasopressin. *Brain Res. 139*: 131-139.

Jenkins, J. S., Mather, H. M., and Ang, U. (1980). Vasopressin in human cerebrospinal fluid. *J. Clin. Endocrinol. Metab. 50*: 364-367.

Kovacs, G. L., Bohus, B., Versteeg, D. H. G., de Kloet, R., and de Wied, D. (1979). Effect of oxytocin and vasopressin on memory consolidation: sites of action and catecholaminergic correlates after local microinjection into limbic-midbrain structures. *Brain. Res. 175*: 303-314.

Landgraf, R., Emisch, A., and Heb, J. H. (1979). Indication for a brain uptake of labelled vasopressin and oxytocin and the problem of the blood-brain barrier. *Endokrinologie 73*: 77-81.

Legros, J. J. (1975). The radioimmunoassay of human neurophysins: contribution to the understanding of the physiopathology of neurohypophyseal function. *Ann. N.Y. Acad. Sci. 248*: 281-303.

Legros, J. J. (1978). Urinary excretion of neurophysins in patients with kidney disease. *J. Endocrinol. 76*: 411-415.

Legros, J. J. (1979). The neurohypophyseal peptides: biosynthesis, biological role and prospects of use in neuropsychiatric therapy. *Triangle 18*: 17-30.

Legros, J. J., and Franchimont, P. (1970). Influence de l'oestriol sur le taux de la neurophysine sérique chez l'homme. Comparaison avec la capacité de fixation plasmatique des polypeptides posthypophysaires marqués étudiés "in vitro." *C. R. Soc. Biol. (Paris) 164*: 2146-2150.

Legros, J. J., and Gilot, P. (1979). Vasopressin and memory in the human. In *Brain Peptides: The New Endocrinology*, A. M. Gotto (Ed.). Elsevier/North Holland Biomedical Press, Amsterdam, pp. 347-364.

Legros, J. J., Franchimont, P., and Hendrick, J. C. (1969). Dosage radioimmunologique de la neurophysine dans le sérum des femmes normales et des femmes enceintes. *C. R. Soc. Biol. (Paris) 163*: 2773-2777.

Legros, J. J., and Grau, J. D. (1973). Effect of ethinyl-estradiol on neurohypophyseal active compounds in the rat. *Nature 241*: 247-249.

Legros, J. J., Gilot, P., Seron, X., Claessens, J. J., Adam, A., Moeglen, J. M., Audibert, A., and Berchier, P. (1978). Influence of vasopressin on learning and memory. *Lancet 1*: 41-42.

Legros, J. J., Gilot, P., Smitz, S., Bruwier, M., Mantanus, H., and Timsit-Berthier, M. (1980). Neurohypophyseal peptides and cognitive function: a clinical approach. In *Progress in Psychoneuroendocrinology*, F. Brambilla, G. Racagni, and D. de Wied (Eds.). Biomedical Press, North Holland, Amsterdam, pp. 325-337.

Matthews, E. K., Legros, J. J., Grau, J. D., Nordmann, J. J., and Dreifuss, J. J. (1973). Effects of lanthanum ions on the isolated neurohypophyseal hormones by exocytosis. *Nature 241*: 86-88.

McNeilly, A. S., Martin, M. J., Chard, T., and Hart, I. C. (1972). Simultaneous release of oxytocin and neurophysin during parturition in the goat. *J. Endocrinol. 52*: 213-214.

Nordmann, J. J., Dreifuss, J. J., and Legros, J. J. (1971). A correlation of release of polypeptide hormones and of immunoreactive neurophysin from isolated rat neurohypophyses. *Experimentia 27*: 1344-1345.

Perry, E. K. (1979). Biochemistry of the cholinergic system in Alzheimer's disease. Communication at the workshop on Biochemist of the Dementias, March 29-30, Southampton, England.

Remond, A., and Isard, C. (1978). Electrophysiological effects on nicotin. Elsevier/ North Holland, Amsterdam, p. 254.

Robinson, A. G. (1975). Isolation, assay and secretion of individual human neurophysins. *J. Clin. Invest. 55*: 360-367.

Robinson, A. G., and Zimmerman, E. A. (1973). Cerebrospinal fluid and ependymal neurophysin. *J. Clin. Invest. 52*: 1260-1267.

Scharrer, E., and Scharrer, B. (1954). Hormones produced by neurosecretory cells. *Recent Progr. Horm. Res. 10*: 183-240.

Sitaram, N., Weingartner, H., Caine, E. D., and Gillin, J. C. (1978). Choline: selective enhancement of serial learning and encoding of low imagery words in man. *Life Sci. 22*: 1555-1560.

Sunde, D. A., and Sokol, H. W. (1975). Quantification of rat neurophysin by polyacrilamide gel electrophoresis (PAGE): application to the rat with hereditary hypothalamic diabetes insipidus. *Ann. N.Y. Acad. Sci. 248*: 345-364.

Tanaka, M., Versteeg, D. H. G., and de Wied, D. (1977). Regional effects of vasopressin on rat brain catecholamine metabolism. *Neurosci. Lett. 4*: 321-325.

Telegdy, G., and Kovacs, G. L. (1979). Role of monoamines in mediating the action of ACTH, vasopressin, and oxytocin. In *Central Nervous System Effects of Hypothalamic Hormones and Other Peptides*, Collu (Ed.). Raven Press, New York.

Timsit-Berthier, M., Audibert, A., and Moeglen, J. M. (1978). Influence de la lysine-vasopressine sur l'EEG chez l'homme. Résultats préliminaires. *Neuropsychology 4*: 129-139.

Timsit-Berthier, M., Gerono, A., and Rousseau, J. C. (1979). Poster presented at the 5th International Symposium on Electrical Potentials Related to Motivation, Motor and Sensory Processes (MOSS V), Ulm, Federal Republic of Germany, May 14-18.

Timsit-Berthier, M., Mantanus, H., Jacques, C., and Legros, J. J. (1980). Utilité de la lysine-vasopressine dans le traitement de l'amnésie post-traumatique. *Acta Psychiatr. Belg. 80*: 728-747.

Tinklenberg, J. R., and Berger, P. A. (1981). Behavioral and cognitive effects of ACTH and vasopressin analogues. In *Neurobiology of Aging*,

Urban, I., and de Wied, D. (1978). Neuropeptides: effects on paradoxical sleep and theta rhythm in rats. *Pharmacol. Biochem. Behav. 8*: 51-59.

van Wimmersma-Greidanus, T. B., and Versteeg, D. H. G. (1980). Neurohypophyseal hormones: their role in endocrine function and behavioral homeostasis. In *Behavioral Neuroendocrinology*, C. B. Numeroff and A. J. Dunn (Eds.). Spectrum Publishers, New York, in press.

Vincent, J. D., and Arnauld, E. (1975). Vasopressin as a neurotransmitter in the central nervous system: some evidence from the supraoptic neurosecretory system. In *Hormones, Homeostasis and the Brain*, W. H. Gispen, T. B. van Wimmersma-Greidanus, B. Bohus, and D. de Wied (Eds.). Elsevier, Amsterdam, pp. 57-66.

Waggoner, R. W., Slonim, A. E., and Armstrong, S. H. (1978). Improved psychological status of children under DDAVP therapy for central diabetes insipidus. *Am. J. Psychiatry 135*: 361-262.

Weindl, A., and Sofoniew, M. V. (1979). Immunohistochemistry of neuropeptides. *XIIth Acta Endocrinologica Congress*, June 16-30, p. 414.

Weingartner, H., Gold, T., Ballenger, J. C., Mallberg, S. A., Summers, R., Rubinow, D. R., Post, R. M., and Goodwin, F. K. (1981). Effect of vasopressin on human memory function. *Science 211*: 602-604.

16
Behavioral Medicine

Bernard T. Engel / *National Institute on Aging, National Institutes of Health, Baltimore, Maryland*

INTRODUCTION

There are several definitions of behavioral medicine. However, for purposes of this review, I shall adhere to the one proposed by Blanchard (1977). According to him, behavioral medicine is "the systematic application of the principles and technology of behavioral psychology to the field of medicine, health and illness," (p. 2). Blanchard identifies behavioral psychology primarily with experimental psychology, which he equates with the psychology of learning, social psychology, and physiological psychology. He states further that, "Behavioral psychology . . . is probably most closely tied to the field of the experimental analysis of behavior or operant conditioning" (p. 2). Finally, he includes four broad areas of application within the domain of behavioral medicine:

1. Direct behavioral intervention into traditionally medical problems such as insomnia, headache, or high blood pressure.
2. The use of behavioral procedures to facilitate medical management in such broad areas as adherence to drug regimens prescribed by a physician, or avoidance of habit regimens proscribed by a physician (e.g., cigarette smoking).
3. Modification of physiological behaviors through the use of conditioning technologies (i.e., biofeedback).

4. Behavioral modification used as a preventive procedure to enable patients to avoid or escape unhealthy habits. This is similar to item 2 except that here the applications are preventative, whereas in 2 they are part of a treatment program.

In this chapter I shall consider only therapeutic or rehabilitative applications, and I shall not deal with preventative procedures. This omission is based on two considerations. First, at this stage the benefits of behavioral prevention programs are the subject of considerable research; however, there is little evidence to warrant calling any of these cost effective; and second, to my knowledge, none of the research on prevention has been directed at older people. In his definition Blanchard also excluded the entire area of mental health or psychiatric problems since these are not, strictly speaking, medical problems, although when present they usually create serious problems in medical management of a patient. I shall adhere to this exclusion also, except that I will consider the behavioral management of depression since depression is such a pervasive problem for health care providers of the elderly.

BEHAVIORAL MEDICINE APPLICATIONS TO OLDER OUTPATIENTS

I must begin this section with the caveat that the applications of behavioral medicine to the older patient are no different than they are to the younger patient. The only point worth noting is that certain disorders are more likely to be present in older patients. In this section I will consider some applications to patients with (1) cardiovascular disorders—control of high blood pressure or postmyocardial infarction rehabilitation; (2) neuromuscular disorders—poststroke rehabilitation or the treatment of incontinence; (3) behavioral applications in the control of insomnia; and (4) behavioral applications in the improvement of adherence to drug regimens.

Cardiovascular Disorders

A number of longitudinal studies have shown that blood pressure rises with age (Engel and Malmstrom, 1967; Julius and Schork, 1971; Engel et al., 1981). Thus, older people are more likely to have elevated pressures than younger people. Furthermore, elevated blood pressure is a greater risk factor in older patients than it is in younger patients (Hypertension Detection and Follow-up Program Cooperative group, 1979). There have been a number of reviews of behavioral strategies which might be helpful in the control of high blood pressure (Shapiro et al., 1977; Frumkin et al., 1978; Seer, 1979). Since I will consider drug treatment adherence below, I will not consider this aspect of behavioral control of hypertension here. Broadly speaking, the behavioral applications in the control of hypertension include diet control programs, exercise procedures, relaxation, or biofeedback. However, only the last two include direct, behavioral interventions, and only they will be considered here.

The relaxation procedures are of two kinds: (1) Those in which patients are taught either to relax specific muscles, until eventually most major muscle groups have been trained (Jacobson, 1938); (2) those in which patients are taught a meditative procedure which is designed to create a physiological state incompatible with muscle tension (Benson, 1975). The feedback procedures also are of two kinds: (1) Those which are designed to facilitate relaxation (Stoyva, 1979); (2) those which are designed to influence blood pressure directly (Kristt and Engel, 1975). Most of the studies either of the relaxation procedures or of the feedback procedures are very limited in their relevance. This is so for two reasons: First, most of the studies are based either on relatively few patients or on relatively short follow-up periods, so that the clinical significance is unclear; and second, most of the studies looked either at relaxation or at feedback but not at both, and with one exception, none of the studies explicitly tested the hypothesis that the two procedures might be synergistic (Glasgow et al., in press). Our study was based on a series of 90 borderline hypertensive patients ranging from 30 to 70 years in age. Our findings were that patients could significantly lower and maintain lower blood pressure using the behavioral procedures we taught them. Patients who received both procedures lowered pressure most; however, control patients who merely monitored their pressure for 6 months and who met regularly with the investigator to review these data also sustained lowered pressures. Age was not a significant factor in ability to control blood pressure.

Behavioral procedures are also used in the rehabilitation of patients who have suffered myocardial infarctions. Unfortunately, these procedures are not sufficiently developed to warrant extensive review. The most widely utilized behavioral prescription for these patients is exercise (Mock et al., 1981). The supervision and implementation of these programs have been largely medically controlled because of the potential risks involved (Council on Scientific Affairs, 1981; Hartley, 1981). The most serious problem from a behavioral point of view has been the poor adherence (Carmody et al., 1980). This has been reflected both in low enrollment and high dropout rates. Hopefully, this will be rectified as more behaviorists become involved in the supervision of the programs.

Neuromuscular Disorders

The rehabilitation of poststroke patients has elicited considerable interest among behaviorists who have developed and applied biofeedback technologies as an adjunct to physical therapy (Baker and Wolf, 1979; Baker, 1979) and in the control and treatment of such problems as poststroke foot drop (Basmajian et al., 1975) or spasticity (DeBacher, 1979). Although these problems are complex, and considerable research will be needed before the methods can be made optimal, the evidence is good that the methods now in use are effective, and many physical therapists already utilize them. These findings are especially relevant here since many of the poststroke patients are elderly.

Incontinence is a major problem among the elderly (Milne, 1976; Schuster, 1977). Although urinary incontinence is most common, fecal incontinence is more serious in the sense that it is more likely to result in institutionalization of the patient. Several years ago we (Engel et al., 1974) described a method which could be used to train many fecally incontinent patients to recover bowel control. Subsequent research has shown that the method is highly effective (Cerulli et al., 1977) and that patients of any age can profit from such training. Urinary incontinence has been studied also, and there is good evidence that many such patients can be trained to become continent (Wilson, 1948; Cardozo et al., 1978). My colleague, Dr. William E. Whitehead, and I are now operating a research geriatric continence clinic in which we are seeing older (65 years or greater) outpatients who are incontinent of either stool or of urine. Our experience to date has been encouraging since four of six fecally incontinent and four of five urinary incontinent patients have been treated successfully (i.e., a reduction of incontinent episodes by 70% or better).

Insomnia

Clinical experience suggests that insomnia is a common problem among older people. Some investigators have suggested that this is, in part, attributable to the age-related changes in sleep cycle. As people grow older, the period of slow-wave sleep diminishes and stage REM periods increase. Thus, elderly patients are more vulnerable to disturbance in sleep patterns, especially frequent awakenings and failure to return to sleep. Another major factor in insomnia among the elderly is drug-related. Paradoxically, chronic use of hypnotics which patients use to induce sleep often are the culprits since such medications frequently also reduce slow-wave sleep when used chronically. Spiegel (1981) has reviewed a number of the normal and clinical features of sleep and sleeplessness in the elderly, and Borkovec (1977) has reviewed a number of the behavioral interventions used to control insomnia. In view of the apparent magnitude of the problem among elderly patients, it would be helpful to expand research efforts in this area.

Adherence to Medical Advice

Poor adherence to medical advice is a ubiquitous problem which is aggravated in elderly patients because of the large number of medications which are prescribed. Haynes (1981) has conducted an extensive review of a variety of procedures which have been purported to be effective in improving adherence to treatment for a wide variety of conditions. Among the procedures he reviewed which were designed to improve compliance with long-term medications, *none* of the following were effective: disease instruction, medication instruction, special pill containers, free medications, home visits, convenient care, biological endpoint monitoring, or group discussions. The procedures which *were* effective included a variety of combinations of behavioral methods designed to reinforce compliance. Among these "packages" were home visits by nurses combined with instructions and encouragement to comply, monitoring, counseling, and blood pressure feedback; self-monitoring of blood pressure, professional monitoring, and self-management of drug protocols. All of these effective applications were studied in hypertensive patients. Thus, while the findings are important in the treatment of elderly patients, many of whom are hypertensive, research is needed for other disorders such as arthritis or ischemic heart disease.

Depression

Depression is a pervasive problem among chronically ill patients. It affects a variety of behaviors such as general activity or medication compliance, and can also be seen to affect memory or morale. Hoyer et al. (1975) published an extensive review of the research on behavioral approaches to the management of problem behaviors in the elderly. Many of these behaviors readily can be recognized as concomitants of depression. Baltes and Barton (1977) also argued for the usefulness of behavioral strategies in the treatment of elderly patients. The pervasive problem for behavioral medicine specialists is that depressed patients are inactive. The absence of activity adversely influences metabolic activities and, therefore, interferes with drug metabolism, as well as reducing the opportunity of the patient to obtain reinforcement from the environment. Thus, the major focus of behavioral treatment in depression is an effort to increase the total activity of the patient. Certainly, the judicious use of antidepressant medication is warranted. However, unless such medication is coupled with environmental rewards for maintained behavior, the patient undoubtedly will regress. A proper behavioral treatment program would be scaled. Initially, the emphasis would be placed on getting the patient to engage in self-care activities; subsequently, one would strive to engage the patient in household chores and eventually outdoor programs.

BEHAVIORAL MEDICINE APPLICATIONS TO ELDERLY PATIENTS

For purposes of this section I shall limit my discussion to chronic inpatient or nursing home programs. Acutely ill inpatients who happen to be elderly should be treated no differently from younger, acutely ill patients.

The most serious problems of inpatient, elderly patients are problems of ambulation, incontinence, dementia, and depression. Very often these problems interact so that a patient who cannot get out of bed also will be classified as incontinent although with proper help he could be continent. Such a patient also is likely to become depressed, which is likely to aggravate his medical problems. The first discussion of behavioral management of these patients probably was that by Whitney (1960). Since then a number of cognate programs have been proposed (Baltes and Zerba, 1976; Harris et al., 1977; Drummond et al., 1978; Rinke et al.,

1978). In every case, the focus of the intervention is, first, to get the patient to engage in self-care procedures, and to elaborate these skills into an expansion of activities within the physical capacity of the patient. All of these programs require that the patient be reinforced for his behaviors and that he be supported so that he can function within his physical limitations. The problem one encounters with such programs is that they require rearrangements of the priorities and procedures of the institution. Thus, although many investigators have shown that self-care programs are cost effective, for example, nursing care for incontinent patients (Willington, 1976), institutions are reluctant to change their practices. Clearly, it is important not only to treat the patient but to treat the staff as well. Thus, the primary research need is to develop improved liaison methods since no therapeutic method can be effective if it is thwarted by the administration of the staff.

REFERENCES

Baker, M. P. (1979). Biofeedback in specific muscle retraining. In *Biofeedback: Principles and Practice for Clinicians*, J. B. Basamajian (Ed.). Williams & Wilkins, Baltimore, pp. 81-91.

Baker, M. P., and Wolf, S. L. (1979). *Biofeedback Strategies in the Physical Therapy Clinic*, J. B. Basamajian (Ed.). Williams and Wilkins, Baltimore, pp. 31-42.

Baltes, M. M., and Barton, E. M. (1977). New approaches toward aging: A case for the operant model. *Educational Gerontology: An International Quarterly 2*: 383-405.

Baltes, M. M., and Zerbe, M. B. (1976). Independence training in nursing-home residents. *Gerontologist 16*: 428-432.

Basamajian, J. V., Kukulka, C. G., Narayan, M. G., and Takebe, K. (1975). Biofeedback of foot-drop after stroke compared with standard rehabilitation technique: Effects on voluntary control and strength. *Arch. Phys. Med. Rehabil. 56*: 231-236.

Benson, H. (1975). *The Relaxation Response*. Morrow Press, New York.

Blanchard, E. B. (1977). Behavioral medicine: A perspective. In *Behavioral Approaches to Medical Treatment*, R. B. Williams, Jr. and W. D. Gentry (Eds.). Ballinger, Cambridge, Mass., pp. 1-6.

Borkovec, T. D. (1977). Insomnia. In *Behavioral Approaches to Medical Treatment*, R. B. Williams, Jr. and W. D. Gentry (Eds.). Ballinger, Cambridge, Mass., pp. 25-40.

Cardozo, L., Stanton, S. L., Hafner, J., and Allan, V. (1978). Biofeedback in the treatment of detrusor instability. *Br. J. Urol. 50*: 250-254.

Carmody, T. P., Senner, J. W., Malinow, M. R., and Matarazzo, J. D. (1980). Physical exercise rehabilitation: Long-term dropout rate in cardiac patients. *J. Behav. Med. 3*: 163-168.

Cerulli, M. A., Nikoomanesh, P., and Schuster, M. M. (1979). Progress in biofeedback for fecal incontinence. *Gestroenterology 76*: 742-746.

Council on Scientific Affairs (1981). Physician-supervised exercise programs in rehabilitation of patients with coronary heart disease. *JAMA 245*: 1463-1466.

DeBacher, G. (1979). Biofeedback in spasticity control. In *Biofeedback: Principles and Practice for Clinicians*, J. B. Basmajian (Ed.). Williams and Wilkins, Baltimore, pp. 61-80.

Drummond, L., Kirchhoff, L., and Scarbrough, D. R. (1978). A practical guide to reality orientation: A treatment approach for confusion and disorientation. *Gerontologist 18*: 568-573.

Engel, B. T., and Malmstrom, E. J. (1967). An analysis of blood pressure trends based on annual observations of the same subjects. *J. Chron. Dis. 20*: 29-43.

Engel, B. T., Gaarder, K. R., and Glasgow, M. S. (1981). Behavioral treatment of high blood pressure: I. Analyses of intra- and interdaily variations of blood pressure during a one-month, baseline period. *Psychosom. Med.*, in press.

Engel, B. T., Nikoomanesh, P., and Schuster, M. M. (1974). Operant conditioning of recto-sphincteric reflexes in the treatment of fecal incontinence. *N. Engl. J. Med. 290*: 646-649.

Frumkin, K., Nathan, R. J., Prout, M. F., and Cohen, M. C. (1978). Nonpharmacologic control of essential hypertension in man: A critical review of the experimental literature. *Psychosom. Med. 40*: 294-320.

Glasgow, M. S., Gaarder, K. R., and Engel, B. T. (in press). Behavioral treatment of high blood pressure: II. Acute and sustained effects of relaxation and systolic blood pressure biofeedback. *Psychosom. Med.*

Harris, S. L., Snyder, B. D., Snyder, R. L., and Magraw, B. (1977). Behavior modification therapy with elderly demented patients implementation and ethical considerations. *J. Chron. Dis. 30*: 129-134.

Hartley, L. H. (1981). Use of exercise tests in cardiac rehabilitation: Part 1, prescribing daily activities. *Prac. Cardiol. 7*: 93-102.

Haynes, R. B. (1981). Lowering blood pressure by gaining patients' cooperation. *Cardiovasc. Med. May*: 451-458.

Hoyer, W. J., Mishara, B. L., and Riebel, R. G. (1975). Problem behaviors as operants. *Gerontologist 15*: 452-456.

Hypertension Detection and Follow-up Program Cooperative Group (1979). Reduction in mortality of persons with high blood pressure, including mild hypertension. *JAMA 242*: 2562-2578.

Jacobson, E. (1938). *Progressive Relaxation*, 2nd ed. University of Chicago Press, Chicago.

Julius, S., and Schork, M. A. (1971). Borderline hypertension: a critical review. *J. Chron. Dis. 23*: 723-754.

Kristt, D. A., and Engel, B. T. (1975). Learned control of blood pressure in patients with high blood pressure. *Circulation 51*: 370-378.

Milne, J. S. (1976). Prevalence of incontinence in the elderly age groups. In *Incontinence in the Elderly*, F. L. Willington (Ed.). Academic Press, New York, pp. 9-21.

Mock, M. B., Ringqvist, I., and Frommer, P. L. (1981). NIH reports: Physical conditioning and cardiovascular rehabilitation. *J. Cardiovasc. Med. 6*: 142-146.

Rinke, C. L., Williams, J. J., Lloyd, K. E., and Smith-Scott, W. (1978). The effects of prompting and reinforcement on self-bathing by elderly residents of a nursing home. *Behav. Ther. 9*: 873-881.

Schuster, M. M. (1977). Constipation and anorectal disorders. *Clin. Gastroenterol.* *6*: 643-658.

Shapiro, A. P., Schwartz, G. E., Ferguson, D. C. E., Redmond, D. P., and Weiss, S. M. (1977). Behavioral methods in the treatment of hypertension. A review of their clinical status. *Ann. Intern. Med. 86*: 626-636.

Seer, P. (1979). Psychological control of essential hypertension: Review of the literature and methodological critique. *Psychol. Bull. 86*: 1015-1043.

Spiegel, R. (1981). *Sleep and Sleeplessness in Advanced Age*. Spectrum Publications, New York.

Stoyva, J. M. (1979). Guidelines in the training of general relaxation. In *Biofeedback: Principles and Practice for Clinicians*, J. B. Basmajian (Ed.). Williams & Wilkins, Baltimore, pp. 99-111.

Whitney, L. (1966). Operant learning theory: A framework deserving nursing investigation. *Nurs. Res. 15*: 229-235.

Willington, F. L. (1976). In *Incontinence in the Elderly*, F. L. Willington (Ed.). Academic Press, New York, pp. 3-8.

Wilson, T. S. (1948). Incontinence of urine in the aged. *Lancet 2*: 374-377.

17
Drug Management in the Elderly

Dan Blazer / *Duke University Medical Center, Durham, North Carolina*

INTRODUCTION

The elderly consume more drugs than any other age group in the United States. Though medications are frequently bought over the counter, a significant percentage of these drugs are prescribed by physicians. The value of our improved pharmacopeia for extending life and alleviating the pain and suffering of illness in the elderly cannot be overestimated. Unfortunately, the misuse, overuse, and abuse of drugs in late life are major health problems. This chapter addresses important issues relevant to the pharmacological treatment of the aged. After a brief overview of the scope of drug use by the elderly, the basis and principles of good prescribing in late life will be reviewed. First, good prescribing is grounded in a thorough knowledge of physiology and pharmacology of aging. Second, good prescribing requires a working knowledge of the psychology and sociology of drug use by the elderly. Finally, good prescribing is based on the application of certain guidelines by the clinician in the office and institution.

EPIDEMIOLOGY OF DRUG USE IN THE ELDERLY

Older persons use 25% of the nation's prescription drugs (FDA, 1968). The annual cost of medications for older people may be as high as 2.5 billion dollars in out-ofpocket expenses. Eighty-five percent of the ambulatory elderly and ninety-five percent of institutionalized elderly receive prescription drugs (Law and Chalmers, 1976). Lamy and Vestal (1976) estimate that over 12 prescriptions are written per person each year for those aged 65 and older.

Among the different groups of medications that are prescribed, cardiovascular drugs account for the highest proportion of use by outpatients. Psychotropic medications are by far the most frequently used drugs by the institutionalized elderly (Ray et al., 1980). Chlorpromazine is the most common drug prescribed in the institution. The level of use of this potent antipsychotic agent in one nursing home study was enough, in and of itself, to suggest that the drug was being misused (Ray et al., 1980).

The misuse, overuse, and abuse of drugs in late life is a major health problem for at least three reasons. First, older persons are at greater risk for medication errors (Lundin, 1978). Even if the patient fully intends to follow the physician's instructions to the letter, the probability of significant medication error increases as age increases. Second, and probably responsible for many of the problems suggested above, the altered physical status of the older person makes usual prescribing directions inadequate (Rossman, 1980). Third, the potential for drug interactions increases geometrically as the number of medications prescribed increases. Therefore, older persons who receive multiple medications are at particular risk for adverse drug-drug interactions.

Fortunately, our knowledge of the physiology and pharmacology of late life has increased dramatically over the past few years. Clinicians now have available, at least potentially, the knowledge and guidelines to ensure a more effective and safe pharmacotherapy for the elderly. A brief review of this working knowledge is presented below.

PHARMACOKINETICS OF AGING

Aging is a dynamic process which not only changes through time but displays its diversity in different structures and functions within the body. Drugs pass through the body in a sequence of events that reflects this same dynamic framework. The term pharmacokinetics refers to the process concerned with the distribution of drugs in the body, their absorption, excretion, and metabolism. These processes are essential to the concentration of therapeutic agents at their respective sites of action. The basic processes of pharmacokinetics of greatest importance to the clinician are as follow.

1. Absorption: Most therapeutic agents are taken by mouth, broken down in the alimentary tract, and absorbed into the bloodstream. The rate at which a drug is absorbed and the site of the absorptive activity depends upon changes within the gastrointestinal tract over time plus the chemical and physical properties of the drug. The most common changes in the absorptive capacity of older persons

are an elevated gastric pH secondary to a decreased secretion of hydrochloric acid, a reduced gastrointestinal blood flow, and a reduction in gastrointestinal mobility (Rossman, 1980). There is little evidence that any significant change occurs in the absorption of most drugs by the gastrointestinal tract with aging (Gorrod, 1974). It has been suggested that the shift toward a more alkaline gastric milieu may effect the ionization and solubility of some acidic drugs (Goth, 1974). For example, chlorazepate, a minor tranquilizer from the class of benzodiazepines, has a chemical structure that requires a low gastric pH for proper absorption. Therefore, the prescription of this drug to a very old person instead of another benzodiazepine must be questioned.

Delayed gastric emptying could potentially lead to increased absorption of drugs primarily absorbed from the stomach and decreased absorption of drugs absorbed from the intestine. Lowered L-dopa serum levels have been correlated with this abnormality in at least one study (Bianchine et al., 1971).

2. Distribution of tissue deposit of drugs: A change in body weight and composition with aging can be associated with changes in drug distribution. With aging, the proportion of body fat to the total body weight increases as the proportion of muscle tissue decreases. Other changes include a reduced total body water, decreased protein synthesis, and a reduced serum albumin (Rossman, 1980). Associated with the changing albumin concentrations is an age-related change of protein binding. Most drugs which enter the bloodstream bind with plasma proteins, usually albumin. A decreased albumin level is associated with decreased binding and has been noted to be associated with adverse reactions to phenytoin (Boston Collaborative Drug Surveillance Program, 1973). Psychotropic drugs most often prescribed to older persons for anxiety and depression are typically stored in body fat. Because of the increased proportion of fat tissue, these drugs would be expected to have a longer duration of action secondary to their fat solubility (Vestal, 1978). This increased capacity to store lipophilic drugs may lead to an increased risk of toxicity as the drugs accumulate.

3. Drug metabolism: From the time of absorption, drugs begin undergoing the process of metabolism. Drugs can be metabolized either to active or inactive forms. In general, drugs are metabolized to a form which can be excreted more readily (Poe and Holloway, 1980). Drug metabolism occurs primarily in the liver. Hepatic cells decrease and hepatic blood flow diminishes with aging. Hepatic activity in the elderly is also reduced through the life cycle (Rossman, 1980). Changes in the hepatic microsomal enzyme system also occur with the aging process, which may significantly affect the liver's ability to metabolize drugs (Crooks, 1976). In general, therapeutic agents are metabolized slower in late life and therefore remain in the body for a longer period of time in their active state (Vestal, 1978). Antipyrine, which is extensively metabolized by the liver, has a definitely prolonged half-life in older patients. Yet, these age-related changes can be influenced considerably by the variability of individuals and by environmental influences.

For example, smoking, which increases the activity of certain hepatic enzymes, may be associated with an increased metabolic rate in older persons.

4. Excretion: Drugs are primarily excreted by the kidney and through the gastrointestinal tract via the liver. The rate of glomerular filtration decreases with aging as does renal blood flow (Rowe et al., 1976). In fact, the kidney is the body organ most susceptible to the loss of functioning cells with aging. Fortunately, older persons can normally experience a sharp reduction in renal function without the appearance of symptomatology. Yet, this is misleading. For example, the serum creatinine may be within normal limits in late life, whereas the 24-hr creatine clearance is only 50% of that at earlier stages of the life cycle. Therefore, serum creatinine alone is not a good laboratory screen for kidney functioning. Since lithium carbonate is excreted almost exclusively by the kidney, and has the potential for significant toxic effects at dose levels very close to those levels required for a therapeutic response, an assessment of creatinine clearance is essential before the drug is prescribed.

The excretion of drugs through the biliary tract is much less understood. It had been documented that the biliary excretion of indomethacin is increased in the elderly, resulting in a lower proportion of the unchanged free drug in the body (Traeger et al., 1973).

5. Drug response: Receptor sensitivity changes with aging. For example, there is a decreased number of receptor cells coupled with a reduced binding of these cells (Roth, 1975). Therefore, an increase in variation in the therapeutic response of an older person to a standard dose from these alterations and adverse drug reactions are more common (Vestal, 1978). Receptors in late life may also be more subject to the adverse effects of continual drug use. Tardive dyskinesia resulting from prolonged use of antipsychotic agents is more prevalent in the elderly. This may not only reflect an increased use of these agents in late life but also an altered sensitivity to their continued use, leading to changes in the receptors which are generally accepted as being the primary cause of the difficulties in this condition.

6. Drug interactions: As noted above, adverse drug-drug interactions are frequent in late life. Potential for such interactions not only includes the interaction of prescribed agents, but also the potential interaction of prescribed and over-the-counter agents. These interactions may occur at various points in the pathway of the drug's passage through the body. For example, aluminum hydroxide interferes with the absorption of tetracycline; the sulfonamides diminish plasma protein binding of phenylbutazone; coumarin increases metabolism of the barbiturates; the thiazide diuretics, through their effect on sodium, interfere with the excretion of lithium carbonate; and methyldopa diminishes the number of receptor sites for adrenergic drugs and for other antihypertensive agents (Poe and Holloway, 1980). A frequent problem is the additive effectives of drugs with anticholinergic properties. Another is the interaction of guanethidine and the tricyclic antidepressants, the antidepressant interfering with the antihypertensive activity of guanethidine.

PSYCHOSOCIAL FACTORS AND DRUG USE IN THE ELDERLY

Psychosocial factors influence the effectiveness and potential toxicity of medications prescribed to older adults at least as often as the change in anatomy and physiology accompanying aging. The character traits of the patients, along with acute psychological problems, may affect both the way patients approach medications and their reactions to chemotherapy (Baldessarini, 1977). For example, obsessional patients worry over the details of their treatment and the reactions to it, thus provoking a string of controversies, arguments, or conversations about their treatment. An impulsive or hysterical patient may react to the expected side effects in an exaggerated manner, or may be inclined to abuse the medication. A patient with paranoid ideation may cooperate poorly because of suspiciousness and/or even delusions about the treatment. The social setting surrounding the prescription of medications may also significantly affect the prescription and the effectiveness of the patient to comply with the prescription. Five psychosocial factors will be discussed below as examples of psychosocial influences on drug use by the elderly.

Noncompliance

Blackwell (1973) estimated that complete failure to take medications may occur in up to 50% of patients. Although this figure appears to be exaggerated, physicians undoubtedly overestimate patient adherence to drug prescription. There is no evidence at present, however, that the elderly comply either more or less than patients at other stages of the life cycle to prescription regimens (Lundin, 1978).

The reasons for noncompliance in late life, however, are important for the clinician to recognize (Lamy, 1980). First, the patient may lack practical information and instructions on proper drug use. In the fast-paced and frequently distracting environment of a clinician's office, information transfer about the proper use of medications is often lacking. Older patients may be hesitant to ask questions about medications that are prescribed, even though they do not understand the physician's initial instruction. If instructions are printed on the pill bottle, older patients who have problems with eyesight may not be able to read the small print. Pills and capsules that look alike can be confused. A common practice by older persons who take multiple medications is to carry one pill bottle with them when they go shopping or visiting. All of their medications are placed within this container, and the potential for a mix-up is great. At other times, instructions on dose schedule may be ambiguous. For example, medications may be prescribed with meals, but the older person may eat only one meal a day and thus take only one-third the amount intended by the prescribing physician.

Many older patients receive medical care from a number of physicians. They may neglect to inform the prescribing physician that medicines have also been prescribed by others and, therefore, the potential for dangerous drug interactions is increased. Frequent visits to multiple caretakers also increase the probability that instructions by any given caretaker about a particular medication will be forgotten. It has been known for many years that error frequency is a definite function of the number of drugs prescribed (Vere, 1965) and the number of times per day the drug is prescribed. At other times, drugs are not taken at all because either the medications are too costly or the patient has difficulty in opening a child-proof pill bottle.

Other older adults may cease taking medication because of adverse side effects. As will be explained below, continued compliance in taking a medication, in spite of side effects, can be facilitated when potential side effects are explained to the patient at the time the prescription is written. Contrary to popular belief, most older adults do not choose to continue taking drugs indefinitely. Therefore, medications that have been prescribed for indefinite periods may be stopped spontaneously by the older adult because he or she no longer feels a need for the medication.

Sharing and Swapping of Medications

Older people enjoy talking with their friends and family about their physical ills and their treatments. Frequently, older persons who are friends, roommates, or married will be treated for similar problems by two different physicians. They inevitably compare notes on the effectiveness of the individual treatments prescribed. If the older person discovers someone else has received a benefit from a particular medication, finances often preclude seeking a second opinion from a physician or investing in a new prescription. Therefore, medications are shared or swapped.

Most older adults do not appreciate the danger in taking pills from another person's prescription. Not only are they unaware of the legal implications of such action (though it is doubtful that an older person would actually be prosecuted for this behavior), they have very little appreciation of the potential danger from drug interaction. The problem is further complicated because the older adult may not inform the attending physician of this swapping practice.

Experimentation with Drugs by Older Adults

Closely akin to sharing and swapping behavior is experimentation. Prescription of a drug at a particular time of day or in a certain dose does not ensure that the older adult will consciously choose to comply with that prescription. Many times older adults fancy themselves to be excellent personal pharmacists and choose to experiment with varied drug regimens, combinations, and dose schedules. Stimulants may be taken at bedtime, sedatives in the midafternoon, and so forth, depending on the whim of the older adult.

Over-the-Counter Drugs

In the Western world, 45-60% of the population in any country use prescription drugs, and an additional 25-40% use over-the-counter drugs in late life. Chaiton et al. (1976) found that nearly 60% of one elderly population had used at least one over-the-counter drug within 48 hr of being surveyed during a community survey. Most of these individuals did not consult their physician about the use of the drugs. Commonly used over-the-counter drugs in late life are internal analgesics and drugs to treat gastrointestinal symptoms, such as constipation.

Many dangers can arise from self-medications with over-the-counter agents. First, older patients who are financially impaired may seek to medicate themselves for conditions that require expert medical care (with or without prescription medications). Second, many of these over-the-counter medications interact with prescription drugs. For example, salicylates can increase the anticoagulant effects of coumadin and increase the hypoglycemic effects of the oral hypoglycemic agents. Third, over-the-counter medications further increase the number of agents being taken and therefore increase the likelihood that prescription drugs will not be taken in proper dose or on the proper schedule.

"Do-Something" Prescribing

Most older persons expect something to be done for them when they seek the consultation of a physician. Though visiting the physician's office may be a pleasant, social occasion for the older adult, the payment of money (however small) for this occasion usually implies that the patient receives something in return. A prescription has been the common means by which the physician has assured the patient that something has been done. Unfortunately, this approach to medical care in late life has greatly increased the likelihood that older persons will encounter the toxic side effects of medication. Such an interchange also reinforces a pattern of medical care which discourages the physician from talking with the older adult about a particular problem and empathizing with pain and suffering that may be encountered without experiencing the necessity of taking action where action will be of no benefit.

Defensive Prescribing

Physicians who cover long-term care facilities or hospital practices are frequently called upon by nursing staff and family to control certain physical symptoms or behavior. Against their better judgment, physicians may prescribe medications to reassure staff and family. The recognition of this defensive prescribing behavior is not an indictment against the care given by physicians as much as it is a symptom of a very difficult situation. For example, the management of the acutely agitated patient suffering from an organic mental disorder in a nursing home where staff is limited can press the staff to perform beyond its capabilities. In less stressful circumstances, the entire health care team is better capable of putting into practice those techniques for managing the disturbed elderly which have been learned in training programs.

Understanding the physiological pharmacokinetic, and psychosocial factors associated with aging should contribute to a more rational state and effective therapy of older adults. Although specific recommendations regarding each medication dose regimen for all age groups are not available, there are a number of general guidelines which can be applied by the physician working with the older adult (Blazer and Friedman, 1979).

1. *Obtain a thorough history of the patient's present drug intake*: Obtaining an accurate account of the drug intake of a patient, either at present or during a past time interval, is not an easy task. At least three procedures can benefit this process. First, the physician should encourage each patient to bring all medications that are currently being taken to the office or hospital at the initial evaluation. Each pill bottle should be examined, and the patient should be asked when the medication was prescribed and how often the patient takes the medication; for example, is the medicine taken continuously, intermittently, or rarely. If the patient does not bring the pill bottles to the initial evaluation, the physician may aid in the identification of certain medications by using the color charts of the *Physician's Desk Reference* (1980). It would be helpful if the color charts could be arranged in such a way that the physician could ask about different categories of medications, such as medications for the gastrointestinal tract, sleep, anxiety, depression, and so forth. Third, and possibly the most important technique, the physician should question a close family member to determine how well the account of the patient and family member's perception of drugs intake corroborate. Because of the time-consuming nature of getting a thorough medication history, physicians may wish to delegate this task to office personnel and paraprofessionals. The difficulty in obtaining the information should not preclude its acquisition, however.

2. *Identify target symptoms*: Whenever a medication is prescribed, the physician must be cognizant of those symptoms which are likely to be reversed following its administration. For example, the symptoms of peptic ulcer disease may be alleviated by cimetidine. Yet, both physician and patient may be unclear as to which particular symptoms can be best alleviated by the medication.

A depressed affect, a frequent symptom in late life, is treated with antidepressant medications. Occasionally, physicians forget that those symptoms most likely to be reversed, at least initially, are sleep disturbances, appetite disturbances, and agitation or retardation, as opposed to a reduction in the depressed affect itself. To ensure that the effectiveness of a medication can be determined, symptoms and severity should be carefully documented at the initial evaluation and, thereafter, periodically reassessed to determine whether the medication in fact has reversed or alleviated particular symptoms. Not only does the physician benefit from this documentation, but he or she may also avoid a potential malpractice suit if prescribing practices are ever challenged.

3. *Use smaller doses of medications and increase these dosages at a slower rate*: As a general rule, dosages of medications used to treat older persons should be

adjusted downward to accommodate the various anatomical, physiological, and pharmacokinetic decrements that predominate in this age group. This downward adjustment is especially important when computing dosages for drugs with known cumulative tendencies.

4. *Simplify the therapeutic regimen*: Whenever possible, medications should be prescribed in the simplest dose regimen. Unfortunately, the potential side effects of certain medications require that the drug be given in divided doses throughout the day, as opposed to a single dose. When instructing the patient, the physician should use easily understood language, avoiding such common medical jargon as "b.i.d." or "p.r.n." Whenever possible, verbal instructions should be complemented by written instructions. The instructions should be repeated and the patient asked to repeat the instructions back to the physician.

To avoid potential errors in compliance to a suggested regimen, the physician should inform both the patient and relative or friend of the dose schedule of a particular medication. This practice is especially helpful when the older adult is suffering from a memory disturbance or is considered to be a poor risk for compliance. Compliance can frequently be enhanced by the use of a medication calendar or diary. Such aids range from a simple partitioned container for each day of the week to more complicated dispensers, such as those used to dispense birth control pills.

Prescribing must be coordinated with the local pharmacist. The pharmacist can frequently inform the physician that competing medications have been prescribed by another doctor or may discover a potential toxic drug interaction which slipped the physician's attention. Pill containers should be labeled so that they can be read by the older adult when distributed by the pharmacist.

5. *Regularly review compliance to prescribed drugs and test for plasma levels when appropriate*: The patient should not be pressured to take medication, for there appears to be a negative relationship between the amount of pressure exerted by the physician and the amount of compliance on the part of the patient in taking medications (Davidson, 1976). Nevertheless, each time the patient returns to the physician's office, a careful review of medication compliance and change in symptoms should take place. A significant breakthrough in recent years is the availability of blood level determinations for many medications, such as dilantin, digitalis, and the tricyclic antidepressants. Therapeutic blood levels in the older adult may be quite different from levels at other stages of the life cycle, so the interpretation of these results must be age-adjusted.

6. *Monitor for side effects*: Side effects for some medications may occur long after the drug has initially been prescribed. A gradual accumulation may lead to the appearance of side effects long after the drug is prescribed and may, in turn, be misinterpreted. One of the more common side effects secondary to prescription of medications to older persons is the appearance of anticholinergic effects. Dry mouth, constipation, urinary retention, tachycardia, blurred vision, exacerbation of acute narrow-angle glaucoma, inhibition of sweating, and occasional secondary

impotence result from the anticholinergic effects of a variety of drugs. Many antihistamines, tricyclic antidepressants, phenothiazines, antiparkinson agents, and so forth produce anticholinergic effects. More serious side effects secondary to these anticholinergic actions include confusion and increased agitation, precipitation of a bundle branch block, or the development of a central anticholinergic syndrome. The latter condition usually consists of psychotic thoughts accompanied by significant confusion and agitation, flushing, and dryness of the skin.

7. *Withdraw unnecessary medications without proven efficacy*: Whenever the physician faces a complicated clinical picture in an older patient on many medications, the first step in proper prescribing should be to withdraw all medications without proven therapeutic efficacy. Nevertheless, these drugs must be withdrawn slowly, for abrupt withdrawal may lead to serious and difficult symptoms.

REFERENCES

Baldessarini, R. J. (1977). *Chemotherapy in Psychiatry*. Harvard University Press, Cambridge, Mass.

Bianchine, J. R., Calimlim, L. R., Morgan, J. P., Dujuvne, C. A., and Lasagne, L. (1971). Metabolism and absorption of L-3, 3-dihydroxy-phenylalanine in patients with Parkinson's disease. *Ann. N.Y. Acad. Sci. 179*: 126-140.

Blackwell, B. (1973). Patient compliance. *N. Engl. J. Med. 289*: 249.

Blazer, D. G., and Friedman, S. W. (1979). Depression in late life. *Am. Fam. Phys. 20*: 91-96.

Boston Collaborative Drug Surveillance Program (1973). Diphenylhydrantoin side effects and serum albumin levels. *Clin. Pharmacol. Ther. 14*: 529.

Chaiton, A., Spitzer, W. O., Roberts, R. S., and Delmore, T. (1976). Patterns of medical drug use—a community focus. *Can. Med. Assoc. J. 114*: 33.

Crooks, J., O'Malley, K., and Stevenson, I. H. (1976). Pharmacokinetics in the elderly. *Clin. Pharmacokinetics 1*: 280-296.

Davidson, P. (1976). Therapeutic compliance. *Can. Psychol. Rev. 17*: 247.

Food and Drug Administration (1968). Task Force on Prescribing Drugs. U.S. Government Printing Office, Washington, D.C.

Gorrod, J. W. (1974). Absorption, metabolism, and excretion of drugs in geriatric subjects. *Gerontol. Clin. 16*: 30.

Goth, A. (1974). *Medical Pharmacology. Principles and Concepts*, 7th ed. C. V. Mosby, St. Louis.

Lamy, P. P. (1980). *Prescribing for the Elderly*. PSG Publ. Co., Littleton, Mass.

Lamy, P. P., and Vestal, R. E. (1976). Drug prescribing for the elderly. *Hosp. Prac. 11*:111.

Law, R., and Chalmers, C. (1976). Medicines and elderly people: A general practice survey. *Br. Med. J. 1*: 565.

Lundin, D. V. (1978). Medication-taking behavior of the elderly: A pilot study. *Drug. Intell. Clin. Pharm. 12*: 581.

Physicians' Desk Reference, 34th ed. (1980). Oradell, N.J. Medical Economics Company.

Poe, W. D., and Holloway, D. A. (1980). *Drugs in the Aging*. McGraw-Hill, New York.

Ray, W. A., Federspiel, C. F., and Schaffner, W. (1980). A study of antipsychotic drug use in nursing homes: Epidemiologic evidence suggesting misuse. *Am. J. Public Health* 70: 485-491.

Rossman, I. (1980). Bodily changes with aging. In *Handbook of Geriatric Psychiatry*, E. W. Busse and D. G. Blazer (Eds.). Van Nostrand and Reinhold, New York.

Roth, G. S. (1975). Altered hormone binding and responsiveness during aging. *Proc. 10th Int. Congress Gerontol. 1*: 44-45.

Rowe, J. W., Andres, R., Tobin, J. D., Norris, A. H., and Shock, N. W. (1976). Age adjusted standards for creatinine clearance. *Ann. Int. Med. 84*: 567.

Traeger, A., Kunze, M., Stein, G., and Ankerman, H. (1973). Zur pharmakokinetik von indomethazin bei alten menschen. *Z. Alternsforsch. 27*: 151.

Vere, D. W. (1965). Errors of complex prescribing. *Lancet 1*: 370.

Vestal, R. E. (1978). A review of pharmacology and aging. *Drugs 16*: 358-382.

18

Age-Related Changes in Sympathetic Function

Keith V. Kuhlemeier / *University of Alabama in Birmingham, Birmingham, Alabama*

INTRODUCTION

The autonomic nervous system plays an involuntary but powerful role in the maintenance of homeostasis during several forms of stress, hence the "fight-or-flight" characterization of the sympathetic portion of the autonomic nervous system. It is widely accepted that the mammalian body's ability to maintain a constant internal environment for the cells in the face of changes in the external environment generally declines with increasing age. Since the sympathetic nervous system is intimately involved with the maintenance of homeostasis, it is possible that a decline in the power of the sympathetic nervous system is responsible for the reduced efficacy of the physiological responses to stress as aging progresses.

This report will examine the role of the sympathetic nervous system in maintaining homeostasis during two types of stress: exercise and thermal (both hot and cold). Data from humans will be presented whenever possible, and animal data will be presented primarily when human data is inadequate, a situation which is distressingly frequent. In the interest of brevity, the literature cited will be representative rather than exhaustive.

AGE-RELATED CHANGES IN BASAL CATECHOLAMINE LEVELS

Activation of the sympathetic nervous system results in the release of both norepinephrine and epinephrine. The source of epinephrine is apparently the adrenal medulla exclusively, whereas norepinephrine is secreted both by the adrenal medulla and the nerve terminals of the autonomic nervous system. There are a multitude of possible fates of the neuron-secreted norepinephrine. It may be released to the blood, catabolized locally, taken up by the secreting neuron, or bound to a postsynaptic neuron. Therefore, blood levels of norepinephrine are obviously a very imperfect index of sympathetic activity. Epinephrine levels may be more indicative of sympathetic function since epinephrine is secreted into the blood and thereby travels from the site of synthesis to the target organs in classic endocrine fashion.

One must remember that blood levels reflect the balance between hormone release and hormone removal, whether that removal be by reuptake, catabolism, or excretion. Metabolites of both norepinephrine and epinephrine appear in urine, so urinary levels of these metabolites are often used as an index to sympathetic activity. A major disadvantage to using urinary metabolite levels is that a confounding factor, kidney function, is introduced. This factor becomes important in aging research since kidney function clearly declines with increasing age.

With these reservations in mind, let us first examine indices of sympathetic activity in man. Dalmaz et al. (1979) examined urinary levels of catecholamine metabolites in humans from birth to middle age. In general, the levels of the compounds studied (dopa, dopamine, norepinephrine, epinephrine, and others) were very low during the first year of life, increased slowly through childhood, increased at a more rapid rate during the pubertal period, and reached the highest levels during adulthood. Unfortunately, no measurements were made in senescent adults. Examination of these data shows a highly variable range of levels, so determining normal levels is exceedingly risky. Ziegler et al. (1976) also found a significant, positive correlation between plasma levels of norepinephrine and age in the range of 10-65 years in resting, apparently healthy, normotensive volunteers. Patients with hypothyroid disease show a more dramatic increase in plasma norepinephrine with advancing age than do normal subjects (Christensen, 1973); this interaction points out the importance of considering the interdependency between the autonomic nervous system and other endocrine systems in aging research.

In rats, epinephrine levels in the adrenal gland rise progressively 2-600 days of age. Norepinephrine levels are relatively constant for the first week and increase suddenly about the second week of life. They remain fairly constant until 120 days of age and then rise progressively until the 600th day of life (Kvetansky et al., 1978).

While data from other species as well as data on synthesis, turnover, and reuptake rates as a function of aging in all species are still needed, current evidence suggests that basal blood catecholamine levels increase with advancing age.

SECRETION OF CATECHOLAMINES IN RESPONSE TO STRESS AS A FUNCTION OF AGING

Rhythmic Work

In general, there is a positive correlation between blood catecholamines and the severity of rhythmic work. The rise in norepinephrine levels in blood is nearly linear at low levels of exercise, but is exponential during moderate and heavy exercise (Haggendal et al., 1970; Vendsalu, 1960). Increases in epinephrine levels in response to exercise are more modest. Some investigators report a linear increase in epinephrine levels with increasing levels of work, whereas others have found that epinephrine excretion (not blood levels) increases during moderate work (50% of maximal aerobic capacity) but does not increase further when the work load is increased (Howley, 1976).

The catecholamine responses to work can be altered by training (Cousineau et al., 1977). Postinfarct patients who trained for 27 weeks at 65-75% of their symptom-limited maximal work capacity showed significantly lower norepinephrine levels both at rest and immediately following a standard work bout (McCrimmon et al., 1976). However, another study (Cronan and Howley, 1974) found no differences in urinary norepinephrine or epinephrine excretion as a result of 8 week's training. The subjects in the latter study were younger and healthier than those of the former study, which may explain part or all of the discrepancy. Moreover, it is difficult to compare blood levels of catecholamines with urinary excretion rates.

There is little information on the effects of age on epinephrine and norepinephrine levels in blood or urine during rhythmic exercise. One report (Blimkie et al., 1978) states that epinephrine and norepinephrine blood levels during a hockey game are greater in 16- and 23-year-olds than in 11- and 13-year-old boys. Marshall and Berrios (1979) found that L-dopa increased the vigor of swimming in 24 to 27-month-old rats but not in 3 to 4-month-old rats.

The consensus is that blood and urine levels of catecholamines increase with exercise, but the effect of age on this response has not received adequate attention. The work of Marshall and Berrios may have important implications for future aging research. Obviously, more work is needed in this critical area.

Static Work

That profound cardiovascular responses are elicited by prolonged static (isometric) work is unquestioned. Moreover, it is widely accepted that the cardiovascular responses elicited depend largely on the effort involved expressed as a fraction of maximal isometric strength and are almost completely independent of muscle mass. It is thought that these responses are elicited because the intramuscular tension produced by the isometrically contracting muscle impinges on the capillaries and precludes the washout of accumulated metabolites into the circulating blood. Nor is there an opportunity for additional nutrients to be delivered to the muscle as occurs during the relaxation phase in rhythmically contracting muscle. Therefore, it is not surprising that there are qualitative and quantitative differences between responses to isometric contraction and rhythmic contractions brought about, perhaps, by differences in sympathetic responses to these types of exercise. The parasympathetic nervous system is also involved in the response to static exercise; it has been suggested (Petro et al., 1970) that a major portion of the response to static exercise is a consequence of vagal withdrawal.

The literature is divided on whether blood catecholamine levels are increased during static exercise. Kozlowski et al. (1973) reported that both norepinephrine and epinephrine levels increased when their subjects (six males and two females, ages 30-40 years) performed a 30% maximal voluntary contraction (MVC) with a hand dynamometer for "as long as possible." Norepinephrine levels tripled whereas epinephrine levels doubled. Since the output of the adrenal medulla is primarily epinephrine, this suggests that the noradrenergic nerve endings of the sympathetic nervous system responded more than the adrenal medulla.

The effect of age on the sympathetic response to static work has been examined more closely than the response to rhythmic work. Few et al. (1975) had 12 subjects aged 20-60 years perform a 50% MVC with their legs and measured total plasma catecholamines. The increase in plasma catecholamine level was 2.31 nmol/ 1, which the authors described as "no marked change" and "significant at the 0.1% level," a point confusing to this author. They found no obvious relationship between blood pressure increases and age, initial blood pressure, or rise in catecholamine concentration. McDermott et al. (1974) found that total plasma catecholamines increases significantly during a 33% MVC in older (mean age 47 years) but not in younger (mean age 25 years) men. This increase was primarily a result of higher epinephrine levels since norepinephrine levels did not increase significantly. Norepinephrine levels in the younger men did not increase during the static contraction proper, but were significantly higher 5 min after cessation of static work than during the control period. However, the mean heart rate and blood pressure responses of the two age groups were not significantly different. Palmer et al. (1978) also examined the plasma norepinephrine responses of old (mean age 53 years) and young (mean age 14 years) people to a 5-min 30% MVC. They found that resting levels were higher in the old group than in the young group (424 pg/ml vs. 240 pg/ml), and that the increase in norepinephrine levels over resting levels in response to static exercise was greater in the old subjects (534 pg/ml) than in the young subjects (336 pg/ml).

The heart rate response (which depends in part on the level of sympathetic activity) to static work declines with advancing age. Petrofsky and Lind (1975) reported that the heart rate response to sustained handgrip decreased with increasing age up to 62 years. Their older subjects had higher systolic blood pressure than their younger subjects, and this difference increased during the hypertension elicited by the static work. Ordway and Wekstein (1979) confirmed the heart rate observations in still older men, one group aged 65-70 years and another group aged 73-91 years. They also found that the diastolic, but not systolic, blood pressure increased more in their youngest subjects (aged 21-42 years) than in their oldest patients. Kino et al. (1975) also found a smaller cardioacceleratory response to static work in old normals aged 54-78 than in young normals.

Many of the available data suggest that the blood catecholamine response to static exercise tends to be greater in older persons than in younger persons. The decrease in the cardioacceleratory response to static work in older humans may be due to a decrease in tissue sensitivity to catecholamines as aging progresses (see below).

Thermal Stress

Considering the importance of the sympathetic nervous system in maintaining homeothermy in mammals, the paucity of data, especially from humans, on age-related changes in thermoregulatory function is somewhat surprising. It seems that much descriptive information remains to be gathered in some areas of physiology, despite (or perhaps due to) the current vogue for elucidating molecular mechanisms of physiological action in health and disease.

Responses to Heat

One of the earliest investigations on the results of high ambient temperature on sympathetic function was made by Saito in 1928. He cannulated the adrenal vein of dogs and measured epinephrine excretion (by a bioassay) while they were unanesthetized. He noted a rise in epinephrine output in hyperthermia with a "fairly long" after-action. Fiorica et al. (1967) exposed unanesthetized dogs to varying levels of ambient temperature ranging from 38-49°C but found no consistent effect on plasma catecholamines even though rectal temperatures exceeded 41°C in some of the dogs. Symbas et al. (1964) heated anesthetized dogs and found that catecholamine levels in arterial blood were increased, often dramatically. His studies, coupled with the work of Saito and Fiorica et al., suggest that the role of anesthesia may be of considerable importance.

In unanesthetized man, sympathetic activity is generally increased by heat. Huikko et al. (1966) reported that norepinephrine excretion in humans rose by 50% in the course of a Finnish sauna bath. Epinephrine excretion rose from 7.0 ng/min prior to the bath to 9.6 ng/min during the bath. Vanilmandelic acid excretion increased but not significantly. Arvela and Huikko (1969) later found that propranolol prevented the tachycardia associated with sauna and that urinary norepinephrine, but not epinephrine, excretion was enhanced by propranolol administration. On the other hand, Iisalo et al. (1969) found that propranolol inhibited, but did not prevent, the expected increase in heart rate on exposure to sauna temperature. Responses to guanethidine treatment did not differ from responses to placebo treatment. Hussi et al. (1977) also found that plasma catecholamines were elevated during a sauna and that oxprenolol, a beta blocker, did not alter the plasma catecholamine patterns but did lower the heart rate. Plasma epinephrine levels decreased to resting values after 5 min in 22°C water following the sauna, but norepinephrine levels remained elevated or increased even further. Lammintausta et al. (1976) found that vanilmandelic acid levels were not affected by a sauna bath, suggesting that there was no increase in the rate of catecholamine degradation. Work in a 40°C environment results in higher plasma epinephrine and norepinephrine levels than does similar work in a 22°C environment, although resting catecholamine levels are not different in the two environments (Kowlowski et al., 1972).

There are other scattered data (in addition to the canine data mentioned above) relating levels of sympathetic function to increased ambient temperature in nonhuman mammals. Baldwin et al. (1969) found that increasing the ambient temperature from 25-35°C slightly decreased norepinephrine excretion but had no effect on epinephrine excretion in pigs. Stefanovic et al. (1970) reported that a 33°C environment increased urinary vanilmandelic acid in pigs. Shum et al. (1969) concluded that norepinephrine synthesis in rats was inversely proportional to ambient temperature. Cattle increase their urinary excretion of norepinephrine, but not epinephrine, in response to heat (Alvarez and Johnson, 1970). Jones and Musacchia (1975, 1976) found that in 2 to 3-month-old hamsters, heart and kidney tissue levels of norepinephrine increased with heat (34°C) exposure compared with levels in animals maintained at 22°C. However, adrenal catecholamines decreased with hot exposure of 5-week duration. Norepinephrine turnover of heart tissue was lower in heat-acclimated animals than in control animals. Norepinephrine turnover rates of splenic tissue were decreased by heat exposure.

The most obvious generalization to be made from the above data, regarding the effects of heat on age-related changes in sympathetic drive, is that more research is urgently needed. Present evidence does suggest, however, that heat stress does result in elevated levels of plasma catecholamines, provided the stress is of sufficient magnitude.

Responses to Cold

It is widely known that catecholamine production increases in response to cold stress. The earliest direct measurements of sympathoadrenal activity during cold exposure were made by Saito (1928), who failed to find an increase in epinephrine secretion with a modest reduction of core temperature in dogs. Wada et al. (1935) induced deeper hypothermia (30°C or less) in dogs and found a "definite conspicuous increase lasting an hour or more" in epinephrine output from cannulated adrenal veins.

In young hamsters, heart and kidney levels of norepinephrine decrease whereas adrenal catecholamine levels increase with chronic cold exposure (Jones and Musacchia, 1975, 1976). Chronic cold exposure also increased norepinephrine turnover in heart tissue but not in splenic tissue. Cattle increase their urinary excretion of norepinephrine, but not epinephrine, in response to cold (Alvarez and Johnson, 1970). Pigs have an increased urinary excretion of both epinephrine and epinephrine in cool environments (Baldwin et al., 1969). LeBlanc and Nadeau (1961) found that catecholamine excretion was increased by cold acclimatization in rats.

Several investigators report that sympathetic activity in humans increases during cold exposure. Arnette and Watts (1960) exposed six lightly dressed, resting men aged 22-40 years, to 6.5°C for 1 hr and found that epinephrine excretion increased from 0.21 µg/hr in the control period (23°C) to 0.38 µg/hr during cold exposure, a highly significant difference; increases in norepinephrine excretion were modest—from 0.61 µg/hr during the control exposure to 0.78 µg/hr during cold exposure—but still statistically significant. Lamke et al. (1972) measured norepinephrine and epinephrine excretion in nude men who remained in a 15°C environmental chamber for 72 hr. Norepinephrine increased from 22.0 ng/min in a warm (28°C) environment to 58.1 ng/min at the end of the cold exposure. Comparable values for epinephrine were 0.93 ng/min and 4.66 mg/min. The effect of cold-water immersion on plasma levels of norepinephrine of 23 to 48-year-old men were measured by Johnson et al. (1977), who reported that norepinephrine levels rose from preimmersion levels of 359-642 pg/ml after 2 min immersion to 1171 pg/ml after 45-min immersion. The correlation between rectal temperature and plasma norepinephrine was highly significant. Immersion of a single hand to the wrist in ice water also markedly increases blood levels of norepinephrine (Winer and Carter, 1977). LeBlanc et al. (1979) found that plasma epinephrine and norepinephrine levels rose during a cold pressor test.

None of the above studies directly examined the effect of age on the sympathetic response to cold. There is, however, some indirect evidence relating age to sympathetic responses to cold. Schulze and Burgel (1977) exposed adult (6-8 months old) and old (26-30 months old) rats to cold environments, the temperature of which could be behaviorally modified by lever pressing by the animals. They found that in preset ambient temperatures ranging from – 8° to +4°C the older rats maintained their body temperatures by selecting warmer ambient temperatures than did the younger animals. At 0 and 4°C the younger rats not only maintained but actually increased their body temperature significantly. Phentolamine (an alpha-adrenergic blocker) administration, 30 min before placement of the rats in a room that was – 4°C at the onset of the experiment, resulted in a fall of core temperature in both older and younger animals, the larger fall being in the older animals, even though the drug caused the older animals to select chamber temperatures that were warmer than the temperatures selected by the younger animals. Moreover, small rats (180 g) raise their urinary norepinephrine from control levels of 2.79-13.89 ng/kg/min when exposed to 3°C for 24 hr (Leduc, 1961). Increases in epinephrine levels are smaller. Larger and presumably older rats (400 g) increase their urinary norepinephrine from a control level of 3.19-16.68 ng/kg/min after 210 days at 10°C (LeBlanc and Naudeau, 1961). Segall and Timiras (1975) found that old rats subjected to ice-water immersion had a greater drop in colonic temperature than young rats, and that the return of core temperature to baseline levels after the animals were removed from the water required more time in the older animals. Moreover, this age-related decline in the ability to maintain body temperature could be retarded by manuevers which retard aging. Rommelspacher et al. (1975) gave phentolamine to older (13 months) and younger (3 months) rats and placed them in cold (4°C) environments. They reported that after 4 hr, the core temperature of the older rats decreased from control values of 37.4-32.9°C, whereas the core temperatures of younger rats dropped from 37.5-35.7°C. They found that in this environment the older rats increased their oxygen consumption to a greater extent than the younger rats, and whereas older rats decreased their metabolic rates in 31°C environments, the younger animals did not. In summary, whereas it is known that cold activates the sympathoadrenal system, the effect of age on this response remains largely a matter of conjecture.

Responses of Aging Animals to Adrenergic Stimulation

There is considerable evidence that while blood levels of catecholamines increase with advancing age (see above), the responses to catecholamines decline as animals age. This topic has recently been reviewed (Lakatta, 1980; Rowe and Troen, 1980) and will not be dealt with here, except to state Lakatta's observation that "the results of *each* of *several different* types of investigation are *all* compatible with the interpretation that the effectiveness of adrenergic stimulation declines with advancing age" (his emphasis).

Age and the Effectiveness of Adrenergic Systems in Maintaining Homeostasis

We (Lewin et al., unpublished observations) attempted to determine the integrated efficacy of the sympathetic nervous system and the organs it innervates by applying a common stress and then measuring how well the animals compensates for the stress at various ages. If sympathetic nervous system function declines with advancing age, then pharmacological blockade should have less effect in older animals than in younger animals. If the sympathetic nervous system becomes totally ineffective, either because of receptor changes or decreased levels of neurotransmitter synthesis or release, then blockade should have no effect on the animal's reaction to the stress. We chose to test the ability of rats to maintain their core temperature in the face of extreme thermal stress. The homeostatic regulation of temperature was chosen because: (1) it is a common stress that animals must face in their natural habitat; (2) core temperature is one of the most tightly regulated physiological variables; and (3) temperature measurements can be made accurately, precisely, rapidly, and inexpensively. Two groups of male Long-Evans rats were used. At the beginning of the study, one group was 5 months of age and the other group was 15 months old. The animals were temperature-stressed by placing them in a snug acrylic restraint and immersing them up to the nose in ice water for 2 min. At the end of the 2-min immersion period, the animal was removed from the restraint and placed in a sawdust-filled cage. Colonic temperatures were measured just prior to immersion and during recovery after immersion. The animals were pretreated with 6 mg/kg phentolamine or vehicle carrier 30 min prior to immersion each month for 5 months.

Figures 1 and 2 show the time course of temperature change for the youngest (5 months) and oldest (20 months) animals after injection of phentolamine or vehicle carrier. In the 5-month rats given vehicle carrier, the temperature decreased from 38.7°C to a minimum of 34.8°C at 10 min postimmersion. Phentolamine administration resulted in a larger decrease in colonic temperature (from 38.9-33.5°C) and delayed the point at which the temperature drop was maximal. In the 20-month-old animals, phentolamine pretreatment had little effect on colonic temperature in the immediate postimmersion period. Maximal temperature drops occurred in both control and drug-treated animals at about the same time, and there was only 0.3°C (33.1 vs. 32.8°C) difference in the colonic temperature between control and phentolamine-treated animals. There was little difference between the recovery rates of the younger rats and older animals in the absence of phentolamine. Thus, in the early postimmersion period, the difference in maximal temperature decrease between phentolamine-treated younger animals and older control animals was only 0.4°C. The responses of the phentolamine-treated younger animals were very much like the responses of the older animals given vehicle carrier. The younger animals respond as if they have aged when their alpha-adrenergic receptors are blocked.

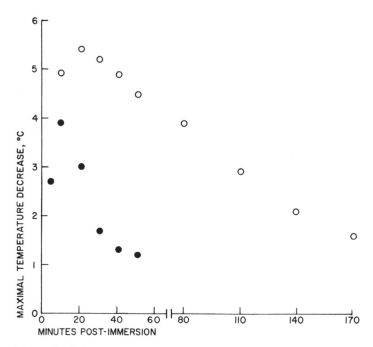

Figure 1 Colonic temperature change in 6-month-old animals given vehicle carrier (closed circles) or phentolamine (open circles) prior to a 2-min ice-water immersion.

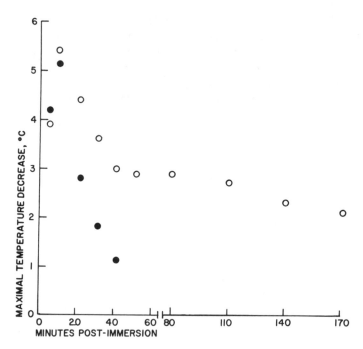

Figure 2 Colonic temperature changes in 20-month-old animals given vehicle carrier (closed circles) or phentolamine (open circles) prior to a 2-min ice-water immersion.

In the later (greater than 20 min) postimmersion period, there was little difference between older and younger animals given vehicle carrier, but phentolamine prolonged the time that temperatures remained depressed for both older and younger animals. In the 20 to 112-min postimmersion period, the body temperatures of the phentolamine-treated younger animals were considerably lower than comparably treated older animals. The reason for these lower body temperatures in the younger animals is unclear. One possibility is that the older animals may develop nonadrenergic physiological mechanisms for coping with cold. It is known, for example, that older animals increase their oxygen consumption more than younger animals on exposure to cold (Rommelspacher et al., 1975). Another possibility is that the larger body fat stores of the older animals (sedentary male rats fed ad libitum continuously increase their stores of body fat) retain the body heat more effectively in the older rats. This may be especially important since the normal vasocontriction of skin vessels in response to cold may be prevented by alpha-adrenergic blockade.

Figure 3 shows that the maximal temperature drop in younger (5-10 month old) rats given vehicle carrier was less than in the older 15 to 20-month-old rats.

Phentolamine administration resulted in a larger decrease in colonic temperature regardless of age, but generally, the control-phentolamine difference was greater in the younger animals than in the older animals. The data shown in Figs. 1 and 2 suggest that there are at least two components to be considered, an early component (vascular?), which is of more importance in younger animals than in old animals, and a later component (metabolic?), which is of more equal importance in the two groups of animals. Because the number of animals tested was small (seven younger, four older), these results must be interpreted with caution, but they do suggest that the efficacy of the sympathetic nervous system in maintaining homeothermy declines with increasing age. Unfortunately, these experiments do not tell

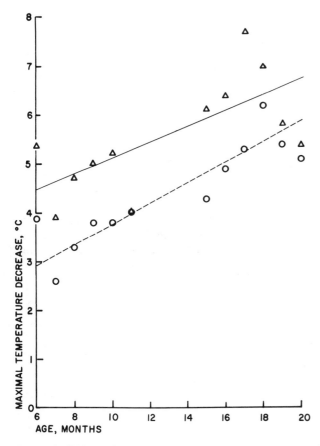

Figure 3 Effect of age on maximal colonic temperature responses of animals given vehicle carrier (circles) or phentolamine (triangles) prior to a 2-min ice-water immersion. Line are least squares regression lines for control (dotted line) and phentolamine-treated (solid line) animals.

us whether this decline in function is due to changes in neurotransmitter biochemistry (sensory, central, or effector) or to changes in neurotransmitter receptors.

These results are consistent with the literature which suggests that circulating levels of catecholamines increase with age but that catecholamine receptor activity declines with advancing age. There are exceptions to this generality, however, and much further study is needed to elucidate the mechanisms of this important system.

REFERENCES

Alvarez, M. B., and Johnson, H. D. (1970). Urinary excretion of adrenaline and noradrenaline in cattle during heat and cold exposure. *J. Dairy Sci. 53*: 928-930.

Arnette, E. L., and Watts, D. T. (1960). Catecholamine excretion in men exposed to cold. *J. Appl. Physiol. 15*: 499-500.

Arvela, P., and Huikko, M. (1969). Effect of propranolol on plasma FFA levels and urinary excretion of catecholamines during Finnish sauna bath. *Acta Physiol. Scand. (Suppl.) 330*: 129.

Baldwin, B. A., Ingram, D. L., and LeBlanc, J. (1969). The effects of environmental temperature and hypothalamic temperature on excretion of catecholamines in the urine of the pig. *Brain Res. 16*: 511-515.

Blimkie, C. J. R., Cunningham, D. A., and Leung, F. Y. (1978). Urinary catecholamine excretion during competition in 11 to 23 year old hockey players. *Med. Sci. Sports 10*: 183-193.

Christensen, N. J. (1973). Plasma noradrenaline and adrenaline in patients with thyrotoxicosis and myxoedema. *Clin. Sci. Mol. Med. 45*: 163-171.

Cousineau, D., Ferguson, R. J., deChamplain, J., Gauthier, P., Cate, P., and Bourassa, M. (1977). Catecholamines in coronary sinus during exercise in man before and after training. *J. Appl. Physiol. 43*: 801-806.

Cronan, T. L., and Howley, E. T. (1974). The effect of training on epinephrine and norepinephrine excretion. *Med. Sci. Sports 6*: 122-125.

Dalmaz, Y., Peyrin, L., Sann, L., and Dutruge, J. (1979). Age-related changes in catecholamine metabolites of human urine from birth to adulthood. *J. Neural. Transm. 46*: 153-174.

Few, J. D., Imms, F. J., and Weiner, J. S. (1975). Pituitary-adrenal response to static exercise in man. *Clin. Sci. Mol. Med. 49*: 201-206.

Fiorica, V., Iampietro, P. F., Huggins, E. A., and Moses, R. (1967). Sympathicoadrenomedullary activity in dogs during acute heat exposure. *J. Appl. Physiol. 22*: 16-20.

Haggendal, J., Hartley, L. H., and Saltin, B. (1970). Arterial noradrenaline concentration during exercise in relation to the relative work levels. *Scand. J. Clin. Lab. Invest. 26*: 337-342.

Howley, E. T. (1976). The effect of different intensities of exercise on the excretion of epinephrine and norepinephrine. *Med. Sci. Sports 8*: 219-222.

Huikko, M., Jouppila, P., and Karki, N. T. (1966). Effect of Finnish bath (sauna) on the urinary excretion of noradrenaline, adrenaline and 3-methoxy-4-hydroxy-mandelic acid. *Acta Physiol. Scand. 68*: 316-321.

Hussi, E., Sonck, T., Poso, H., Remes, J., Eisalo, A., and Janne, J. (1977). Plasma catecholamines in Finnish sauna. *Ann. Clin. Res. 9*: 301-304.

Iisalo, E., Kanto, J., and Pihlajamaki, K. (1969). Effects of propranolol and guanethidine on the circulatory adaptation to the Finnish sauna. *Ann. Clin. Res. 1*: 251-255.

Johnson, D. G., Hayward, J. S., Jacobs, T. P., Collis, M. L., Eckerson, J. D., and Williams, R. H. (1977). Plasma norepinephrine responses of man in cold water. *J. Appl. Physiol. 43*: 216-220.

Jones, S. B., and Musacchia, X. J. (1975). Tissue catecholamine levels of the golden hamster (Mesocricetus auratus) acclimated to 7, 22, and 34°C. *Comp. Biochem. Physiol.* (C) *52*: 91-94.

Jones, S. B., and Musacchia, X. J. (1976). Norepinephrine turnover in heart and spleen of 7, 22, and 34°C acclimated rats. *Am. J. Physiol. 230*: 564-568.

Kino, M., Lance, V. Q., Shahamatpour, A., and Spodick, D. H. (1975). Effects of age on responses to isometric exercise. *Am. Heart J. 90*: 575-581.

Kozlowski, S., Brzezinska, Z., Nazar, K., Kowalski, W., and Franczyk, M. (1973). Plasma catecholamines during sustained isometric exercise. *Clin. Sci. Mol. Med. 45*: 723-731.

Kozlowski, S., Soltysiak, J., Tomaszewska, L., Brzezinska, Z., and Kowalski, W. (1972). Activity of the adrenergic system in humans during physical effort at high environmental temperature. *Acta Physiol. Pol. 23*: 827-833.

Kvetnansky, R., Jahnova, E., Torda, T., Strbak, V., Balaz, V., and Macho, L. (1978). Changes of adrenal catecholamines and their synthesizing enzymes during ontogenesis and aging in rats. *Mech. Ageing Dev. 7*: 209-216.

Lakatta, E. G. (1980). Age-related alterations in the cardiovascular response to adrenergic mediated stress. *Fed. Proc. 39*: 3173-3177.

Lamke, L.-O., Lennquist, S., Liljedahl, S.-O., and Wedin, B. (1972). The influence of cold stress on catecholamine excretion and oxygen uptake of normal persons. *Scand. J. Clin. Lab. Invest. 30*: 57-62.

Lammintausta, R., Syvalahti, E., and Pekkarinen, A. (1976). Change in hormones reflecting sympathetic activity in the Finnish sauna. *Ann. Clin. Res. 8*: 266-271.

LeBlanc, J. A., and Nadeau, G. (1961). Urinary excretion of adrenaline and noradrenaline in normal and cold-adapted animals. *Can. J. Biochem. Physiol. 39*: 215-217.

LeBlanc, J. A., Cote, J., Jobin, M., and Labrie, A. (1979). Plasma catecholamines and cardiovascular responses to cold and mental activity. *J. Appl. Physiol. 47*: 1207-1211.

Leduc, J. (1961). Catecholamine production and release in exposure and acclimation to cold. *Acta. Physiol. Scand.* (*Suppl. No. 183*) *53*: 1-101.

Lewin, M. B., Hudson, D. B., Timiras, P. S., and Kuhlemeier, K. A. (1980): unpublished observations.

Marshall, J. R., and Berrios, N. (1979). Movement disorders of aged rats: reversal by dopamine receptor stimulation. *Science 206*: 477-479.

McCrimmon, D. R., Cunningham, D. A., Rechnitzer, P. A., and Griffiths, J. (1976).

Effect of training on plasma catecholamines in post myocardial infarction patients. *Med. Sci. Sports 8*: 152-156.

McDermott, D. J., Stekiel, W. J., Barboraik, J. J., Kloth, L. C., and Smith, J. J. (1974). Effect of age on hemodynamic and metabolic response to static exercise. *J. Appl. Physiol. 37*: 923-926.

Ordway, G. A., and Wekstein, D. R. (1979). The effect of age on selected cardiovascular responses to static (isometric) exercise. *Proc. Soc. Exp. Biol. Med. 161*: 189-192.

Palmer, G. J., Ziegler, M. G., and Lake, C. R. (1978). Response of norepinephrine and blood pressure to stress increases with age. *J. Gerontol. 33*: 482-487.

Petro, J. K., Hollander, A. P., and Bouman, L. N. (1970). Instantaneous cardiac acceleration in man induced by a voluntary muscle contraction. *J. Appl. Physiol. 29*: 794-798.

Petrofsky, J. S., and Lind, A. R. (1975). Isometric strength, endurance, and the blood pressure and heart rate responses during isometric exercise in healthy men and women, with special reference to age and body fat content. *Pflugers Arch 360*: 49-61.

Rommelspacher, H., Schulze, G. W., and Bolt, V. (1975). Ability of young, adult and aged rats to adapt to different ambient temperatures. In *Temperature Regulation and Drug Action*, P. Lomax, E. Schonbaum, and J. Jacob (Eds.). Karger, Basel, pp. 192-201.

Rowe, J. W., and Troen, B. R. (1980). Sympathetic nervous system and aging in man. *Endocrinol. Rev. 1*: 167-179.

Saito, S. (1928). Influence of application of cold or heat to the dog's body upon the epinephrine output rate. *Tohoku J. Exp. Med. 11*: 544-567.

Schulze, G., and Burgel, P. (1977). The influence of age and drugs on the thermoregulatory behavior of rats. *Nauyn. Schmiedebergs. Arch. Pharmacol. 298*: 143-147.

Segall, P. E., and Timiras, P. S. (1975). Age-related changes in thermoregulatory capacity of tryptophan-deficient rats. *Fed. Proc. 34*: 83-85.

Shum, A., Johnson, G. E., and Flattery, K. V. (1969). Influence of ambient temperature on excretion of catecholamines and metabolites. *Am. J. Physiol. 216*: 1164-1169.

Stefanovic, M. P., Bayley, H. S., and Slinger, S. J. (1970). Effect of stress on swine: heat and cold exposure and starvation on vanilmandelic acid output in the urine. *J. Anim. Sci. 30*: 378-381.

Symbas, P. N., Jellinek, M., Cooper, T., and Hanlon, C. (1964). Effect of hyperthermia on plasma catecholamines and histamine. *Arch. Int. Pharmacodyn. Ther. 150*: 132-136.

Vendsalu, A. (1960). Studies on adrenaline and noradrenaline in human plasma. *Acta Physiol. Scand. (Suppl.) 49*: 1-123.

Wada. M., Seo, M., and Abe, K. (1935). Further study of the influence of cold on the rate of epinephrine secretion from the suprarenal glands with simultaneous determination of blood sugar. *Tohoku J. Exp. Med. 26*: 381-411.

Winer, N., and Carter, C. (1977). Effect of cold pressor stimulation on plasma norepinephrine, dopamine beta hydroxylase, and renin activity. *Life Sci. 20*: 887-894.

Ziegler, M. G., Lake, C. R., and Kopin, I. J. (1976). Plasma noradrenaline increases with age. *Nature 261*: 333-335.

19
Drug and Hormonal Modification of Sleep Rhythms in Female Rats: Changes in Aging

Sadao Yamaoka / *Saitama Medical School, Moroyama-cho, Saitama, Japan*

INTRODUCTION

There are a number of physiological and behavioral changes that occur with aging in the human such as alterations in sleep, mood, total motor activity, endocrine function, and memory. A number of studies indicate that in humans, as well as experimental animals, deficiencies in brain monoaminergic systems also occur with aging (Estes and Simpkins, 1980; Finch, 1979; Govani et al., 1977; Greenberg and Weiss, 1978; McGeer and McGeer, 1980; Severson and Finch, 1980; Simpkins et al., 1977; Weiss et al., 1979), and these changes may lead to reproductive dysfunction (Clemens and Bennett, 1977; Everett, 1980; Gerall et al., 1980; Riegle et al., 1977; Steger and Peluso, 1979; Wise and Ratner, 1980). These studies suggest that decreases in the enzymes that synthesize neurotransmitters and their products represent a neuroendocrine mechanism for reproductive dysfunction in aging rodents (Huang and Meites, 1975; Linnoila and Cooper, 1976; Quadri et al., 1973; Walker et al., 1980; Wilkes et al., 1979).

Previously (Yamaoka, 1978, 1980), we found that the circadian rhythm for sleep (especially for paradoxical sleep) varied over the estrous cycle and was correlated with changes in ovarian steroid levels in the blood. However, relatively little is known of the relationship between the age-related changes in circadian rhythmicity and loss of reproductive cycles in aging rats.

In this chapter, the possibility that neuroendocrine changes affecting reproductive system development and senescence also affect the circadian rhythm of
sleep are discussed.

METHODS

The animals used in these studies were raised in our breeding colony (original
source: Sprague-Dawley strain, Charles River, Japan) and were maintained under
controlled humidity (45-55%), temperature ($24 \pm 0.5^{\circ}$C), and lighting conditions
(lights on, 0500-1900 hr, and lights off, 1900-0500 hr). All rats were implanted
with electrodes for recording EEGs from the frontal cortex, limbic cortex, and
pontine reticular formation, and for EMG from the dorsal neck muscle.

Based upon visual inspection and using a Sleep Pattern Analyzer (Diamedical
System Co.), polygraphic records were taken at slow paper speeds (1 mm/sec) and
divided into three stages according to the characteristic changes in EEG and EMG
activity. These stages or categories included alertness (A), slow-wave sleep (SWS),
and paradoxical sleep (PS). The total duration of SWS and PS episodes was calcu-
lated for each 2 hr and expressed as the mean ($\pm$SEM) duration of SWS and PS.
The mean ($\pm$SEM) of PS for 4 hr during peak times was also recorded and graphed
for each group. Data were analyzed using Student's t-test.

SLEEP RHYTHMS IN THE YOUNG-ADULT RAT

Intact Female Albino Rats

Circadian changes in sleep-wakefulness patterns of female albino rats shown by
long-term EEG recordings have been reported by several investigators (Colvin et
al., 1968; Yamaoka, 1978). These investigators showed that PS is decreased on
proestrus in the intact cycling female albino rat. The characteristics of SWS and
PS rhythms during the estrous cycle are shown in Fig. 1. In the bihourly mean distribution of SWS and PS, the peak periods of SWS were 0600-0800 hr and 1200-
1400 hr, whereas the trough period of SWS was 2000-2200 hr. The peak period of
PS was 1200-1400 hr or 1400-1600 hr, and the trough period of PS was 0400-
0600 hr. A small PS peak which normally occurred during the dark phase between
2200-2400 hr on the days of diestrus and estrus was not seen on proestrus.

These changes in PS and SWS over the estrous cycle seem to be strain-specific
since Long-Evans hooded rats did not show any significant changes during the estrous cycle, whereas Wister wild hooded rats showed estrous cycle-dependent
changes similar to Sprague-Dawley rats. However, the SWS peak (0600-0800 hr)
in the Wistar rats was accompanied by a PS peak on every day except estrus.
Otherwise, the sleep rhythms of both Sprague-Dawley and Wistar albino rats was
not different.

SLEEP RHYTHM AND SEXUAL CYCLE IN FEMALE RAT

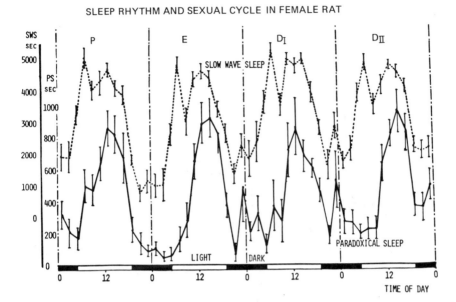

Figure 1 The mean amount of bihourly distribution of slow-wave sleep (SWS) (●- - - -●) and paradoxical sleep (PS) (●————●) during the same time zone on the day showing the same vaginal cycle and their standard errors in six regularly cycling female albino rats. The ordinate indicates 2-hr amounts of SWS and PS and the abscissa indicates the time of day. P, proestrus; E, estrus; D, diestrus.

Effect of Ovariectomy and Sex Steroid Treatment

Colvin et al. (1969) demonstrated that estradiol (E_2) decreased night PS in ovariectomized (OVX) rats. Later, Branchey et al. (1971) showed that progesterone (P) given with E_2 decreased SWS as well as PS in the OVX rat. These findings suggest that decreased total sleep in female rats on proestrus resulted from the elevated level of sex steroids on that day. However, these studies did not define the mechanisms controlling this phenomenon. In our previous study (Yamaoka, 1980), we found that the increase in night PS after gonadectomy in male or female rats is associated with the loss of the negative feedback influence of gonadal steroids. On the other hand, elimination of night PS on proestrus in intact rats or after treatment of OVX rats with E_2 correlates with the positive feedback mechanism of E_2 and not with changes in gonadotropins.

In the present study, night PS rapidly increased on the day of ovariectomy. Treatment of OVX rats with E_2 did not block the increase in night PS until 78 hr after OVX (see Fig. 2). Ramirez and Sawyer (1974) demonstrated that some residual influence from the gonads seems to restrain LH output for at least 78 hr

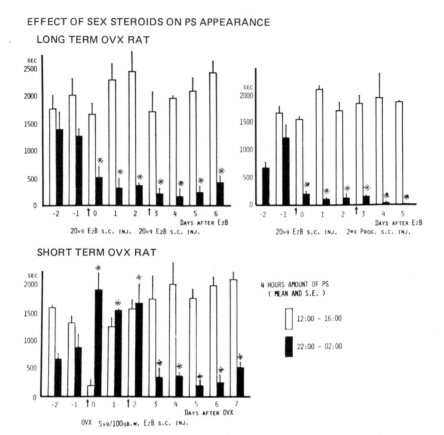

Figure 2 Effect of sex steroids on PS appearance in ovariectomized (OVX) rats. Graphs are showing the 4-hr mean amounts of PS with standard errors in six rats of each during peak time (daytime peak, 1200-1600 hr, open bars; nighttime peak, 2200-0200 hr, black bars). The top two graphs represent the alteration of PS appearance during peak time in long-term OVX (4 or more weeks after OVX) rats. E_2B (estradiol benzoate) 20 μg was injected at 1200 hr on day 0 and 20 μg E_2B or Prog. (progesterone) was injected at 1200 hr on day 3. Bottom graph represents the alteration of peak time PS appearance in short time OVX (ovariectomized on day 0) rats. E_2B was injected on day 2. The mark (✵) indicates the statistically significant difference from the data before treatment ($p < 0.05$).

after OVX. Therefore, this finding could indicate the involvement of a positive feedback effect of E_2 in this response. However, in the long-term OVX rat (i.e., 1 or more months), E_2 treatment eliminated night PS on the day of E_2 injection, and this effect continued about 1 week. A second E_2 or P injection 72 hr later did not alter this elimination of night PS (see Fig. 2). According to Caligaris et al. (1971a,b) a single injection of E_2, given 72 hr after an initial priming dose of E_2

causes daily LH surges. However, if P, instead of E_2, is given at 72 hr, only one LH surge occurs. Therefore, unlike the differential effect of these steroids on LH, they did not have opposite effects on night PS.

In contrast to our finding in albino rats, Branchey et al. (1971) reported that treatment of E_2-primed, OVX, Long-Evans hooded rats with P enhanced the effect of E_2 on night PS. As mentioned before, the estrous-cycle-dependent alterations in sleep rhythm may be strain-specific in rats. Therefore, we performed the same experiment in Long-Evans OVX female rats and confirmed their results. Possibly these strain differences in sleep rhythms may be due to strain differences in the brain's sensitivity to estrogen.

In contrast to these findings in female rats, E_2 plus P treatment did not eliminate night PS in orchidectomized male rats or ovariectomized, neonatally testosterone-treated female rats that do not show the positive feedback response of sex steroids (see Fig. 3). These results suggest that the positive feedback system must be intact for E_2 to eliminate night PS.

Modification of Sleep Rhythms by Sex Steroids: Central Mechanisms

To elucidate the neural mechanisms of the above-mentioned hypothesis, the relationship between the gonadal steroids feedback system and sleep circadian rhythm was studied. Kawakami et al. (1976) suggested that the medial amygdala and bed nucleus of the stria terminalis are implicated in the mechanism controlling the positive feedback response of estradiol. Carrer and Taleisnik (1970) demonstrated that the mesencephalic tegmental area also influences ovulation and LH release. In our previous study (Yamaoka, 1978), we found that bilateral lesions or horizontal deafferentation above the medial preoptic area (MPO-roof cuts) in intact rats increased night PS, an effect which was similar to OVX. On the other hand, posterior deafferentation of the medial basal hypothalamus (PDM) eliminated night PS and abolished the estrous-cycle-dependent changes in sleep circadian rhythm (see Fig. 4). Further studies were performed on ovariectomized rats bearing brain lesions or deafferentation. MPO-roof cuts or septal lesions in OVX rats prevented the effect of E_2 and/or progesterone on night PS, whereas the effect of E_2 on nighttime PS was delayed for 1 or 2 days in OVX-PDM rats (see Fig. 5). The results suggest that changes in night PS correlate with the feedback effects of steroids in the brain. The increase in night PS correlates with the loss or decrease of steroid negative feedback and/or damage to forebrain limbic structures which play an important role in sex steroid feedback mechanisms. The decrease of night PS, however, correlates with the ability of an animal to show positive feedback effects to gonadal steroids, especially E_2.

Central Monoaminergic Mechanisms in Sleep Rhythms

An extensive literature is concerned with the relationship between central monoaminergic systems and feedback responses to gonadal steroids. The effect of PDM

EFFECT OF SEX STEROIDS ON PS APPEARANCE

OVX TP TREATED RAT

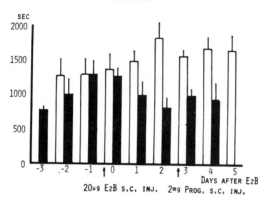

20µg E2B s.c. INJ.   2mg PROG. s.c. INJ.

ORCHIDECTOMIZED MALE RAT

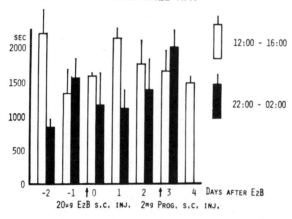

20µg E2B s.c. INJ.   2mg PROG. s.c. INJ.

Figure 3 Effect of sex steroids on peak time PS appearance in OVX rats treated with 50 µg testosterone propionate on the third day of life and in orchidectomized male rats. See Fig. 2. for details.

on PS may be due to the deafferentation of catecholaminergic tracts. This is supported by the finding that intraventricular administration of 6-hydroxydopamine (6-OHDA) reduces night PS and abolishes estrous-cycle-dependent changes in sleep patterns. Furthermore, as shown in Fig. 6, E_2 administration to OVX-6-OHDA rats does not promptly eliminate night PS. To elucidate the role of monoaminergic mechanisms in this phenomenon, neuropharmacological studies were performed. The administration of L-dopa (L-β-3,4-dihydroxyphenylalanine) or DL-DOPS (DL-threo-3,4,-dihydroxyphenylserine) to pargyline-pretreated OVX rats reduced night

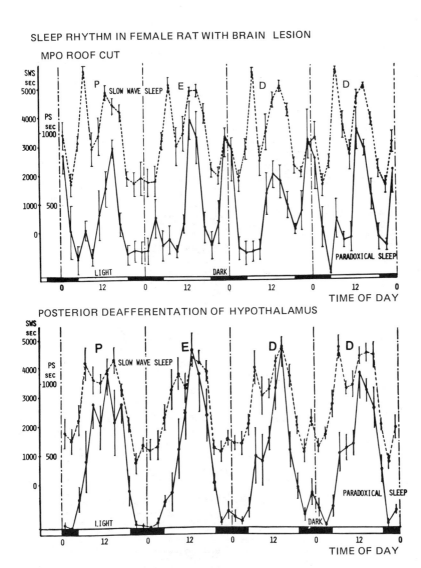

Figure 4   The mean amount of bihourly distribution of SWS and PS in six female rats with horizontal deafferentation above the medial preoptic area (top) and with posterior deafferentation of medial basal hypothalamus at the level of retromamilliary area (bottom). See Fig. 1 for details.

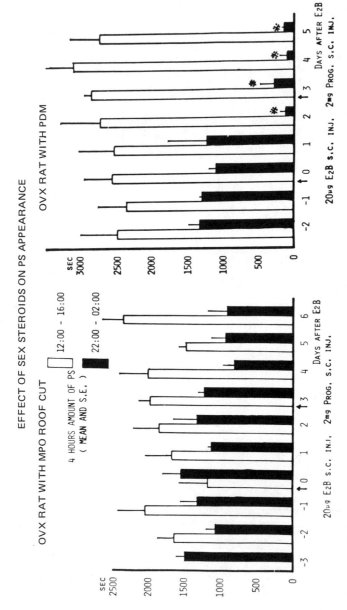

Figure 5 Effect of sex steroids on peak time PS appearance in OVX rats with MPO-roof cut and posterior de-afferentation of medial basal hypothalamus. See Fig. 2 for details.

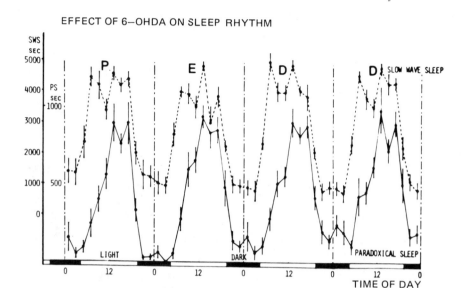

EFFECT OF 6–OHDA ON SLEEP RHYTHM

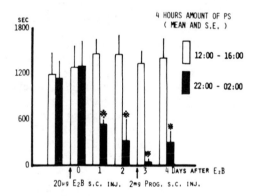

EFFECT OF SEX STEROIDS ON PS APPEARANCE
IN OVX & 6–OHDA TREATED RAT

Figure 6 Effect of 6-OHDA on sleep rhythm and changes in peak time PS appearance by sex steroids. The twice intraventricular administration of 250 mg 6-hydroxydopamine within 24 hr was performed on 10 days before experiment. See Figs. 1 and 2 for details.

PS, whereas 5-HTP (5-hydroxytryptophan), administered with pargyline, did not affect night PS (Fig. 7). These findings using the amine precursors are similar to the above results in which surgical (PDM) and chemical (6-OHDA) procedures were used.

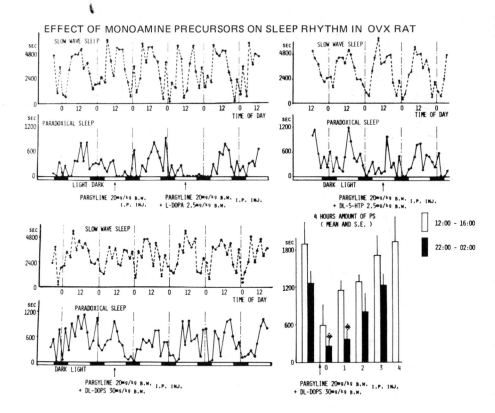

Figure 7 Effect of monoamine precursors on sleep rhythm in OVX rats. Three pairs of line graphs shows the sequential data of sleep records. Arrows under each graph of PS rhythm represent the injection of drugs with their dosages. A bar graph shows the changes in peak time PS appearance by DL-DOPS. See Fig. 2 for details of bar graph and see text for abbreviations of drugs.

We also investigated the effect of aminergic blocking agents on steroid modification of sleep patterns. The beta-adrenergic receptor blocker propranolol given to OVX rats treated with E_2 blocked the ability of the steroid to eliminate night PS. On the other hand, the alpha-adrenergic receptor blocker phenoxybenzamine did not block the elimination of night PS by E_2. The administration of the dop-amine-receptor blocker pimozide prevented the elimination of night PS by E_2, but this drug also caused a marked decrease of PS 0-6 hr after injection, as well as a marked increase in SWS (Fig. 8). Yanase (1977) demonstrated that intraperitoneal administration of adrenalin enhanced the ability of E_2 to induce lordosis behavior in OVX rats. Adrenalin also alters the response of sleep rhythms to steroids. For example, 2 μg E_2 and 1 mg P did not affect the sleep rhythm in five or eight OVX rats, whereas 50 μg adrenalin, given with 2 μg E_2, blocked the appearance of night PS on the day of P treatment in all five rats (Fig. 9). These results suggest that the elimination of night PS by E_2 requires the activation of postsynaptic beta-adren-ergic receptors and that a posterior catecholaminergic pathway may be involved in the effect of E_2 on night PS. Furthermore, adrenalin, given with E_2, may augment the E_2 sensitivity of P-induced night PS elimination.

SLEEP RHYTHMS IN THE IMMATURE ALBINO RAT

It is known that sexual maturation occurs as the result of a number of physiological events occurring in several brain areas (especially the hypothalamus), as well as in the pituitary and gonads. Ramirez and McCann (1965), Odell and Swerdloff (1976), and Smith et al. (1977) indicated that the hypothalamopituitary axis of the im-mature rat is more sensitive to inhibition by gonadal steroids than the hypothal-amus of the adult rat. Raum et al. (1980) postulated that norepinephrine turnover in the hypothalamus of immature rats is inhibited by gonadal steroids and that these inhibitory effects diminish with age. Harden et al. (1977) reported that the density of beta-adrenergic receptors increased markedly 7 and 14 days after birth, but cerebral cortical norepinephrine stores developed slowly, reaching adult levels at approximately 2 months of age. As demonstrated above, sleep rhythms are re-sponsive to steroid hormone feedback and changes in central monoamine function. Therefore, the sleep rhythm was examined during the immature period when steroid and monoamine systems are developing. Sieck et al. (1976, 1978) reported that wakefulness was increased, whereas both SWS and PS were decreased at puberty. In the current study, EEG records were taken beginning at 29 days of age. At 30 days of age, the SWS rhythm showed a circadian pattern similar to that in adult rats, whereas the bihourly distribution of PS showed a semicircadian pat-tern. The peak periods of PS were at 1000-1200 hr or 1200-1400 hr (daytime peak), and at 2200-2400 hr or 0000-0200 hr (nighttime peak). These peaks did not show any significant difference (see Fig. 10). Total amounts of PS were sig-nificantly greater in immature rats than in adults (Table 1). Treatment of immature rats with pregnant mares serum (PMS) at 30 days of age induced precocious pu-berty. However, the treatment decreased the daytime PS peak and increased the nighttime PS peak. When puberty occurred spontaneously, the nighttime PS peak

EFFECT OF AMINERGIC BLOCKERS ON SLEEP RHYTHM

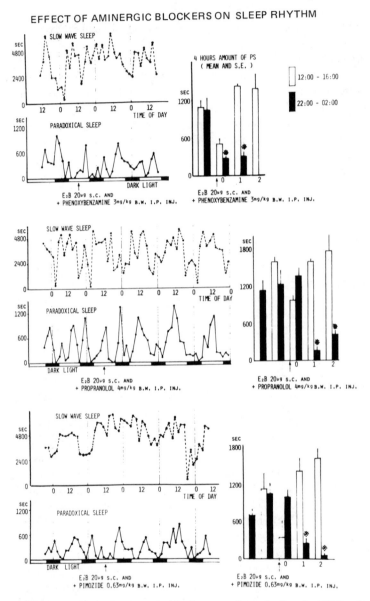

Figure 8 Effect of aminergic blockers on sleep rhythm in OVX rats. Left graphs shows the sequential data of sleep records. Right graphs shows the changes in peak time PS appearance by aminergic blockers and E_2. E_2 was injected at 1200 hr and aminergic blockers were injected within 2 hr after E_2. See Fig. 7 for details.

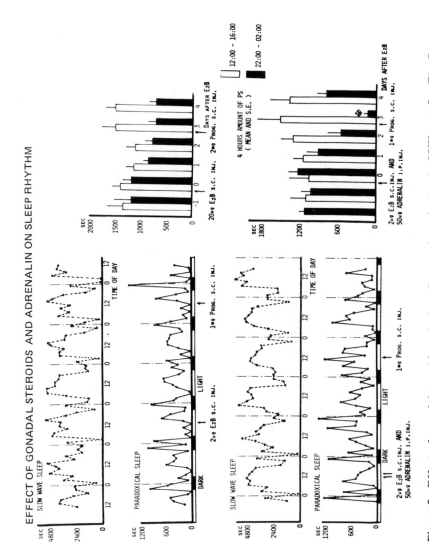

Figure 9 Effect of gonadal steroids and adrenaline on sleep rhythm in OVX rats. See Fig. 7 for details.

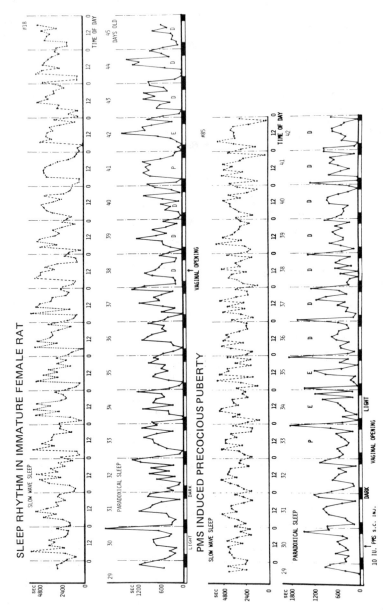

Figure 10 Sleep rhythm in immature female rats. Top graph shows an example of consecutive sleep records (bihourly amounts of SWS and PS) from 29 to 45-day-old spontaneously maturing female rats. Bottom graph shows a consecutive sleep record in a rat with precocious puberty induced by PMS (pregnant mare serum gonadotropin).

Table 1 Sleep in Various Conditions or Treatments (12 hr segments)

Condition or treatment	Slow-wave sleep			Paradoxical sleep		
	0600-1800(sec)	1800-0600 (sec)	Total (sec)	0600-1800 (sec)	1800-0600 (sec)	Total (sec)
Intact	P 25753 ± 702(18)[a]	8124 ± 853(18)[c]	33882 ± 1130(18)	3982 ± 394(18)	554 ± 116(18)[f]	4517 ± 428(18)
	E 23137 ± 1343(19)	12224 ± 1067(18)[d]	35976 ± 1206(18)	3433 ± 229(21)	1304 ± 198(18)[g]	4784 ± 358(18)
Female	D 25622 ± 817(17)	12636 ± 873(17)	38259 ± 1285(17)	3667 ± 320(16)	1729 ± 208(18)	5376 ± 353(18)
	D 26008 ± 707(17)	14613 ± 877(16)	40506 ± 1257(16)	3253 ± 254(16)	1997 ± 262(15)	5320 ± 362(15)
OVX	24651 ± 678(33)	14478 ± 516(33)	38614 ± 1076(26)	2666 ± 163(33)[b]	3099 ± 159(33)[h]	5609 ± 247(26)
PDM	E 23498 ± 1104(9)	9443 ± 850(8)[e]	32689 ± 1992(8)	5497 ± 843(9)	1005 ± 263(8)	6688 ± 1122(8)[l]
Immature female	23064 ± 235(41)	14919 ± 467(41)	37878 ± 547(37)	3468 ± 122(42)[b]	3375 ± 95(43)[i]	6908 ± 137(38)[m]
Aging SPE	26071 ± 487(42)	14759 ± 513(44)	41066 ± 931(39)	3161 ± 108(39)[l]	1075 ± 70(45)[j]	4197 ± 124(40)
Immature female PSP	25168 ± 799(16)	15568 ± 780(18)	40810 ± 1479(16)	1845 ± 220(16)[m]	2894 ± 201(17)[k]	4685 ± 360(16)
Induced PSP	24778 ± 635(24)	16429 ± 568(23)	40839 ± 1073(18)	2817 ± 119(25)	2103 ± 103(23)	4966 ± 202(18)

[a] Mean ± standard error (days of record).

[b] No significant difference between 0600-1800 and 1800-0600. Significant difference between following pairs (p < 0.05): c vs. d, d vs. e, f vs. g.

Values of h, i, g, and k are significantly higher than others (p < 0.01). Value of m is significantly lower than others (p < 0.01). Value of m is significantly higher than others except l (p = 0.001).

P, proestrus; E, estrus; D, diestrus; OVX, ovariectomized female; PDM, posterior deafferentation of medial basal hypothalamus; SPE, spontaneous persistent estrus; PSP, pseudopregnancy. Induced PSP, pseudopregnancy induced by cervical stimulation in young-adult rats.

decreased gradually and showed the estrous-cycle-dependent changes when adulthood was reached. These changes in the sleep rhythm strongly correlate with developmental changes in steroid feedback and central monoaminergic mechanisms.

SLEEP RHYTHMS IN THE OLD FEMALE ALBINO RAT

Sleep Rhythms and the Vaginal Cycle

As they approach the end of their first year of life, female rats tend to show irregular estrous cycles. Afterward, their regular estrous cycle ceases and they show a persistent estrous state (SPE). SPE, which may last for weeks or months, is often followed by pseudopregnancy (PSP). PSP may last for about 1 year and then may be replaced by chronic anestrus (Aschheim, 1961, 1965a,b; Clemens and Meites, 1971; Ingram, 1959; Mandl and Shelton, 1959; Thung et al., 1956). It has been suggested that these age-related changes in the estrous cycle reflect a defect in hypothalamic regulation and not a failure of ovarian function (Clemens and Bennett, 1977; Peng and Huang, 1972). Also, ovulation can be induced in old SPE rats by electrical stimulation of the hypothalamus (Clemens et al., 1969), LH administration (Aschheim, 1965a,b), injections of progesterone (Everett, 1940), a variety of centrally acting compounds (including epinephrine, L-dopa, and CA agonists), adrenocorticotropic hormone (ACTH), ether stress (Quadri et al., 1973; Huang and Meites, 1975; Linnoila and Cooper, 1976; Huang et al., 1976; Everett, 1980), and even exposure to constant darkness (Aschheim, 1965a,b). On the other hand, it is generally accepted that the suprachiasmatic nucleus (SCN) is a critical component of the central mechanism of circadian rhythm generation and entrainment in rodents. SCN lesions abolish circadian rhythmicity in a variety of physiological and behavioral functions, including estrous cycles, and cause a persistent estrous state similar to that in old rats. Mosko et al. (1980) found altered circadian rhythmicity of locomotor activity and drinking behavior in reproductively senescent rats.

In the present study, age-related changes in circadian rhythmicity were investigated by comparing SWS and PS rhythms in old SPE and PSP rats with those of young adults showing regular estrous cycles. The SWS rhythm in old SPE rats was similar to that in young-adult cycling rats, but the PS rhythm, which showed a single peak during daytime, lacked the night PS peak in four out of six old SPE rats (11-15 months old). Two old SPE rats showed the ultradian PS rhythm (see Fig. 11). Persistent estrus can be induced by testosterone propionate treatment neonatally (days 0-5 of life; TP-PE), or by SCN lesions (SCN-PE). The sleep rhythm in both TP-PE and SCN-PE rats was compared with that observed in old SPE rats. The SWS rhythm in TP-PE rats showed two peaks at 0400-0600 hr and 1000-1200 hr in the bihourly mean distribution, but the first peak was variable. The bihourly PS distribution also showed two peaks at 0200-0400 hr (small night PS peak) and

1400-1600 hr, but the daytime PS peak was delayed 4 hr from the SWS peak. SCN-PE rats showed the ultradian SWS and circadian PS rhythm. Therefore, the sleep rhythm in these PE rats was different from that in old SPE rats (see Fig. 12).

In old PSP rats (13-18 months old), the SWS rhythm was also similar to that in young-adult cycling rats, but the PS rhythm showed two or three peaks over 24 hr. The nightime peak was often higher than the daytime peak (see Fig. 11). This PS rhythm in old PSP rats was similar to that in prepubertal rats and in rats made PSP by cervical stimulation.

Modification of Sleep Rhythms in Old OVX Rats by Sex Steroids

The rise in LH after OVX is diminished in old, noncycling female rats, but E_2 treatment suppresses LH levels to the same degree as in young cycling rats (Howland and Preiss, 1975; Peluso et al., 1977; Shaar et al., 1975). Peluso et al. (1977) showed that the positive feedback response to estrogen is severely impaired in old female rats, despite the fact that the negative feedback system is intact. We previously showed that estrous-cycle-dependent or sex-steroid-induced changes in the sleep rhythm are related to the steroid feedback mechanisms (Yamaoka, 1980). In order to determine the effect of endocrine changes with age on the steroidal modification of sleep rhythms, we investigated the effect of hormone treatment in old OVX rats. After OVX, both SPE and PSP rats showed irregular or ultradian PS rhythms and SWS rhythms that were similar to those in young OVX rats. Twenty micrograms of E_2, given to old OVX rats, increased the circadian rhythm of PS and did not immediately alter night PS. However, night PS decreased significantly on the second night of E_2 treatment. This decrease was less than in comparably treated young OVX rats. On the other hand, 2 mg of P, 72 hr after E_2, totally eliminated night PS in old OVX rats. This response was different from that in young-adult OVX rats in which P administration did not alter E_2 effects (see Fig. 13). In contrast to these findings in the female rat, E_2 and P treatment did not show any effects in rats with impaired positive feedback systems such as orchidectomized males, OVX-TP females, and OVX-roof cut females. However, in old OVX rats, the E_2 effect was diminished and the P effect remained intact. Therefore, it is possible that the positive feedback system of E_2 but not P is impaired in old OVX rats.

Central Monoaminergic Mechanisms in Sleep Rhythms

It is generally accepted that various brain areas in aging rats show decreased monoamine content. Furthermore, the density of beta-adrenergic receptors also declines with age in the pineal gland, corpus striatum, and cerebellum of rats (Greenberg and Weiss, 1978). On the other hand, Walker et al. (1980) reported that pCPA (p-chlorophenylalanine) placed locally in the rostral suprachiasmatic area of young-adult female rats during diestrus 2 mimicks the condition seen in old SPE rats. In

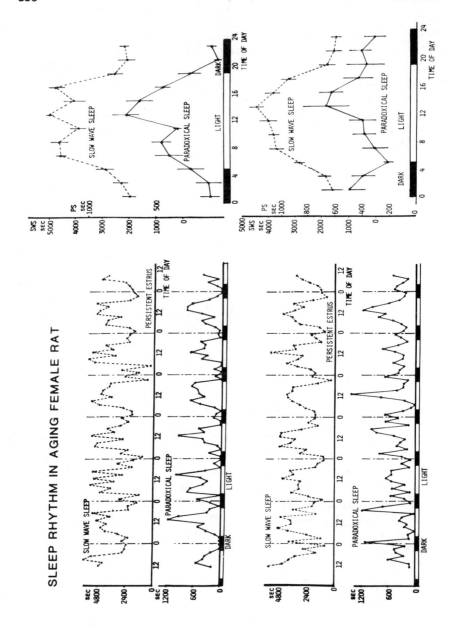

SLEEP RHYTHM IN AGING FEMALE RAT

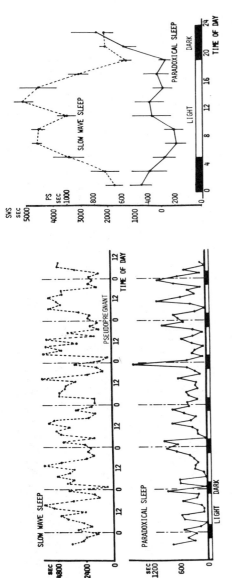

Figure 11   Sleep rhythm in aging female rats. Left graphs show examples of consecutive 7 to 9-day records in old persistent estrous rats (top and middle) and in old pseudopregnant rats (bottom). Right graphs show the mean amount of bihourly distribution of SWS and PS during the same time zone and their standard errors in each rat. Middle graph shows an example of sleep records in four old SPE rats showing the ultradian or irregular PS rhythm.

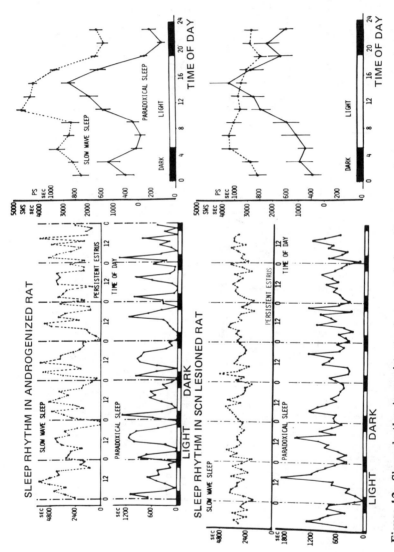

Figure 12   Sleep rhythm in persistent estrous rats induced by neonatal testosterone treatment of suprachiasmic lesion. See Fig. 11 and text for details.

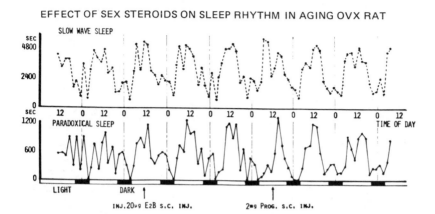

EFFECT OF SEX STEROIDS ON SLEEP RHYTHM IN AGING OVX RAT

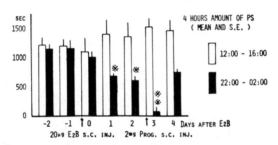

Figure 13 Effect of sex steroids on sleep rhythm in aging OVX rats (see Fig. 7 for details). The mark ( ) indicates the statistically significant difference from the data after E_2 treatment (day 1 or 2).

the present study, alterations of sleep rhythms were investigated by administering pCPA and a-MT (alpha-methyl-p-tyrosine) via indwelling cannulae to the rostral SCN of young-adult rats during diestrus 2. From 2 to 30 hr after pCPA was given, the SWS rhythm fluctuated, showing multiple peaks with 4-hr periods. This change was followed by restored regular SWS rhythms. Ten to fourteen hours after pCPA treatment, PS increased and showed a large peak. After this initial PS increase, the PS rhythm became ultradian until the estrous cycle reappeared (10-20 days after pCPA treatment). On the other hand, a-MT treatment abolished the circadian periodicity of both SWS and PS for 2-3 days. Afterwards, regular circadian rhythms of both sleep patterns returned; however, estrous cycles remained irregular with 3 to 5-day estrous intervals. These results suggest that pCPA treatment was more effective than a-MT in producing changes in sleep patterns in young rats that resemble the patterns present in old SPE rats, but neither was as effective as PDM or

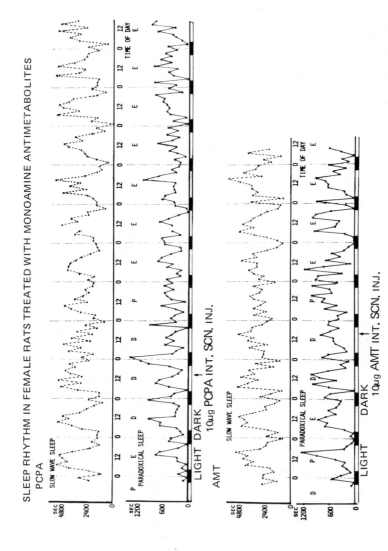

Figure 14 Sleep rhythm in female rats treated with monoamine antimetabolites. pCPA (p-chloro-phenylalanine) 10 μg or α-MT (α-methyl-p-tyrosine) were administered into rostral suprachiasmatic nucleus through indwelling cannulae at 1600 hr during diestrus 2 in cycling female rats.

6-OHDA treatment in this regard. However, the PDM and 6-OHDA rats showed regular estrous cycles, and total PS appearance of PDM rats was higher than in old SPE rats.

It has been shown that the denervation of noradrenergic tracts causes post-synaptic supersensitivity of beta-adrenergic receptors (Sporn et al., 1976). However, old rats show decreased noradrenalin content and decreased density of beta-adrenergic receptors in the brain. This apparent discrepancy of decreased receptor and transmitter content requires more experimental investigation.

The sleep rhythm of old PSP rats is very similar to that of PSP rats induced by cervical stimulation. Both induced and old PSP rats show high prolactin concentration in serum and low dopamine concentration in the pituitary stalk (Gudelsky et al., 1977). Furthermore, Clemens and Bennett (1977) reported that lesions of the medial preoptic area induced repeated PSP of variable duration. These PSP rats showed high serum prolactin levels which were suppressed by lergotrile mesylate (a dopamine agonist). Our preliminary results with PSP rats resulting from medial preoptic lesions indicate that a similar pattern of sleep rhythm occurs in old PSP and cervically stimulated PSP rats. The sleep rhythms of old PSP rats may result from an impairment of dopaminergic neurons arising or passing through the medial preoptic area.

CONCLUSION

Despite considerable research on aging, little is known about the neuroendocrine mechanisms controlling age-related changes in circadian rhythmicity. Possibly the results presented in this chapter are a first step in elucidating the neuroendocrine mechanisms of age-related changes in sleep circadian rhythms. It has been shown that the sleep rhythm, especially involving PS, often reflects gonadal steroid feedback conditions. This is supported by the findings that sleep rhythms are modified by gonadal steroids or centrally acting drugs in adult female rats.

In immature rats, the development of sleep rhythms correlates with the developmental changes in aminergic systems. The increased night PS in developing rats seems to reflect the immature state of the positive feedback system, as well as the low content of norepinephrine and the low numbers of beta-adrenergic receptors in these animals. The sleep rhythms of old female rats showed patterns that were different from those observed in young-adult female animals, and these differences appeared to be a consequence of age-related changes in ovarian function. The data suggest that low night PS in the old SPE rats results from supersensitivity of beta-adrenergic receptors during the early SPE. After disturbances of hypothalamic aminergic systems (that can be mimicked by pCPA administration into the SCN), PS rhythm may change to ultradian rhythms (four SPE rats). The sleep rhythm of PSP rats may result from a decreased dopamine content in brain or an impairment in the dopaminergic neurons originating from or passing through the medial preoptic area. However, to elucidate these highly speculative considerations, much experimental work remains to be done.

ACKNOWLEDGMENTS

The author thanks Mr. T. Onodera for his technical assistance. The work described in this chapter was supported in part by a Grant-in-Aid for Scientific Research from the Ministry of Education, Science, and Culture of Japan.

REFERENCES

Aschheim, P. (1961). La pseudogestation à repetition chez les rattes seniles. *Comptes Rendus Hebdomadaires des Seances de L'Academie des Sciences 253*: 1988-1990.

Aschheim, P. (1965a). La reactivation de l'ovarie des rattes seniles en oestrus permanent au moyen d'hormones gonatropes de la mise à l'obscurité. *Comptes Rendus Hebdomadaires des Seances de L'Academie des Sciences 260*: 5627-5630.

Aschheim, P. (1965b). Resultats fournis par greffe heterochrome des ovaries dans l'étude de la régulation hypothalamo-hypophyseo-ovarience de la ratte. *Gerontologia (Basel) 10*: 67-75.

Branchey, M., Branchey, L., and Nadler, R. D. (1971). Effects of estrogen and progesterone on sleep patterns of female rats. *Physiol. Behav. 6*: 743-746.

Caligaris, L., Astrada, J. J., and Taleisnik, S. (1971a). Release of luteinizing hormone induced by estrogen injection into ovariectomized rats. *Endocrinology 88*: 810-815.

Caligaris, L., Astrada, J. J., and Taleisnik, S. (1971b). Biphasic effect of progesterone on release of gonadotropin in rats. *Endocrinology 89*: 331-337.

Carrer, H. F., and Taleisnik, S. (1970). Effect of mesencephalic stimulation on release of gonadotrophins. *J. Endocrinol. 48*: 527-539.

Clemens, J. A., and Bennett, D. R. (1977). Do aging changes in the preoptic area contribute to loss of cyclic endocrine function? *J. Gerontol. 32*: 19-24.

Clemens, J. A., and Meites, J. (1971). Neuroendocrine status of old constant estrous rats. *Neuroendocrinology 7*: 247-256.

Clemens, J. A., Amenomori, Y., Jenkins, T., and Meites, J. (1969). Effects of hypothalamic stimulation, hormones and drugs on ovarian function in old female rats. *Proc. Soc. Exp. Biol. Med. 132*: 561-563.

Colvin, G. B., Whitmoyer, D. I., and Sawyer, C. H. (1969). Circadian sleep-wakefulness patterns in rats after ovariectomy and treatment with estrogen. *Exp. Neurol. 25*: 616-625.

Colvin, G. B., Whitmoyer, R. D., Lisk, R. D., Walter, D. O., and Sawyer, C. H. (1968). Changes in sleep-wakefulness in female rats during circadian and estrous cycles. *Brain. Res. 7*: 173-181.

Estes, K. S., and Simpkins, J. W. (1980). Age-related alterations in catecholamine concentration in discrete preoptic area and hypothalamic regions in the male rat. *Brain Res. 194*: 556-560.

Everett, J. W. (1940). The restoration of ovulatory cycles and corpus luteum formation in persistent-estrous rats by progesterone. *Endocrinology 27*: 681-686.

Everett, J. W. (1943). Further studies on the relationship of progesterone to ovulation and luteinization in the persistent-estrous rat. *Endocrinology 32*: 285-292.

Everett, J. W. (1980). Reinstatement of estrous cycles in middle-aged spontaneously persistent estrous rats: Importance of circulating prolactin and the resulting facilitative action of progesterone. *Endocrinology 106*: 1691-1696.

Finch, C. E. (1979). Neuroendocrine mechanisms and aging. *Fed. Proc. 38*: 178-183.

Gerall, A. A., Dunlap, J. L., and Sonntag, W. E. (1980). Reproduction in aging, normal and neonatally androgenized female rats. *J. Comp. Physiol. Psychol. 94*: 556-563.

Govani, S., Loddo, P., Spano, P. F., and Trabucchi, M. (1977). Dopamine receptor sensitivity in brain and retina of rats during aging. *Brain Res. 138*: 565-570.

Greenberg, L. H., and Weiss, B. (1978). β-adrenergic receptors in aged rat brain: Reduced number and capacity of pineal gland to develop supersensitivity. *Science 201*: 61-63.

Gudelsky, G. A., Nansel, D. D., and Porter, J. C. (1981). Dopaminergic control of prolactin secretion in the aging male rat. *Brain Res. 201*: 446-450.

Harden, T. K., Wolfe, B. B., Sporn, J. R., Perkins, J. P., and Molinoff, P. B. (1977). Ontogeny of β-adrenergic receptors in rat cerebral cortex. *Brain Res. 125*: 99-108.

Howland, B. E., and Preiss, C. (1975). Effect of aging on basal levels of serum gonadotropins, ovarian compensatory hypertrophy and hypersecretion of gonadotropins after ovariectomy in female rats. *Fertil. Steril. 26*: 271-276.

Huang, H. H., and Meites, J. (1975). Reproductive capacity of aging female rats. *Neuroendocrinology 17*: 289-295.

Huang, H. H., Marshall, S., and Meites, J. (1976). Induction of estrous cycles in old non-cyclic rats by progesterone, ACTH, ether stress or L-dopa. *Neuroendocrinology 20*: 21-34.

Ingram, D. K. (1959). The vaginal smear of senile laboratory rats. *J. Endocrinol. 19*: 185-188.

Kawakami, M., Kimura, F., and Konda, N. (1976). Role of forebrain structure in the regulation of gonadotropin secretion. In *Neuroendocrine Regulation of Fertility*, T. C. Anand Kumar (Ed.). Karger, Basel, pp. 101-113.

Linnoila, M., and Cooper, R. L. (1976). Reinstatement of vaginal cycles in aged female rats. *J. Pharmacol. Exp. Ther. 199*: 477-482.

Mandl, A. M., and Shelton, M. (1959). A quantitative study of oocytes in young and old multiparous laboratory rats. *J. Endocrinol. 18*: 444-450.

McGeer, E. G., and McGeer, P. L. (1980). Aging and neurotransmitter systems. In *Ergot Compounds and Brain Function: Neuroendocrine and Neuropsychiatric Aspect*, M. Goldstein, D. B. Calne, A. N. Lieberman, and M. O. Thorner (Eds.). Raven Press, New York, pp. 304-314.

Mosko, S. S., Erickson, G. F., and Moore, R. Y. (1980). Dampened circadian rhythm in reproductively senescent female rats. *Behav. Neurol. Biol. 28*: 1-14.

Odell, W. D., and Swerdroff, R. S. (1976). Etiologies of sexual maturation: a model based on the sexually mature rat. *Recent Prog. Horm. Res. 32*: 245-288.

Peluso, J. J., Steger, R. W., and Hafez, E. S. E. (1977). Regulation of LH secretion in aged female rats. *Biol. Reprod. 16*: 212-215.

Peng, M. T., and Huang, H. H. (1972). Aging of hypothalamic-pituitary-ovarian function in the rat. *Fertil. Steril. 23*: 535-542.

Quadri, S. K., Kledzik, G. S., and Meites, J. (1973). Reinitiation of estrous cycles in old constant-estrous rats by central-acting drugs. *Neuroendocrinology 11*: 248-255.

Ramirez, V. D., and McCann, S. M. (1965). Inhibitory effect of testosterone on luteinizing hormone secretion in immature and adult rats. *Endocrinology 76*: 412-417.

Ramirez, V. D., and Sawyer, C. H. (1974). Differential dynamic responses of plasma LH and FSH to ovariectomy and to a single injection of estrogen in the rat. *Endocrinology 94*: 987-993.

Raum, W. J., Glass, A. N., and Swerdloff, R. S. (1980). Changes in hypothalamic catecholamine neurotransmitters and pituitary gonadotropins in the immature female rat: Relationships to the gonadostat theory of puberty onset. *Endocrinology 106*: 1253-1258.

Riegle, G. D., Meites, J., Miller, A. E., and Wood, S. M. (1977). Effect of aging on hypothalamic LH-releasing and prolactin inhibiting activities and pituitary responsiveness to LHRH in the male laboratory rat. *J. Gerontol. 32*: 13-18.

Severson, J. A., and Finch, C. E. (1980). Reduced dopaminergic binding during aging in the rodent striatum. *Brain Res. 192*: 147-162.

Shaar, C. J., Euker, J. S., Riegle, G. D., and Meites, J. (1975). Effects of castration and gonadal steroids on serum LH and prolactin in old and young rats. *J. Endocrinol. 66*: 45-51.

Sieck, G. C., Ramaley, J. A., Harper, R. M., and Taylor, A. N. (1976). Sleep-wakefulness changes at the time of puberty in the female rat. *Brain Res. 116*: 346-352.

Sieck, G. C., Ramaley, J. A., Harper, R. M., and Taylor, A. N. (1978). Puberty related alteration in the organization of sleep-wakefulness states: differences between spontaneous and induced pubertal conditions. *Exp. Neurol. 61*: 407-420.

Simpkins, J. W., Mueller, G. P., Huang, H. H., and Meites, J. (1977). Evidence for depressed catecholamine and enhanced serotonin metabolism in aging male rat: possible relation to gonadotropin secretion. *Endocrinology 100*: 1672-1678.

Smith, E. R., Damassa, D. A., and Davidson, J. M. (1977). Feedback regulation and male puberty: testosterone luteinizing hormone relationships in the developing rat. *Endocrinology 101*: 173-180.

Sporn, J. R., Harden, T. K., Wolfe, B. B., and Molinoff, P. B. (1976). β-adrenergic receptor involvement in 6-hydroxydopamine-induced supersensitivity in rat cerebral cortex. *Science 194*: 624-625.

Steger, R. W., and Peluso, J. J. (1979). Hypothalamic-pituitary function in the old irregularly cycling rat. *Exp. Aging Res. 5*: 303-317.

Thung, P. J., Boot, L. M., and Muhlbock, O. (1956). Senile changes in the estrous cycle and in ovarian structure in some inbred strains of mice. *Acta Endocrinol. (Kbh.) 23*: 8-32.

Walker, R. F., Cooper, R. L., and Timiras, P. S. (1980). Constant estrus: role of rostral hypothalamic monoamines in development of reproductive dysfunction in aging rats. *Endocrinology 107*: 249-255.

Weiss, B., Greenberg, L., and Cantor, E. (1979). Age-related alterations in the development of adrenergic denervation supersensitivity. *Fed. Proc. 38*: 1915-1921.

Wilkes, M. M., Lu, K. H., Hopper, B. R., and Yen, S. S. C. (1979). Altered neuroendocrine status of middle-aged rats prior to the onset of senescent anovulation. *Neuroendocrinology 29*: 255-261.

Wise, P. M., and Ratner, A. (1980). LHRH-induced LH and FSH responses in the aged female rat. *J. Gerontol. 35*: 506-511.

Yamaoka, S. (1978). Participation of limbic-hypothalamic structures in circadian rhythm of slow wave sleep and paradoxical sleep in the rat. *Brain Res. 151*: 255-268.

Yamaoka, S. (1980). Modification of circadian sleep rhythm by gonadal steroids and the neural mechanisms involved. *Brain Res. 185*: 385-398.

Yanase, M. (1977). A possible involvement of adrenaline in the facilitation of lordosis behavior in the ovariectomized rat. *Endocrinol. Jap. 24*: 507-512.

20
Aging and Temporal Organization

Harvey V. Samis and Leslie Zajac-Batell / *Veterans Administration Medical Center, Bay Pines, Florida*

INTRODUCTION

Recognition and acceptance of the importance of environmental cycles in human health and well-being date from the time of Hippocrates (Stupfel, 1975). It is, nevertheless, only with the relatively recent technological improvements in the environmental sciences and the advent of computer analysis, that the temporal aspects of biological processes have become recognized as vital aspects of organismic functional capacity and well-being by modern scientists and physicians. It is now incontrovertible that a wide variety of biological processes and functions are as much organized and integrated in time as they are in space. The success and effectiveness of systems and processes, moreover, appear to derive from or depend upon their continued and coherent juxtaposition in time. With the importance of temporal order well established, it is reasonable for gerontologists to extend their investigations and explanations of the deterioration of biological function which accompanies or defines aging to this dimension of biological organization—the organization of processes in time. Indeed, the notion was soon preferred (Samis, 1968) that aging may be due, at least in part, to a deterioration in temporal organization.

The argument at that time was, as it is now, logically limited to studies based on observed age-related changes. No assertions can be made as to the cause and effect relationships between changes in temporal organization and advancing age. In that the mechanisms, direct or indirect, by means of which longevity or its limits are regulated remain to be elucidated, it is necessary to concentrate on the correlates of aging and their physiological consequences, while remaining mindful that correlates of aging need not be related to its cause or causes, nor necessarily its effects; they may well be nothing more than responses to changes in external factors such as diet or the levels and nature of environmental insults.

This chapter is intended as an examination of the possible relationships between changes in temporal organization and aging; specifically, those correlates of advancing age which either effect or are affected by altered temporal organization, and which appear to change or have a reasonable potential to effect change in the functional capabilities and adaptive capacity of the organism. Evidence as to the functional importance of processes being organized in time will be provided, as well as that concerning the functional consequences of biological processes becoming disorganized in time or with respect to the periodic changes in the environment. In the framework of correlational rather than causal relationships, aging may be dealt with in terms of chronopathology, chronopharmacodynamics, and chronotoxicology. Using this approach, chronobiological data not directly related to aging may be marshalled as evidence that the manipulation or disruption of temporal organization can result in the generation of changes similar to many of the deleterious age-related changes which hallmark aging throughout the biome. Furthermore, this approach may be helpful in the development of potentially fruitful new avenues of inquiry, if not in uncovering the cause or causes of senescence, then possibly in optimizing both the quality and duration of useful and healthy life, as well as leading to more efficacious methods for the management and treatment of aging individuals.

CIRCADIAN RHYTHMS

Biological processes of living organisms have been found to present a wide range of rhythmic fluctuations or oscillations that range from approximations of the seasons of the year to periods of a second or less (Aschoff, 1979). There are, roughly speaking, two classes of biological rhythms which are distinguished by their probable derivations: those which reflect passive responses to periodic changes in the environment (exogenously derived rhythms) and those which have their genesis within the organism (endogenously derived rhythms). Under normal environmental conditions, the latter type may be entrained to environmental cues or synchronized with respect to them as well as to one another. A rhythm that persists in the absence of any external cues as to the passage of time and continues to approximate the period of the cyclic environmental cues is said to be free-running. Halberg (1959) introduced the term circadian (circa = about, dias = day) for those rhythms which continue to approximate the 24-hr diel cycle to which they are normally synchronized after the external cues have been removed. Free-running circadian rhythms have been observed in eukaryotic, unicellular, and multicellular organisms, and evidence for them in prokaryotic cells has also been reported (Halberg and Conner, 1961; Sturtevant, 1973). They exhibit the following properties: (1) a free-running period of approximately 24 hr; (2) ubiquity, at least among eukaryotes; (3) entrainability to environmental changes or cues of light or temperature; (4) persistence under constant environmental conditions; (5) phase-shiftability by light or temperature signals; and (6) a temperature-independent period (Edmunds, 1975, 1978).

Parameters of biological temporal organization are often described mathematically in terms of a type of wave analysis known as cosiner analysis, a statistical method of fitting a cosine wave form to data by least squares. This method, developed by Halberg (1959), confers on the fitted rhythmic function a number of descriptive elements which permit comparison of rhythmic processes as to period, amplitude, mean value of the fitted curve (mesor), peak amplitude, time of occurrence of peak amplitude (acrophase), and a measure of variability in the time of occurrence of the peak amplitude, usually expressed in terms of the 95% confidence interval (Fig. 1). Diagrams of the relationships between the various rhythmic functions can also be constructed. They graphically illustrate the temporal organization in terms of the acrophases of the processes or function and the 95% confidence limits for those characteristics of the fitted curves (Fig. 2).

The preponderance of evidence indicates that the temporal profiles of organisms reflect genetically determined characteristic relationships which serve the adaptive functions of internally ordering biological processes and behaviors in time, as well as coordinating them with periodic environmental changes. The highly characteristic nature of the temporal arrangements of molecular and physiological properties in particular species and strains of organisms led Ehret in 1974 (Ehret, 1974) to coin the word "chronotype" for the array of rhythms which represents an individual's temporal profile, as exemplified by the acrophase map of the human circadian system shown in Fig. 2. If one were to compare group acrophase maps of one species with another, or individual acrophase maps within a species, one would find both species specificity and interindividual variability for many functions. Healthy individuals of any particular species, however, would be expected to exhibit similar relationships between the timing of rhythmic characteristics of certain activities, such as body temperature, steroid excretion, and feeding behavior, and the appearance of light/dark cues to which they are entrained. For directly linked processes such as DNA synthesis and mitosis, the importance of a closely maintained temporal relationship is intuitively obvious in that DNA synthesis within a given cell is necessary for the completion of the mitotic event (Samis, 1968). Similarly, it may be inferred that temporal coordination between urine volume and excretion of urinary constituents K^+, Na^+, Ca^{2+} (Aschoff and Wever, 1976) serves an adaptive function in the maintenance of electrolyte balance. The implications of maintaining other temporal relationships such as those which normally obtain among brain 5-hydroxytryptamine levels, phagocytic index, and liver

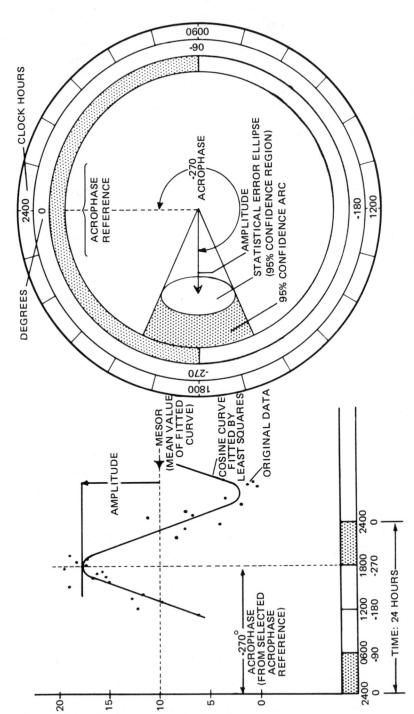

Figure 1 Relationship between cosine function drawn through hypothetical data and the cosinor analysis of those data. (Redrawn courtesy of Halberg and Nelson, 1978.)

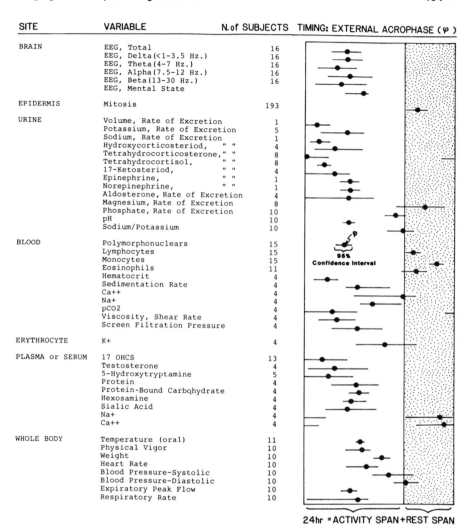

SITE	VARIABLE	N. of SUBJECTS
BRAIN	EEG, Total	16
	EEG, Delta(<1-3.5 Hz.)	16
	EEG, Theta(4-7 Hz.)	16
	EEG, Alpha(7.5-12 Hz.)	16
	EEG, Beta(13-30 Hz.)	16
	EEG, Mental State	
EPIDERMIS	Mitosis	193
URINE	Volume, Rate of Excretion	1
	Potassium, Rate of Excretion	5
	Sodium, Rate of Excretion	1
	Hydroxycorticosteriod, " "	4
	Tetrahydrocorticosterone," "	8
	Tetrahydrocortisol, " "	8
	17-Ketosteriod, " "	4
	Epinephrine, " "	1
	Norepinephrine, " "	1
	Aldosterone, Rate of Excretion	4
	Magnesium, Rate of Excretion	8
	Phosphate, Rate of Excretion	10
	pH	10
	Sodium/Potassium	10
BLOOD	Polymorphonuclears	15
	Lymphocytes	15
	Monocytes	15
	Eosinophils	11
	Hematocrit	4
	Sedimentation Rate	4
	Ca++	4
	Na+	4
	pCO2	4
	Viscosity, Shear Rate	4
	Screen Filtration Pressure	4
ERYTHROCYTE	K+	4
PLASMA or SERUM	17 OHCS	13
	Testosterone	4
	5-Hydroxytryptamine	5
	Protein	4
	Protein-Bound Carbohydrate	4
	Hexosamine	4
	Sialic Acid	4
	Na+	4
	Ca++	4
WHOLE BODY	Temperature (oral)	11
	Physical Vigor	10
	Weight	10
	Heart Rate	10
	Blood Pressure-Systolic	10
	Blood Pressure-Diastolic	10
	Expiratory Peak Flow	10
	Respiratory Rate	10

TIMING: EXTERNAL ACROPHASE (φ)

95% Confidence Interval

24hr = ACTIVITY SPAN + REST SPAN

Figure 2 Acrophase diagram of human circadian rhythms. (From Halberg and Nelson, 1978.)

RNA metabolism are less clear, as are the possible consequences of the disruption of the relationships between them. It may be that the relationships between some activities depend on common denominators such as substrate or cofactor availability. These, in turn, may depend on the periodic ingestion and assimilation of necessary nutrients. A wide range of diverse processes, remote from environmental events such as cyclic periods of light and darkness, may be linked through complex metabolic processes and neurohormonal feedback mechanisms to effect an internal coordination in time.

It is widely reasoned that most biological rhythms have evolved in response to specific selective pressure. Certain rhythms, such as the spike frequency transfer of information within the CNS and the pulsar pump functions of the heart and lungs, appear to primarily serve specific functions within the organism. All circadian rhythms, however, regardless of the internal process they reflect, also serve to coordinate the organism with its environment. The incorporation by the organism into its own organization of the external time structure (in this case a 24-hr cycle of light/dark) gives rise to what are often referred to as the biological clocks which, in turn, enable the organism, at each point in time, to prepare for imminent, regular, and periodic changes in the environment (Edmunds, 1978). The requisite synchrony between the internal clocks and the environmental cycles they mimic is induced by periodic changes in the environment. It seems likely that these periodic changes were probably among the imposed conditions which were evolutionarily selected for in the establishment of the 24-hr clock, but the evidence indicates that they no longer provide the immediate basis for these rhythms. Instead, the environmental changes serve as cues or *zeitgebers* (time givers) that synchronize the organism's endogenous self-sustaining oscillations with the environment.

The regulatory roles of these internal oscillations or endogenous pacemakers have been the subject of several studies. One study (Brownstein and Axelrod, 1974) of the 24-hr rhythms in norepinephrine turnover in the pineal gland demonstrates the complex interrelationships which can exist between exogenous and endogenous pacemakers. These investigators observed that the endogenous diurnal cycles in the concentrations of serotonin N-acetyltransferase (NAT) and serotonin which exist in sighted rats, although shifted, persisted in blinded rats and those placed in constant darkness. The rhythmic changes in pineal indoleamines which persisted in blinded rats, however, were abolished by interrupting nerve impulses from the brain to the superior cervical ganglia (a major source of pineal innervation), which suggested the presence of an endogenous pacemaker "clock" in the central nervous system. These workers, along with Moore and Klein (1974) and Pittendrigh (1974), suggested that the suprachiasmatic nucleus of the hypothalamus acts as the central endogenous pacemaker, a theory which continues to receive support (Stetson, 1978; Zucker et al., 1976; Halberg and Nelson, 1978).

As stated previously, there are virtually no tissues or functions which do not exhibit periodic changes, usually related to and cued by light-dark cycles. Under normal circumstances, the diverse rhythms within an organism usually maintain distinct phase relationships to each other and to the zeitgebers to which they are entrained. The entire rhythmic array presents a high degree of temporal organization, and available evidence indicates that for many rhythms interdependence takes the form of a hierarchical order, the maintenance of one rhythm being essential for the proper ordering of another. The maintenance of temporal organization between the interrelated and juxtaposed rhythms which make up an organism's time structure, moreover, appears to be critical to the optimal functioning of the organism and, thereby, to its biological success.

For the majority of biological processes and physiological and psychological variables which demonstrate circadian periodicity, age-related changes have not yet been rigorously or systematically investigated. There are, however, a number of studies which have focused on the importance of maintenance of temporal organization to optimal functioning and well-being, as well as on the often deleterious effects of alterations or deficits in biological time structure, both of which may be directly applicable to considerations of biological rhythms and aging.

Many of the areas in which temporal organization has been found to play a significant role, among them cancer chemotherapy (Scheving et al., 1980; Halberg et al., 1980), cardiovascular disease (Millar-Craig et al., 1978), manic-depressive illness (Kripke et al., 1978; Halberg et al., 1977, 1978; Curtis, 1972; Klein et al., 1970), and psychological and cognitive performance (Klein et al., 1970, 1972; Tapp and Holloway, 1981), are also areas with which geriatric medicine must be concerned. The increased incidence of illness and the increased drug consumption by the elderly, as well as their often declining mental acuity, are all potentially affected by age-related alterations in biological time structure. This suggests that information concerning biological temporal organization may be applied to problems of aging to reveal possible bases for many disorders, as well as the means for achieving the most efficacious treatments of them.

The majority of information concerning the effects of altered temporal organization on organismic function derives from investigations concerning the effects of zeitgeber manipulation on various parameters of biological processes. Typically, entraining cues are either removed, presented at abnormal times or in abnormal juxtapositions, or subjected to shifts in phase. As a result, a wide range of behaviors and functions are altered. When maintained under constant environmental conditions, a variety of organisms exhibit characteristic changes in their behaviors and constituent functions; eclosion in *Drosophila* becomes aperiodic (Bruce, 1960), tissue damage develops in tomatoes (Hillman, 1956), running rhythms in the mouse first lengthen and then become increasingly aperiodic (Pittendrigh, 1960), rats exhibit aperiodic feeding behavior and cortisol concentrations (Krieger and Hauser, 1978), and hamsters move from concurrent free-running rhythms of locomotor activity and estrus cyclicity to locomotor arrhythmicity and persistent estrus (Stetson, 1978). Similarly, under conditions of inverted lighting regimens or lighting regimens with abnormal periods, a general shift occurs in the phase of many biological functions such as urine flow, excretion of sodium and potassium, body temperature (Gerritzen, 1962; Lobban, 1965; Aschoff and Wever, 1976), sleep and wakefulness, and urinary excretion of cortisol, adrenaline, and noradrenaline (Aschoff and Wever, 1976). Performance variables such as computation speed (Aschoff and Wever, 1976), pilot flight control accuracy (Klein et al., 1970, 1972), and task performance following passive avoidance training (Tapp and Holloway, 1981) are deleteriously affected by abnormal lighting cycles. Alteration of other zeitgebers such as feeding schedules and composition of the diet are also capable of causing marked phase shifts in functions such as plasma corticosteroid levels (Krieger and Hauser, 1978) and liver glycogen and serum glucose levels (Phillippens et al., 1977).

The administration of certain chemicals may also induce alterations in biological rhythms. Ehret et al. (1978) referred to such compounds as "chronobiotics" because their administration affects a resetting of the phase of a biological oscillation. Pentobarbital, theophylline, and caffeine, when delivered in punctuate fashion, have all been reported to cause phase advances or delays in the timing of certain plant and animal functions (Ehret et al., 1975; Mayer and Scherer, 1975). When administered chronically, theophylline and caffeine cause a marked dose-dependent lengthening of circadian period in neurospora (Feldman, 1975), and chronic administration of phenobarbital causes circadian dyschronism (the absence of a strong rhythm where normally one is found).

Consonant with notions concerning events or changes which may be involved with aging processes across time is the observation that phase shifts which result from alterations in zeitgebers do not occur immediately after the phase shifts in zeitgebers or to the same degrees; moreover, they need not necessarily have deleterious consequences for the organism. The mechanisms by which temporal order is maintained are highly adaptive in nature and capable of accommodating a significant degree of zeitgeber variability, as illustrated by the daily resetting of the biological clock by environmental cues. It is possible, however, that the effects of repeated, even though intermittent, disruptions of zeitgebers and their entrained rhythmic functions may be additive over time, resulting in a progressive loss of organization. Although rhythmic biological processes are normally integrated, they are not irrevocably coupled to each other or to the same environmental cues and endogenous pacemakers. They are, in fact, mutable and, to varying degrees, vulnerable to dissociation and, in some cases, desynchronization. Aschoff and Wever (1976) clarified this distinction, stating that during the transition phase between prior entrainment and free-run the circadian rhythms of an organism may run with different periods until they reach a new "mutual phase relationship." This they termed internal dissociation. However, in certain instances, a new stable phase relationship is not reached, and the rhythms continue to run with different frequencies. In this case, the organism is said to be in a state of internal desynchronization, the consequences of which are deleterious in many instances.

Alterations in the normal phase relationships between functions have been implicated in the occurrence of a number of diseases and pathologies, many of which increase in incidence and severity with advancing age. Of the numerous potentially deleterious effects of altered time structure, one of the most interesting reports (Kripke et al., 1978) is that concerning the circadian rhythms of circular manic-depressives. In five of seven subjects studied there was evidence that the circadian rhythms exhibited free-run periods greater than the 24-hr period of environmental zeitgeber to which the patients were exposed. A similar observation had previously been made by Pflug et al. (1976). In that some processes free-ran fast while others remained synchronized to the 24-hr day, internal desynchronization of body functions was postulated to have resulted. According to Kripke et al., both mania and depression were possible results, depending on the internal phase-angle relationships among the functions. The finding in five of seven patients that lithium treatment slowed the circadian oscillators is particularly intriguing, as is the demonstration that lithium also slows or delays circadian rhythms in plants (Engelmann, 1973; Engelmann et al., 1976). In the two patients classified as lithium nonresponders, rhythms were observed to be abnormally slow or acrophases to have peaked late compared with control patients. This is consistent with the theoretical prediction that patients with slow oscillators would not respond positively to a drug which further slows the oscillators.

Available evidence suggests that this type of internal desynchronization may be induced by environmental factors. Pittendrigh (1974) produced cyclic switches in the activity patterns of rodents which resemble manic-depressive cycles simply through the manipulation of light cycles. Other factors are also capable of promoting internal desynchronization among circadian oscillators. Experiments with laboratory animals have shown that stress may cause certain oscillators to free-run (Calhoun, 1977; Regal, 1975); and air travel and isolation (Wever, 1975a), artificial lighting (Wurtman, 1975), and social factors (Wever, 1975a) have also been cited as promoting desynchronization, theoretically with the potential for producing depression. Not every subject who experiences internal desynchronization experiences depression of clinical severity, however, nor need even recognize the existence of depression. The suggestion has been made that there may be other factors, genetically determined, which predispose particular individuals to express the effects of desynchronization more severely than others. However, it seems highly probable that a subclinical depression resulting from mild desynchrony might easily be implicated as an invisible predisposing factor in such illnesses as cancer, heart disease, and sleep disorders, in which depression is a suspected contributing factor in susceptibility, morbidity, and mortality.

Both the genetic and age-related features of circadian oscillators have a certain degree of consistency with aspects of manic-depressive illness. Investigations using *Drosophila* (Konopka and Benzer, 1971) indicate that various alleles on the X chromosome control circadian frequency with incomplete dominance. Although the lack of homology between *Drosophila* and humans makes any comparison tenuous, it may be noted that susceptibility to manic-depressive illness also appears to be X-linked (Mendlewicz et al., 1972).

More directly pertinent to considerations of aging is the evidence that (1) in some cases circadian oscillators seem to free-run progressively faster with advancing age (Pittendrigh and Daan, 1974; Samis and Zajac-Batell, unpublished); (2) older persons are more likely to experience internal desynchronization (Wever, 1975b); and (3) there is a marked increase in the incidence of affective symptoms among older persons (Kripke et al., 1978). Work by Halberg et al. (1978) provides one experimental model in support of this theory, as well as an anatomical basis. Following disruption of the circadian rhythms of temperature via dinuclear suprachiasmatic lesions, the body temperatures of rats were observed to mimic those of depressed patients who experience sleep disruptions.

CIRCADIAN RHYTHMS AND AGING

A relatively small but rapidly growing area of interest centers directly on the relationship between biological time structure and aging. Results of studies which specifically document age-related changes in the rhythmic properties of various functions are shown in Table 1. It appears that two types of age-related change in temporal organization occur. In one, the variable remains rhythmic but some aspect of its rhythmic character, such as the timing of the demonstrable acrophase, is altered. A shift in the acrophase of one variable may then be followed by alterations in the phase relationships between it and other processes with which it is normally linked in time, thus amplifying the effect throughout the biological system. In the other type, the rhythmic character of the variable diminishes to the point where it is no longer discernible or statistically significant. Comparison between the acrophases of the processes shown in the acrophase map for old men (Fig. 3) with those for young men (Fig. 4) demonstrates the occurrence of both types of change, as well as examples of no change, with advanced age. The acrophases for oral temperature in young and old men occur closely in time, whereas those for systolic and diastolic blood pressure do not. Other physiological parameters such as pulse, peak expiratory flow, and performance, as well as certain psychological factors (Fig. 3) which are highly rhythmic in the young group, show no statistically significant rhythms by cosiner analysis in the old group.

In 1970, Erk and Samis (Fig. 5) reported mean survival in populations of *Drosophila melanogaster* imagoes maintained under constant light to be approximately half that of populations subjected to alternating periods of 12 hr of light and 12 hr of darkness, demonstrating that the physiological effects induced by the aberrant lighting, although not necessarily those of aging, were sufficiently deleterious to drastically limit longevity. Subsequent work by Pittendrigh and Minis (1972) showed that *D. melanogaster* maintained on a 24-hr day lived significantly longer than imagoes maintained on a non-24-hr-period day. They interpreted this as evidence that 24 hr is the normal or natural period for eukaryotic systems, and attributed the shorter life spans of non-24-hr-maintained *Drosophila* to systemic lack of effectiveness, which resulted from attempts to "drive" the system at an abnormal period (i.e., one differing from that of 24 hr). In both instances, the deleterious effects of altering the inherent temporal organization of the organism were readily demonstrable, and the link between temporal organization and optimal function was strengthened.

Later investigations by Pittendrigh and Daan (1974) revealed that in the golden hamster and two species of deer mouse the periods of their free-running activity rhythms became progressively shorter as the animals became older. They concluded that if the frequencies of the rhythms change at different rates and in different directions (i.e., becoming longer or shorter) with age, then their mutual phase relations could conceivably change. The result would be a systematic change in the temporal organization of the animal concomitant with age, possibly leading to some of the physiological changes associated with aging.

Recent work in our laboratory (Samis et al., 1981) is consistent with this possibility. Measurements of the circadian rhythms of phototaxis, geotaxis, and catalase activity of *D. melanogaster* as a function of age show that age-related changes that take place in the magnitude of activity, and in its circadian distribution, are different for each of the three functions. A loosening or uncoupling of the temporal order between these processes may be occurring as the organisms age. Similarly, other recent work in this laboratory (unpublished) shows that the temporal organization of locomotor and drinking activity in mice also changes as a function of age. Under free-run conditions of constant light, animals aged 4 months retained well-defined clusters of periodic activity which moved through the 24-hr day at a steady rate, whereas the 12-month-old middle-aged animals exhibited more diffuse activity patterns, particularly for their locomotor activity. The very old animals present the most interesting phenomena. As in the case of the young animals, their activity patterns remained tightly clustered, yet they appeared to shift at a rate almost half that of the young animals. One interpretation, consistent with Pittendrigh's (1974), is that the period of free-running activity rhythms becomes shorter with age in this species of mouse also. It is significant that those mice which have survived to 34 months of age are a very select population. This raises the question as to whether the ability of these animals to maintain well-defined patterns of free-run activity, compared with the 12-month-old animals, is in some manner related to their ability to reach the 10% survival age.

Reinberg et al. (1978) recently reported some findings which may be indicative of the same type of phenomenon. These investigators reported that older shift workers who remain tolerant of continued shift work (subjectively rated) demonstrate a larger amplitude in temperature rhythms and slower adaptation to the new schedule. Reinberg's interpretation of slower adaptation in "successful" older subjects and our observation of shorter periods in those highly select long-lived mice may both be reflective of a phenomenon of more highly maintained, less mutable

Table 1 Summary of Age-Related Effects on Biological Rhythms

Variable	Age-related effect	Reference
Urinary norepinephrine (human)	Decrease in amplitude	Halberg and Nelson (1978)
Urinary epinephrine (human)	Decrease in amplitude	Halberg and Nelson (1978)
LH, esterone, estradiol, 17-hydroxyproges-terone, prolactin (human)	Change in mesors, LH increased, esterogens + 17-hydroxyprogesterone decreased	Nelson et al. (1980)
LH, estradiol, 17-hydroxyprogesterone (human)	LH and estradiol amplitudes, progesterone amplitude	Nelson et al. (1980)
Plasma norepinephrine (human)	Increase in nocturnal amplitude	Prinz et al. (1979)
Pulse, peak expiratory flow, grip strength (human)	Loss of statistically significant rhythm	Scheving et al. (1978)
Time estimations, eye-hand coordination (human)	Loss of statistically significant rhythm	Scheving et al. (1978)
Urinary excretion of sodium, potassium, chloride, 17-ketogenic steroids, epinephrine (human)	Loss of statistically significant rhythm	Scheving et al. (1978)
Plasma cortisol (human)	Shift in acrophase	Serio et al. (1970)
Sleep structure (human)	Shift in phasing of stages 3, 4, and REM; stage 4 decrease in amplitude	Webb (1978)
Serum TSH (rat)	Loses periodicity with no significant difference in mean level	Klug and Adelman (1979)
Plasma corticosterone (rat)	Increase in amplitude	Klug and Adelman (1979)
Plasma prolactin (rat)	Shift in acrophase of surge	Damassa et al. (1980)
Spontaneous locomotor activity (rat)	Shift in phasing	Mohan and Radha (1978) Mohan (1979)
Brain acetylcholine levels (rat)	Decrease in mesor, increase in amplitude, region-specific shifts in acrophase	Mohan and Radha (1978)

Brain acetylcholine-esterase activity (rat)	Region-specific changes in mesor, amplitude; overall decrease in amplitude 25% of mesor; shifts in acrophase	Mohan and Radha (1978)
Brain choline acetylase activity (rat)	Decrease in mesor and amplitude; shift in acrophase	Mohan and Radha (1978)
Inhibition of acetylcholine-esterase activity (rat)	Shift in phasing; increase in amplitude	Mohan and Radha (1978)
Hepatic monoamine oxidase levels (rat)	Decrease in amplitude	Radha (1978)
Hepatic tryptophan pyrolase activity (rat)	Shift in acrophase	Patnaik and Sarangi (1980)
Locomotor and drinking rhythms (rat)	Progressive flattening of spectrum and diminished peak	Mosko et al. (1980)
Body temperature (rat)	Decrease in amplitude	Scheving et al. (1978)
Serum calcium (rat)	Shift in amplitude mesor and phasing	Scheving et al. (1978)
Serum potassium (rat)	Shift in phasing	Scheving et al. (1978)
Serum alkaline phosphatase (rat)	Shift in acrophase	Scheving et al. (1978)
Serum inorganic phosphorous (rat)	Change in phasing, mesor; increase in amplitude	Scheving et al. (1978)
Blood urea nitrogen (rat)	Change in phasing	Scheving et al. (1978)
Serum cholesterol (rat)	Increase in mesor and amplitude; shift in phasing	Scheving et al. (1978)
Energy metabolism (mouse)	Decrease in mesor and amplitude	Sacher and Duffey (1978)
Body temperature (mouse)	Decrease in mesor and amplitude	Sacher and Duffey (1978)
Leukocyte counts (rat)	Decrease in amplitude	Samis (1978)
Locomotor activity (hamster, deermouse)	Progressively shorter periods	Pittendrigh and Daan (1974)

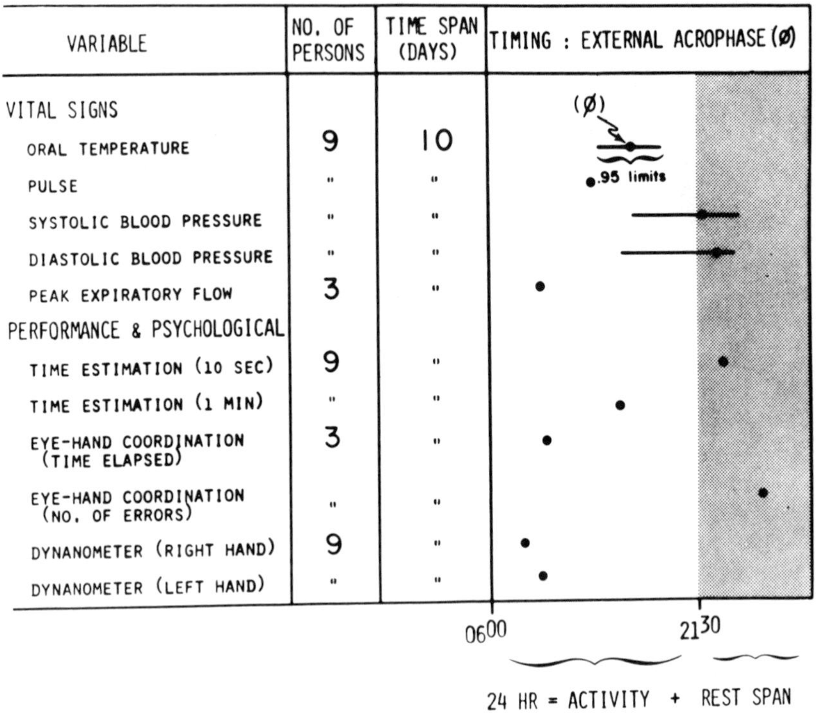

VARIABLE	NO. OF PERSONS	TIME SPAN (DAYS)	TIMING : EXTERNAL ACROPHASE (∅)
VITAL SIGNS			(∅)
ORAL TEMPERATURE	9	10	
PULSE	"	"	.95 limits
SYSTOLIC BLOOD PRESSURE	"	"	
DIASTOLIC BLOOD PRESSURE	"	"	
PEAK EXPIRATORY FLOW	3	"	•
PERFORMANCE & PSYCHOLOGICAL			
TIME ESTIMATION (10 SEC)	9	"	•
TIME ESTIMATION (1 MIN)	"	"	•
EYE-HAND COORDINATION (TIME ELAPSED)	3	"	•
EYE-HAND COORDINATION (NO. OF ERRORS)	"	"	•
DYNAMOMETER (RIGHT HAND)	9	"	•
DYNAMOMETER (LEFT HAND)	"	"	•

0600   2130

24 HR = ACTIVITY + REST SPAN

Figure 3   Acrophase map for a group of nine senior citizens. It should be noted that statistically significant group rhythms were obtained only from data on oral temperature and systolic and diastolic blood pressure. (From Scheving et al., 1978).

temporal organization, which in some manner appears to confer an adaptive advantage upon the older individuals studied in both instances.

In the context of age-related changes in rhythmic functions, perhaps the hypothalamopituitary system has received the greatest amount of attention, in that it constitutes a central mechanism for the regulation of the reproductive system, which exhibits both well-defined rhythmic patterns and predictable senescent changes (Stetson, 1978) and thus provides an integrated model easily amenable to investigation. Nelson et al. (1980) have recently reported that there is a definite age-related effect on the mesors (24-hr means) of the circadian rhythms of the several hormones related to the estrus cycle: luteinizing hormone (LH), prolactin, estrone, estradiol, 17-hydroxyprogesterone (17-OH-progesterone), and dehydroepiandrosterone (DHEA-S), as well as on the circadian amplitudes of LH, estradiol and, to a lesser extent, DHEA-S and aldosterone.

Investigations of age-related changes in reproductive functions by Damassa et al. (1980) have found the 24-hr patterns of prolactin secretion, as reflected by the

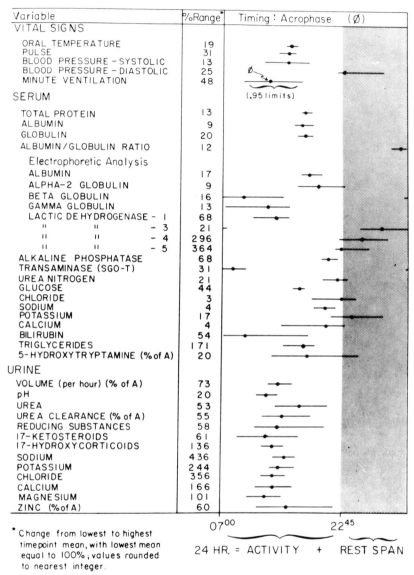

Figure 4 Acrophase map for 13 apparently healthy young men. (From Kanabrocki et al., 1974.)

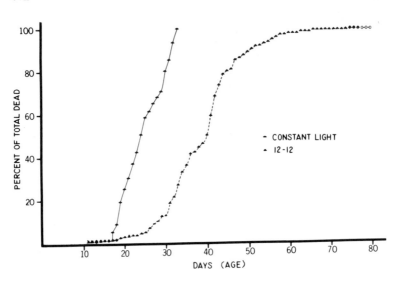

Figure 5 Survival in populations of *Drosophila melanogaster*, Oregon R wild-type males, at 25°C subjected to constant light and to 12 hr of light followed by 12 hr of darkness.

timing of the acrophase of the peak surge, to be almost inverted between constant estrous and pseudopregnant aging female rats. The aging rats in constant estrous exhibited large diurnal surges in prolactin secretion at 1700 hr, compared with nocturnal surges observed at 0200-0500 hr for the pseudopregnant rats. These investigators suggest that the high levels of estrogen and progestin which characterize the constant estrous and pseudopregnant states may be partially responsible for the control of daily prolactin secretion.

Other workers in this area (Klug and Adelman, 1979) have recently reported that the circadian rhythm of serum thyroid-stimulating hormone (TSH) was gradually abolished between 2 and 24 months of age, whereas the average serum TSH concentration remained unchanged. In contrast, the temporal organization of serum corticosterone appears very similar between 2 and 24 months, although plasma levels are significantly higher in the 24-month-old animals. Plasma TSH increased after thyrotropin-releasing hormone (TRH) administration at all ages, but pituitary sensitivity to TRH-mediated TSH secretion was not altered during aging. These investigators speculate that differences in the regulation of TSH during aging may reflect very specific alterations in hypothalamic activity and/or neural functions.

In another study, Finkelstein et al. (1972) found age-related changes in both the spontaneous secretory rate and secretory pattern of growth hormone in human subjects, prepubescent to 62 years of age. During prepubescence, growth hormone was excreted only during sleep, whereas during adolescence, the secretion increased markedly and occurred throughout the 24 hr. The secretion rate then tapered off from young to old adulthood and, although there was some correlation between slow-wave sleep and excretion in old subjects, the high degree of interindividual variability in these subjects obscured any circadian pattern which may have existed. In an interesting study by Patnaik and Sarangi (1980) it was found that, although the mean level of the enzyme tryptophan pyrolase (TP) does not change significantly over the 24-hr day, the activity pattern of this enzyme in the postreproductive rat is almost the direct inverse of that observed in young and adult rats; peak activity occurs at 1800 hr in young and adult, and minimum activity occurs at 1800 hr in the old rats. The possibility was raised by these authors that the inverted pattern of enzyme activity and induction observed in the postreproductive rats may be due to a disturbance of the relationship between levels of TP and the circulating glucocorticoids, as well as changes in the rate of TP degradation.

Work by Dean and Felton (1979) in elderly patients (65-90), however, demonstrated that neither the levels of plasma cortisol nor its pattern of secretion change with age. They concluded that the functional integrity of the hypothalamopituitary-adrenal axis is maintained, even though the adrenal gland itself undergoes tissue atrophy and pigment deposition during the senescent period. Serio et al. (1970) have obtained evidence that although circadian periodicity of the adrenal cortex, as measured by plasma cortisol, persists in persons over 70 years of age, the acrophase of the rhythm shifts with age, appearing later in the day in younger subjects when compared with their older fellows. Thus, although the hypothalamo-pituitary-adrenal axis may remain functional in terms of retaining periodicity, there is also evidence that changes in the structure and organization of that periodicity occur.

Recent work reported by Mosko et al. (1980) on reproductively senescent female rats indicated that the circadian rhythmicity of both locomotor and drinking activities declines with increasing age under both entrained and free-running conditions. As have others, these investigators speculated that aging of the suprachiasmatic nucleus (SCN) could account for many of the age-related changes observed in circadian and cyclic reproductive behavior. In that many of the rhythmic diurnal variations in parameters of immune system processes are thought to be related to rhythmic fluctuations in processes of the neuroendocrine system (Rogers et al., 1979), age-related changes in the SCN may also be involved in the documented age-related changes in immune functions (Makinodan and Yunis, 1977).

Work on sleep patterns and plasma catecholamine levels in the elderly by Prinz et al. (1979) showed that, although both norepinephrine and epinephrine levels continued to exhibit significant diurnal variations in elderly subjects, norepinephrine levels were found to be 28% higher during the day (1100 hr) and 75% higher at night (2200-0900 hr) than those in young subjects. Correlated with the changes in norepinephrine levels was the observation that older subjects slept less well, with 90% shorter stage-4 sleep, 27% less REM sleep, and twice as much night wakefulness as the young. This suggested to the authors that the well-known sleep problems of older persons may be due to increased activity of the sympathetic nervous system. Although these authors did not study the circadian rhythms of the sleep patterns themselves, Rosenberg and Rechtschaffen (1978) reported that the circadian rhythms of waking and non-REM sleep are dampened or absent in senescent male rats, which is consistent with that possibility.

If, as postulated, the SCN serves the function of a central pacemaker or clock, one may suggest, on the basis of the age-related temporal changes which occur in the neuroendocrine functions it regulates, that the temporal organization of the organism as a whole may suffer a deterioration with age, the implications, in terms of function and well-being, becoming increasingly severe as temporal disorganization spreads through the tightly coupled hierarchies of clocks. The evidence available is consistent with the prediction that degenerative changes, which occur in relatively vulnerable sites such as those of the CNS, will be translated through the levels of organization to effect a cascading decline in tissue and cellular functions which will appear as organismic deterioration. In view of the ubiquitousness which characterizes reproductive senescence, there is also reason to consider that the changes postulated to occur in the primary or "master clock" may be, to some extent genetically programmed.

CONCLUSION

There is little or no argument that aging results in a decrease in functional capacity accompanied by an increasing probability of death. Furthermore, this incontrovertible endpoint, death, as a measure of aging, although of little use in the determination of the biological age of an individual, does allow for the estimation of biological aging in populations. As estimated by this endpoint, it is apparent that the rate of aging is species-specific and by some as yet not understood way, genetically determined (Samis, 1978). It is also apparent that the compromised function seen to accompany advancing age, in turn, is often accompanied by changes in the characteristics of the rhythms of these processes (Table 1). The regular and predictable rhythmic fluctuations which characterize the dynamic homeostasis of the young vigorous system may give way to less organized sorts of temporal variations with advancing age. In other instances, organization may be maintained but the pattern may be fundamentally altered. These same alterations in temporal organization, when induced experimentally, result in illness, injury, and poor performance, which at the very least mimic the compromised function of old age. The combined evidence presents a strong case for delineating as many age-related changes in the rhythmic characteristics of clinical parameters as possible when attempting to treat the geriatric patient. This will serve to aid in development of procedures which can maximize the healthfulness and productivity of older persons, and it may well add significantly to our understanding of the aging processes themselves.

REFERENCES

Aschoff, J. (1979). Circadian rhythms: General features and endocrinological aspects. In *Endocrine Rhythms*, D. T. Krieger (Ed.). Raven Press, New York, pp. 1-62.

Aschoff, J., and Wever, R. (1976). Human circadian rhythms: A multi-oscillator system. *Fed. Proc. 35*: 2326-2332.

Brownstein, M. J., and Axelrod, J. A. (1974). Pineal gland: 24-hour rhythm in norepinephrine turnover. *Science 184*: 163-165.

Bruce, V. G. (1960). Environmental entrainment of circadian rhythms. *Quant. Biol. 25*: 29-48.

Calhoun, J. B. (1977). Social modification of activity rhythms in rodents. In *Proc. Intl. Soc. for Chronobiology XII*. II Ponte, Milan, p. 83.

Curtis, G. C. (1972). Psychosomatics and chronobiology: Possible implications of neuroendocrine rhythms. *Psychsom. Med. 34*: 235-256.

Damassa, D. A., Crilman, D. P., Lu, K. H., Judd, H. L., and Sawyer, C. H. (1980). The 24-hour pattern of prolactin secretion in aging female rats. *Biol. Reprod. 22*: 571-575.

Dean, S., and Felton, S. P. (1979). Circadian rhythm in the elderly: A study using a cortisol-specific radio-immunoassay. *Age and Aging 8*: 243-245.

Edmunds, L. N. (1975). Temporal differentiation in Euglena: Circadian phenomena in non-dividing populations and in synchronously dividing cells. In *Les Cycles Cellutains et heir Blocaga chez Plusieurs Protistes*. Collogues Int. CNRS n 240. Centre National de la Rechercha Scientifique, Paris, pp. 53-67.

Edmunds, L. N. (1978). Clocked cell cycle clocks. In *Aging and Biological Rhythms*, H. V. Samis and S. Capobianco (Eds.). Plenum, New York, pp. 125-184.

Ehret, C. F. (1974). The sense of time: Evidence for its molecular basis in the eukaryotic gene-action system. *Adv. Biol. Med. Phys. 15*: 47-77.

Ehret, C. F., Groh, K., and Meinert, J. C. (1978). Circadian dyschronism and chronotypic ecophilia as factors in aging and longevity. In *Aging and Biological Rhythms*, H. V. Samis and S. Capobianco (Eds.). Plenum, New York, pp. 185-213.

Ehret, C. F., Potter, V. R., and Dobra, K. W. (1975). Chronotypic action of theophylline and of pentobarbital as circadian zeitgebers in the rat. *Science 188*: 1212-1215.

Engelmann, W. (1973). A slowing down of circadian rhythms by lithium ions. *Z. Naturforsch 286*: 733-736.

Engelmann, W., Bollig, I., and Hartmann, R. (1976). Effects of lithium ions on circadian rhythms. *Arzneimittel-Forsch 26*: 17.

Erk, F. C., and Samis, H. V. (1970). Light regimines and longevity. *DIS 45*: 148.

Feldman, J. F. (1967). Lengthening the period of a biological clock in Euglena by cycloheximide, an inhibitor of protein synthesis. *Proc. Natl. Acad. Sci. USA 57*: 1080-1087.

Feldman, J. F. (1975). Circadian periodicity in Neurospora: Alteration by inhibitors of cyclic AMP phosphodiesterase. *Science 190*: 789-790.

Finkelstein, J. W., Roffwarg, H. P., Boyar, R. M. Kream, J., and Hellman, L. (1972). Age-related change in the twenty-four hour spontaneous secretion of growth hormone. *J. Clin. Endocrinol. Metab. 35*: 665-670.

Gerritzen, F. (1962). The diurnal rhythm in water chloride sodium and potassium excretion during rapid displacement from east to west and vice versa. *Aerospace Med. 33*: 697-701.

Halberg, F. (1959). Physiologic 24-hour periodicity; general and procedural considerations with reference to the adrenal cycle. *Fermentforsch 10*: 225-296.

Halberg, F., and Conner, R. L. (1961). Circadian organization and microbiology: Variance spectra and a periodogram on behavior of Escherichia coli growing in a fluid culture. *Proc. Minn. Acad. Sci. 29*: 227-239.

Halberg, F., and Nelson, W. (1978). Chronobiologic optimization of aging. In *Aging and Biological Rhythms*, H. V. Samis and S. Capobianco (Eds.). Plenum, New York, pp. 5-56.

Halberg, F., Kabat, H. F., and Klein, P. (1980). Chronopharmacology: A therapeutic frontier. *Am. J. Hosp. Pharm. 37*: 101-106.

Halberg, F., Powell, E. W., Lubanovic, W., Scheving, L. E., Pasley, J. N., Ernsberger, P. R., Sothern, R. B., and Brockway, B. (1978). Chronopharmacologic approach to vigilance: Models and methods for anticircadian dyschronic drug tests based on different kinds of murine thermodyschronism following unilateral or bilateral suprachiasmatic lesions. *Adv. Biosci. 21*: 39-46.

Halberg, F., Powell, E. W., Lubanovic, W., Sothern, R. B., Brockway, B. Pasley, R. N., and Scheving, L. E. (1977). Nomifensine chronopharmacology, scheduleshifts and circadian temperature rhythms in di-suprachiasmatically lesioned rats—modeling emotional chronopathology and chronotherapy. *Chronobiologia 4* (Suppl. 1): 191-197.

Hillman, W. S. (1956). Injury of tomato plants by continuous light and unfavorable photoperiodic cycles. *Am. J. Bot. 43*: 89-96.

Kannabrocki, E. L., Scheving, L. E., Halberg, F., Brewer, R. L., and Bird, T. J. (1974). Circadian variation in presumably healthy young soldiers. *U.S. Dept. Commerce Doc. BP 2248427*, Washington, D.C., p. 56.

Klein, K. E., Bruner, H., Holtmann, H., Rehme, H., Stolze, J., Steinhoff, W. D., and Wegmann, H. M. (1970). Circadian rhythm of pilots' efficiency and effects of multiple time zone travel. *Aerospace Med. 41*(2): 125-132.

Klein, K. E., Wegmann, H. M., and Bonnie, I. H. (1972). Desynchronization of body temperature and performance circadian rhythm as a result of outgoing and homegoing transmeridian flights. *Aerospace Med. 43*(2): 119-132.

Klug, T. L., and Adelman, R. C. (1979). Altered hypothalamic pituitary regulation of thyrotropin in male rats during aging. *Endocrinology 104*(4): 1136-1142.

Konopka, R. J., and Benzer, S. (1971). Clock mutants of Drosophila melanogaster. *Proc. Natl. Acad. Sci. USA 68*: 2112.

Krieger, D. T., and Hauser, H. (1978). Comparison of synchronization of circadian corticosterone rhythms by photoperiod and food. *Proc. Natl. Acad. Sci. USA 75*: 1577-1581.

Kripke, D. F., Mullaney, D. J., Atkinson, M., and Sanford, W. (1978). Circadian rhythm disorders in manic-depressives. *Biol. Psychiatry 13*: 335-351.

Lobban, M. C. (1965). Dissociation in human rhythmic functions. In *Circadian Clocks*, J. Aschoff (Ed.), North Holland, Amsterdam, p. 219.

Makinodan, T., and Yunis, E. (Eds.) (1977). *Immunology and Aging*, Vol. 1, *Comprehensive Immunology*, R. A. Good and S. B. Day (Eds.). Plenum, New York.

Mayer, W., and Scherer, I. (1975). Phase shifting effect of caffeine in circadian rhythm of Phaeolus-Coccineus-L. *Z. Naturforsch. 30c*: 885-856.

Mendlewicz, J., Fleiss, J. L., and Fieve, R. R. (1972). Evidence for x-linkage in the transmission of manic-depressive illness. *JAMA 222*: 1624.

Millar-Craig, M. W., Bishop, C. N., and Raftery, E. B. (1978). Circadian variation of blood pressure. *Lancet 8068*: 795-797, Apr. 15.

Mohan, C. (1975). Behavioral responses of aging rats to cholinergic and adrenergic drugs. In *Proc. Vth Ann. Conf. Ethol Soc. India*, pp. 22-23.

Mohan, C., and Radha, E. (1978). Circadian rhythms in the central cholinergic system in aging animals. In *Aging and Biological Rhythms*, H. V. Samis and S. Capobianco (Eds.), Plenum, New York, pp. 275-299.

Moore, R. Y., and Klein, D. C. (1974). Visual pathway and the central neural control of a circadian rhythm in pineal N-acetyltransferase activity. *Brain Res. 71*: 17-33.

Mosko, S. S., Erickson, G. F., and Moore, R. Y. (1980). Locomotor and drinking activity in reproductively senescent female rats. *Behav. Neural. Biol. 28*: 1-14.

Nelson, W., Bingham, C., Haws, E., Lakatua, D. J., Kawaski, T., and Halberg, F. (1980). Rhythm-adjusted age effects in a concomitant study of 12 hormones in blood plasma of women. *J. Gerontol. 35*(4): 512-519.

Patnaik, S. K., and Sarangi, S. K. (1980). Effects of age and substrate on the circadian rhythm of liver tryptophan pyrrolase of female rats. *Cell. Biol. Intl. Repts. 45*: 471-477.

Peraino, C., Fry, R. J. M., and Staffeldt, E. (1973). Brief communication: Enhancement of spontaneous hepatic tumorigenesis in C3H mice by dietary phenobarbital. *J. Natl. Cancer Inst. 51*: 1349-1350.

Pflug, B., Erikson, R., and Johnsson, A. (1976). Depression and daily temperature. *Acta Psychiatr. Scand. 54*: 254.

Philippens, K. M. H., Mayersbach, H. Von, and Scheving, L. E. (1977). Effects of the scheduling of meal feeding at different phases of the circadian system in rats. *J. Nutr. 107*: 176-193.

Pittendrigh, C. S. (1960). Circadian rhythms and the circadian organization of living systems. *Quant. Biol. 25*: 159-182.

Pittendrigh, C. S. (1974). Circadian oscillations in cells and the circadian organization of multicellular systems. In *The Neurosciences—Third Study Program*, F. O. Schmitt and F. G. Worden (Eds.). MIT Press, Cambridge, Mass., pp. 437-458.

Pittendrigh, C. S., and Daan, S. (1974). Circadian oscillations in rodents: A systemic increase of their frequency with age. *Science 186*: 548-550.

Pittendrigh, C. S., and Minis, D. H. (1972). Circadian systems: Longevity as a function of circadian resonance in Drosophila melanogaster. *Proc. Natl. Acad. Sci. USA 69*(6): 1537-1539.

Prinz, P. N., Halter, J., Bendetti, C., and Raskind, M. (1979). Circadian variations of plasma catecholamines in young and old men: Relation to rapid eye movement and slow wave sleep. *J. Clin. Endocrinol. Metab. 49*(2): 300-304.

Radha, E. (1978). Age related circadian responsiveness of MAO inhibitors. In *Aging and Biological Rhythms*, H. V. Samis and S. Capobianco (Eds.). Plenum, New York, pp. 301-308.

Regal, P. J. (1975). Social synchronization and desynchronization of biological rhythms in the fitness and pathology of vertebrates. *Chronobiologia (Suppl. 1) 1*: 57.

Reinberg, A., Andlaven, P., Guillet, P., and Nicolai, A. (1978). Oral temperature, circadian rhythm amplitude, ageing and tolerance to shift work. *Ergonomics 23*(1): 55-64.

Rogers, M. P., Devendra, D., and Reich, P. (1979). The influence of the psyche and the brain on immunity and disease susceptibility: A critical review. *Psychosom. Med. 41*: 147-164.

Rosenberg, R. S., and Rechtschaffen, A. (1978). Lifespan changes in the diurnal sleep patterns of rats. *Soc. Neurosci. 4*: 378 (abstract).

Sacher, G. A., and Duffey, P. H. (1978). Age changes in rhythms of energy metabolism, activity and body temperature in *Mus* and *Peromyscus*. In *Aging and Biological Rhythms*, H. V. Samis and S. Capobianco (Eds.). Plenum, New York, pp. 105-124.

Samis, H. V. (1968). Aging: The loss of temporal organization. *Perspect. Biol. Med. 12*: 95-102.

Samis, H. V. (1978). Introduction. In *Aging and Biological Rhythms*, H. V. Samis and S. Capobianco (Eds.). Plenum, New York, pp. 1-4.

Samis, H. V., and Zajack-Batell, L. (unpublished). Aging: Locomotor and drinking activity changes in the mouse.

Samis, H. V., Rubenstein, B. J., Zajac, L. A., and Hargen, S. M. (1981). Temporal organization and aging in *Drosphila melanogaster*. *Exptl. Gerontol. 14* (2): 109-117.

Scheving, L. E., Burns, E. R., Pauly, J. E., and Halberg, F. (1980). Circadian bioperiodic response of mice bearing advanced L1210 leukemia to combination therapy with adriamycin and cyclophosphamide. *Cancer Res. 40*: 1511-1515.

Scheving, L. E., Pauly, J. E., and Tsai, T. H. (1978). Significance of the chronobiological approach in carrying out aging studies. In *Aging and Biological Rhythms*, H. V. Samis and S. Capobianco (Eds.). Plenum, New York, pp. 57-96.

Serio, M., Piolanti, P., Romano, S., DeMagistris, L., and Guistri, G. (1970). The circadian rhythm of plasma cortisol in subjects over 70 years of age. *J. Gerontol. 25*(2): 95-97.

Stetson, M. H. (1978). Circadian organization and female reproductive cyclicity. In *Aging and Biological Rhythms*, H. V. Samis and S. Capobianco (Eds.). Plenum, New York, pp. 251-274.

Stupfel, M. (1975). Biorhythms in toxicology and pharmacology. I. Generalities, ultradian and circadian biorhythms. *Biomedicine 22*: 18-24.

Sturtevant, R. P. (1973). Circadian variability in *Klebsiella* demonstrated by cosinor analysis. *Int. J. Chronobiol. 1*: 141-146.

Tapp, W. N., and Holloway, F. A. (1981). Phase shifting circadian rhythms produces retrograde amnesia. *Science 211*: 1056-1058.

Webb, W. B. (1978). Sleep, biological rhythms and aging. In *Aging and Biological Rhythms*, H. V. Samis and S. Capobianco (Eds.). Plenum, New York, pp. 309-323.

Wever, R. (1975a). Autonomous circadian rhythms in man. Singly versus collectively isolated subjects. *Naturwissenschaften 62*: 443.

Wever, R. (1975b). The meaning of circadian rhythmicity with regard to aging man. *Verh. Dtsch. Ges. Pathol. 59*: 169.

Wurtman, R. (1975). The effects of light on the human body. *Sci. Am. 7*: 69.

Zucker, I., Rusak, B., and King, R. G. (1976). Neural bases for circadian rhythms in rodent behavior. *Adv. Psychbiol. 3*: 35-74.

Index